ORTHOPAEDICS AND TRAUMA
FOR MEDICAL STUDENTS AND JUNIOR RESIDENTS

GODWIN IWEGBU

authorHOUSE®

AuthorHouse™
1663 Liberty Drive
Bloomington, IN 47403
www.authorhouse.com
Phone: 1-800-839-8640

While every effort has been made to ensure the accuracy of the content of this book, no responsibility for loss or injury whatsoever occasioned to any person acting or refraining from action as a result of information contained herein can be accepted by the author or publishers.

Published by AuthorHouse 10/19/2012

ISBN: 978-1-4772-6095-1 (sc)
ISBN: 978-1-4772-6094-4 (e)

Library of Congress Control Number: 2012915552

Any people depicted in stock imagery provided by Thinkstock are models, and such images are being used for illustrative purposes only.
Certain stock imagery © Thinkstock.

This book is printed on acid-free paper.

Because of the dynamic nature of the Internet, any web addresses or links contained in this book may have changed since publication and may no longer be valid. The views expressed in this work are solely those of the author and do not necessarily reflect the views of the publisher, and the publisher hereby disclaims any responsibility for them.

Dedicated to:

My grandchildren: Boris, Alexander, Sebastian, Nicholas, Oliver and Ava.

TABLE OF CONTENTS

Preface.. ix

Part I: General Introduction to Orthopaedics

Chapter 1:   General Introduction to Orthopaedics. Anatomy and Physiology of the
             Musculo-skeletal System...1
Chapter 2:   Principles of Classification, Diagnosis and Treatment of Bone Diseases and Injuries 25

Part II: Orthopaedic Diseases

Chapter 3:   Arthritis.. 45
Chapter 4:   Metabolic Bone Diseases.. 59
Chapter 5:   Bone and Joint Infections... 69
Chapter 6:   Congenital and Developmental Abnormalities.. 85
Chapter 7:   Bone Tumours.. 115
Chapter 8:   Back Pain.. 129

Part III: Fractures

Chapter 9:   Introduction to Fractures... 139
Chapter 10:   Diagnosis and Treatment of Fractures.. 149
Chapter 11:   Complications of Fractures and of Fracture Treatment.......................... 173
Chapter 12:   Principles and Management of Soft-tissue and Nerve Injuries............... 191
Chapter 13:   Injuries of the Shoulder and Humerus...207
Chapter 14:   Injuries of the Elbow and Forearm 235
Chapter 15:   Fractures and Dislocations of the Wrist (Carpus) 259
Chapter 16:   Fractures of the Spine and Pelvis..273
Chapter 17:   Dislocations of the Hip Joint and Fractures of the Femur 299
Chapter 18:   Fractures of Tibia and Fibula 321
Chapter 19:   Injuries of the Ankle and Foot 335
Chapter 20:   Sports Injuries...353

Part IV: Miscellaneous Bone Diseases

Chapter 21:   Sickle-cell Disease and the Skeleton... 361
Chapter 22:   Some Other Orthopaedic Diseases 369

Index..385

PREFACE

The curriculum of most universities hardly provides for meaningful teaching or learning of orthopaedics at the undergraduate level. The total time allotted to orthopaedics is not enough to revise the anatomy and physiology of the musculo-skeletal system first studied in the first two years, let alone grasp the principles of fracture and bone diseases management. This book is directed at Medical Students and Junior Residents, who may not have had the opportunity to learn a lot of orthopaedics during their brief introduction to the specialty in the medical school and who may not wish to specialise in orthopaedics but are, nevertheless, required to take care of patients with orthopaedic problems on orthopaedic and non-orthopaedic wards.

The book summarises in four parts the core knowledge needed to diagnose and treat bone injuries and diseases. Part I deals with the basic sciences applied to orthopaedics. Part II discusses the pathology, diagnosis and treatment of the major groups of bone diseases whilst Part III discusses the general principles of diagnosis and treatment of fractures and gives a regional survey of individual fractures. Part IV summarises sickle-cell disease as it affects the skeleton as well as a mixed bag of less well-known orthopaedic diseases. The contents are based on three previous volumes: *Principles and Management of Acute Orthopaedic Trauma (1988; 2004); Orthopaedic Diseases: Summary of Principles and Management (2006)* and *A Patient and Carer's Guide to Bone Diseases and Fractures (2010)*.

Oghara, Nigeria, 2012 CGI

PART I
GENERAL INTRODUCTION TO ORTHOPAEDICS

CHAPTER 1

GENERAL INTRODUCTION TO ORTHOPAEDICS. ANATOMY AND PHYSIOLOGY OF THE MUSCULO-SKELETAL SYSTEM

General introduction

The word "Orthopaedics" derives from two Greek words, "orthos", meaning "straight" and "paedon", meaning "child" and was coined in 1741 by Nicholas Andry, who was then a Professor of Medicine at the University of Paris. This relation of the subject to children arose from the historical fact the orthopaedic practice at that time was preoccupied with the "straightening-up" of children made "crooked" by various crippling diseases, especially poliomyelitis, prevalent at that time. Modern orthopaedics has gone beyond this; it manages all abnormal conditions, including injuries, affecting the musculo-skeletal system.

The adult human skeleton (Fig.1.1.) is made up of over two hundred separate bones of different shapes and sizes, which, with their associated joints, form a complex solid framework for the whole body. Together with attaching muscles and other soft tissues, they form the locomotor system, a system whose complexity beats even the imagination of the cleverest of architects and engineers and whose efficiency is the marvel of all that have studied it. The growing skeleton differs from the adult version by its possession of growth plates and epiphyses (Fig.1.2).

Functions of the skeleton

The skeleton performs a number of important functions in the body:

- It is the basic framework on which the entire body is designed and built.
- It protects the soft tissues of the body such as the brain, the spinal cord and the intrathoracic organs from mechanical injury.
- Together with attached muscles, tendons and ligaments, it makes it possible for the joints and the individual as a whole to move.
- In addition to these mechanical functions, the bone is *a big reservoir of minerals*, especially calcium, phosphorus and magnesium, and

1

- The bone marrow is the main seat of manufacture of blood (*haemopoiesis*)
- It is important to stress that in spite of its compact structure, bone is one of the most reactive of tissues, responding to virtually all the organs of internal secretion and to various other normal and abnormal stimuli.

A few reminders of the structure and function of the locomotor system may help us to understand the subject of orthopaedic trauma. Bone, cartilage and muscle are the main tissues of the locomotor system and all derive from the embryonic mesoderm.

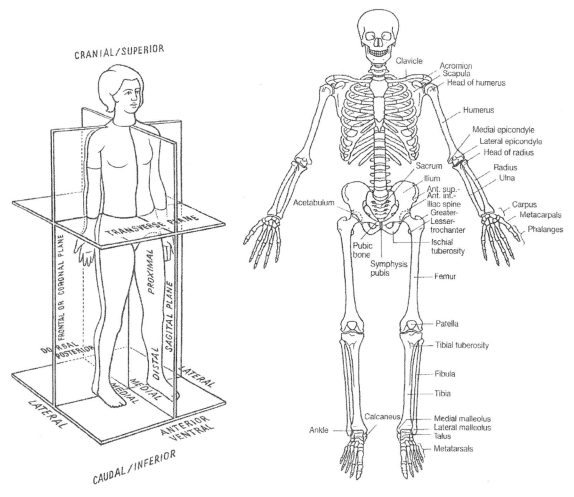

Fig.1.1. Orientation of the Human Body for descriptive purposes and The Human Skeleton (Reproduced with permission from Springer-Verlag)

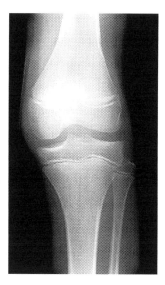

Fig.1.2. The growing skeleton differs from the adult version by its possession of growth plates.

ORIGIN AND DEVELOPMENT OF BONE

Bone originates from the embryonic mesoderm in which it forms by one of two mechanisms - *intramembranous bone formation* or *endochondral ossification*.

Intramembranous Bone Formation

In this mechanism, bone is formed directly by an aggregate of bone forming cells, without a cartilaginous precursor. The cranial vault, facial bones and part of the clavicle and mandible form by this route.

Endochondral Ossification

In this mechanism, from condensations of primitive mesenchymal cells, the framework of the bone first forms in cartilage, the so-called cartilage model, which is then replaced by bone through a series of complicated processes.

It is interesting to note that these two embryonic pathways of bone formation exist in the post-natal period: growth originating at the growth plate is essentially by endochondral ossification while growth originating from the periosteum occurs by intramembranous ossification.

Centres of ossification (Fig.1.3)

Centres of ossification relate to endochondral ossification. There are two of them - primary and secondary.

- *The primary centre of ossification*
  This is the central portion of the cartilaginous model of a long bone. It ossifies by a gradual process of endochondral ossification, beginning in the 7th - 8th week of intrauterine life.

The ossification proceeds from the centre towards both ends of the model, forming the shaft (diaphysis) of the bone.

- ***Secondary centres of ossification***
  These appear at the ends of long bones at different times in infancy and childhood, gradually developing to form the bony eminences at the ends of long bones. Examples of such bony eminences include the tuberosities and the epicondyles of the humerus, the trochanters of the femur and the condyles of the tibia.

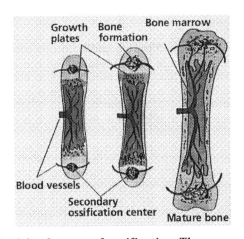

Fig.1.3a. Centres of ossification. The segment occupying most of the shaft is the primary ossification centre. Secondary centres of ossification appear at the ends of the shaft.

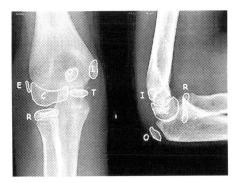

Fig.1.3b. Additional ossification centres around the elbow joint appear at different ages. The mnemonic for remembering this *for the elbow region* is CRITOE: C – Capitulum, R – Radial head, I – Internal (medial) epicondyle, T – Trochlea, O – Olecranon, E – External (lateral) epichondyle, appearing at the ages of 1-3-5-7-9-11 years respectively.

ANATOMY OF BONE

GROSS ANATOMICAL TYPES OF BONE

The human skeleton can be divided into two groups: *axial skeleton*, comprising the bones of the skull, neck, truck and pelvis, and *appendicular skeleton*, comprising the bones of the upper and lower limbs. Based on their shape, size and structure, the bones of major significance to the orthopaedic surgeon fall into one of the following groups: *long, short, flat, irregular* and *sesamoid bones.*

Long Bones

Most of the bones of the limbs belong to this group. Typical examples are the femur, tibia, fibula, humerus, the radius and ulna. A long bone is made up of a shaft, the *diaphysis*, which houses a medullary canal, and two ends, each comprising the *metaphysis* and *epiphysis*.

Short Bones

The bones of the carpus and tarsus are typical examples. They are made of spongy bone surrounded by a thin layer of compact bone.

Flat Bones

These have an outer and inner layer of compact bone between which a layer of spongy cancellous bone is sandwiched. The bones of the skull vault typify this structure even though they cannot really be described as "flat". The sternum, ribs and scapulae are other examples of flat bones.

Irregular bones

Any bones, which cannot be conveniently included in the above groups, are classified as irregular. The vertebrae and bones of the face are examples.

Sesamoid Bones

These are round, spherical or triangular bones, which are embedded in tendons or fascia. They are classically small in size and inconstant in location, but the patella is both large and important.

ARCHITECTURE OF BONE (Fig.1.4)

Bone tissue occurs in two forms - woven (or fibrous) bone and lamellar bone. Their location and arrangement represents an example of perfect architecture, always in harmony with their intended function.

Woven Bone

This is a transient form. It is seen during phases of rapid bone formation such as occurs in embryonic life, at zones of endochondral ossification and at fracture sites during healing. It consists of a loose framework of delicate bone trabeculae which, in a histological section, has the appearance of loosely woven material. It is mechanically inefficient as a structural material and is normally rapidly replaced by the lamellar bone.

Lamellar Bone

This is mature bone. It consists of distinct and regularly arranged layers of bone in which the collagen fibres have a distinct orientation. Lamellar bone occurs in two different structural forms - *cortical* (compact) and *cancellous* (spongy) bone.

- **Cortical Bone**
  This is made up of cylindrical units called *Haversian systems* or *osteones* which, in a long bone, are compactly arranged in successive concentric circles around the medullary canal. Each Haversian system (osteone) consists of up to fourteen concentric circles or lamellae of bone tissue surrounding a central canal which contains blood vessels and nerve fibres. The osteones branch and interweave among themselves, their long axes coinciding with the major lines of stress to which a given bone is subjected.

- **Cancellous Bone**

  This is located in the expanded or bulbous ends of the long bones and also in most of the irregular bones of the skeleton. In orthopaedic practice, the iliac crest is a regular source of cancellous bone for the purpose of bone-grafting. Cancellous bone is lamellar bone arranged in the form of the trabeculae laid down in an orderly manner (Fig 1.4). These trabeculae are always arranged in such a manner as to be maximally able to withstand the stress experienced by a particular bone. A typical example is the proximal femur and the acetabulum in which their arrangement in both bones coincides with the directions of forces acting at the hip joint during weight-bearing.

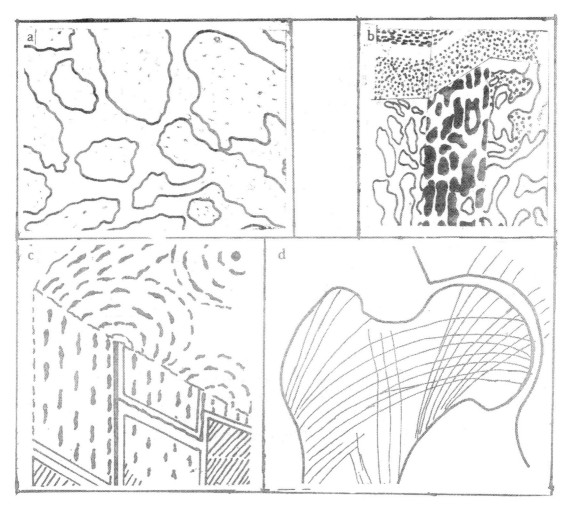

Fig.1.4. The structure of bone

a. Woven bone is a loose framework of delicate immature bone present only at sites of rapid new bone formation

b. Cancellous bone is lamellar bone arranged in the form of trabeculae. It is found at the ends of long bones and at other sites

c   Cortical (or compact) bone forms the cortices of bones. It is made up of large a number of Haversian systems.

d. The orientation of the trabeculae of a given bone always coincides with the lines of forces the bone is functionally subjected to.

MICROSCOPIC STRUCTURE OF BONE

Microscopically, bone is made up of bone cells (*Cellular component*) and matrix (*Extracellular component*). The matrix in turn has an organic fraction and an inorganic fraction.

BONE CELLS

Despite its compact nature, bone is very much alive and made up of living cells. These are the *osteoblasts* which synthesises bone tissue, the *osteocytes* which maintain it and the *osteoclasts* which resorb it (Fig.1.5). They arise from the pluripotential mesenchymal cells inhabiting all bone surfaces and probably from other connective tissues. They are highly differentiated cells, which are incapable of self-reproduction.

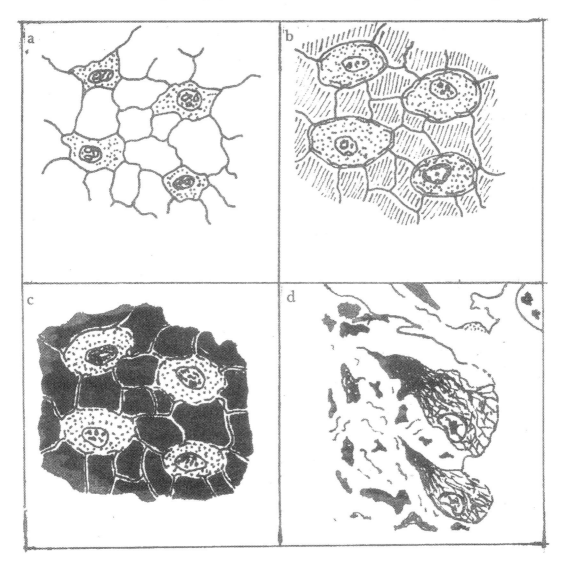

Fig.1.5. Bone cells

   a.   Osteoblasts secreting intercellular substance
   b.   Osteoblasts completely surrounded by secreted intercellular substance
   c.   Ageing osteoblasts imprisoned by calcified intercellular substance are called osteocytes
   d.   Osteoclasts are multinucleated giant cells found on or near bone surfaces undergoing resorption

Osteoblasts

These are plump, single-nucleated cells with characteristic basophilic cytoplasm. Fine cytoplasmic processes connect neighbouring cells, forming continuous networks. They are usually found lying tightly in a single file along active bone-forming surfaces. Osteoblasts are very active cells and are particularly plentiful at sites of active bone formation. They produce and extrude *osteoid*, the organic matrix of bone, which consists of collagen, protein polysaccharides and glycoproteins. Osteoid subsequently becomes mineralised into bone.

Osteocytes

These are "ageing" osteoblasts that have become imprisoned in calcified bone matrix. They metabolise at a slower rate than the osteoblasts and although isolated in lacunae, have an enormous surface contact with bone tissue via their long cytoplasmic processes, which pass through channels called canaliculi. They are considered to maintain the viability of mature bone tissue and to be involved in calcium homeostasis.

Osteoclasts

These are multinucleated giant cells found on or near bone surfaces undergoing resorption. They are derived from haematopoietic monocyte cell precursor and vary greatly in size, from small cells with one or two nuclei to the largest cells in the body with several hundred nuclei. They resorb bone by secreting proteins and lysosomal enzymes. Their "escavating" action on bone is attested to by the presence of "brush border" between them and bone. Like osteocytes, they are considered to play a vital role in calcium homeostasis. Their activity is increased by parathyroid hormone and thyroxine and decreased by calcitonin and oestrogens. Osteoclasts and certain tumour cells are the only cells known to be capable of bringing about the resorption of bone.

BONE MATRIX

This consists of two parts - *organic* and *inorganic*.

Organic Bone Matrix

The organic matrix of bone, otherwise called *osteoid*, consists mainly of Type 1 collagen, with small quantities of protein-polysaccharides (glycosaminoglycans) and glycoproteins. Type I collagen is the most common form of collagen, accounting for 25% of the weight and 38% of the volume of adult bone.

Ninety-five per cent (95%) of the organic matrix consists of collagen, the remaining 5% being made up of the above-named protein complexes. Collagen is made up of bundles of fibrils, which in turn are composed of stacked molecules formed from polypeptide chains arranged in a triple helical pattern. It is a banded structure of specific periodicity - 70nm. The basic molecule is called tropocollagen and the basic fibre unit is called a microfibril. It is common to all connective tissues but in bone it has the unique ability to produce and accumulate minerals in an orderly fashion.

Inorganic Bone Matrix

This is made up of calcium, phosphate and small variable amounts of other ions, notably magnesium, sodium, bicarbonate and fluoride. It is closely associated with collagen, *in the substance of which it is formed.*

Bone mineral occurs in two forms: as amorphous calcium phosphate and as a crystalline structure with an X-ray diffraction pattern characteristic of the apatites. Bone crystals come closest in chemical composition to hydroxyapatite, $Ca10(PO4)6(OH)2$. Amorphous calcium phosphate is formed initially but is gradually transformed into needle-shaped apatite crystals. The crystals then become associated with the periodic banding of collagen and orientated along the collagen axes. Bone crystals are closely associated with water which forms a hydration shell around each of them. This shell contains the ions Na +, Mg ++, Ca++, citrate, carbonate and also trace elements such as strontium, radium, lead and fluoride. Exchange of ions with body fluids occurs at this site.

Mineralisation is catalysed by prophosphatases, which include alkaline phosphatase. *Why does collagen in other connective tissues not calcify?* This is because an inhibitor substance, called inorganic pyrophosphate (PP), is present in these tissues, which inhibits mineralisation in them. In bone, the inhibitory action of this enzyme is first nullified by the pyrophosphatases before they proceed to catalyse mineralisation.

In good health, un-mineralised bone (osteoid) can be found only in minute quantities at sites of bone formation e.g. at a fracture site. This is because mineralisation normally takes place rapidly. However, it is abundant in rickets or osteomalacia in which mineralisation is impaired.

MECHANICAL PROPERTIES OF BONE

The shape, structure and location of each bone are determined by its intended function. In general, bone possesses the physical property of *mechanical strength* which is determined by its *stiffness*. *Stiffness* is a measure of how much a bone deforms under load, *strain* is a measure of the deformity. *Stress* is the force applied to a bone divided by its cross-sectional area. The *stress/strain curve* is graphically illustrates these mechanical properties of bone. On this curve (Fig.1.6a), the *elastic zone* of the material is represented by the almost vertical line. Here, stress is directly proportional to strain, and the *stress/strain ratio* is known as *Young's modulus of elasticity, E*. Beyond the elastic zone is the *plastic zone* which is represented by the almost horizontal part of the curve; increasing the stress in this zone will lead to permanent deformity, followed by breakage. The point of change from vertical to horizontal part of the curve is called the *yield point. Young's modulus of elasticity* for bone compares most favourably with that of other structural materials; it is about ten times that of cast iron!

Wolff's law relates the structure of a given bone to the forces acting upon it: "Bone develops a structure most suited to the forces acting upon it, adapting both the internal architecture and the external conformation to the change in external loading conditions".

The forces a bone could be subjected to include tension, compression and rotational forces. A fracture results if the injuring force exceeds the breaking strain of the bone, and its characteristics e.g. fracture planes, will be determined by those of the injuring force. In general, a tension force will produce a transverse fracture, a compression force will produce an oblique fracture and a bending force, which has a tension and a compression component, will first produce a transverse fracture and then a butterfly fragment from its compression component (Fig.1.6b); a torsional force will produce a spiral fracture.

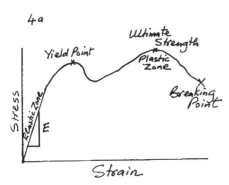

Fig.1.6a Mechanical Properties of Bone
The stress-strain curve and *Young's modulus of elasticity, E.*

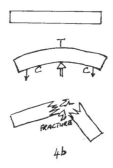

Fig.1.6b. Mechanical Properties of Bone
Bone possesses the mechanical properties of mechanical strength and elasticity. When a bone is subjected to a bending force, the convexity is in tension (T) while the concavity is in compression (C). Bone is weaker in tension than in compression. This, together with the characteristics of the injuring force e.g. the presence or absence of a twisting element, determine the fracture lines should a fracture result.

BASIC ANATOMY AND PHYSIOLOGY OF CARTILAGE, MUSCLE AND JOINT

Introduction

Cartilage is a very important component of the musculo-skeletal system. It has been stated earlier that in the embryonic period, most of the bones of the skeleton were first laid in cartilage before ossification. In the foetus and adult, however, cartilage becomes restricted to three areas - articular surfaces, epiphyseal growth plates and the ribs. Outside of the skeleton, cartilage is found in the framework of the ear and respiratory system.

Cartilage exists in three forms - hyaline, fibrous and elastic cartilage. Hyaline cartilage contains type II collagen. Fibrocartilage contains more fibres than ground substance and elastic cartilage contains elastic and collagen fibrils. Articular and rib cartilage is hyaline cartilage whereas the menisci of the knee joint are made of fibrocartilage. When articular cartilage heals following injury, fibrocartilage forms in its place. Elastic cartilage contains a relatively large amount of elastin; it is yellow in colour and is found in the structure of the ear and the epiglottis.

STRUCTURE AND FUNCTION OF CARTILAGE

Cartilage consists of cells (chondrocytes and chondroblasts) and matrix (collagen, protein polysaccharides and water).

THE CELLS OF CARTILAGE

These are chondrocytes and chondroblasts. The chondrocyte is the principal cell of cartilage. Its size and shape vary with its location in cartilage and its function at that site. Usually it is a plump, circular cell with large rounded nucleus filling the lacuna within the cartilage matrix but it may be flat as in the superficial zone of articular cartilage. In the proliferative zone of epiphyseal cartilage, it is smaller in size, flattened and may show mitotic figures. Here it is referred to as a chondroblast.

Mature chondrocytes have a low turnover of cells. Ageing chondrocytes have shrunken nuclei and disorganised intracellular organelles such as mitochondria and endoplasmic reticulum but cellular activity in the form of matrix production continues throughout life. Chondrocytes have a limited capacity to repair large defects such as may result from injury or disease.

Cartilage Matrix

Chondrocytes and chondroblasts are responsible for the production of cartilage matrix, which is made up of collagen, protein polysaccharides (proteoglycans) and water. The principal protein polysaccharides in cartilage are chondroitin sulphates and keratan sulphate.

The Structure of Articular Cartilage (Fig.1.7)

Articular cartilage is hyaline cartilage. It is composed of water (75%), type II collagen (12.5%) and proteoglycans (12.5%). The high water content is made possible by the hydrophilic properties of the proteoglycans. This composition of articular cartilage gives it the mechanical properties of being able to deform and recover its shape after the cessation of the deforming force. Articular cartilage also acts as a damper or shock absorber, reducing the damaging effect of sudden load on bone ends.

The Four Zones of Articular Cartilage

Articular cartilage is a highly organised structure. This is necessary in order to enable it to serve the mechanical functions outlined above. Starting from the surface, the four zones are:

Superficial zone. This is a narrow zone in which collagen fibres are abundant, closely packed and arranged parallel to the joint surface. The chondrocytes here are discoid in shape with their long axes parallel to the surface.

Intermediate zone. This is thicker than the superficial zone. In it the collagen fibres form an irregular interlacing mesh. The chondrocytes here are larger, rounder and more evenly spaced.

Deeper zone. Here the collagen fibres are arranged perpendicular to the underlying bone and the chondrocytes are disposed in columns parallel to the collagen fibres.

Calcified zone. This is a narrow calcified zone lying just above the underlying bone.

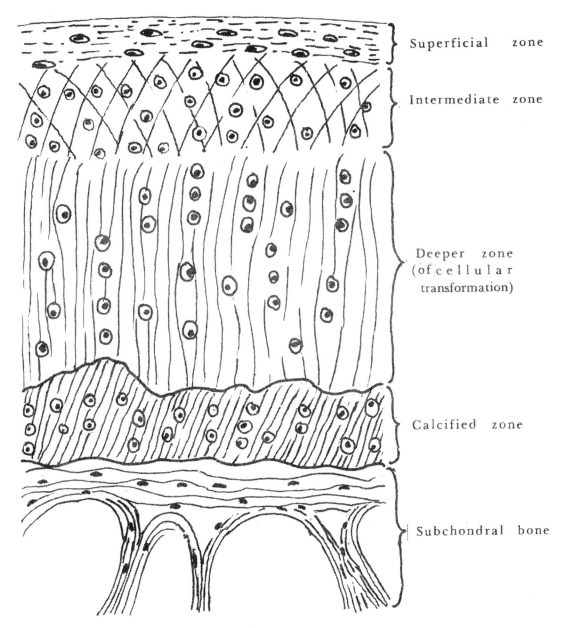

Superficial zone

Intermediate zone

Deeper zone (of cellular transformation)

Calcified zone

Subchondral bone

Fig.1.7 . The structure of articular cartilage

The Structure of the Epiphyseal Growth Plate (Fig.1.8)

The growth plate is a band of hyaline cartilage separating the epiphysis of a long bone from the metaphysis. Accordingly, each long bone has two growth plates. The growth plate is responsible for growth of the bone mainly in length but also contributes to its growth in width. The rate of growth in the two growth plates of a bone usually differs. For example, in the femur, the distal growth plate accounts for 70% of the growth in length while the proximal plate accounts for only 30%.

Starting from the epiphyseal end, the growth plate can be divided into three main zones - zone of growth, zone of cartilage formation and zone of ossification. Each zone can be subdivided into layers of cells or sub-zones at different levels of cellular activity.

There is a tendency to conceptualise the zones only in terms of their cellular components. This is incorrect because the cartilage matrix and the changes occurring in it in the different sub-zones are equally important.

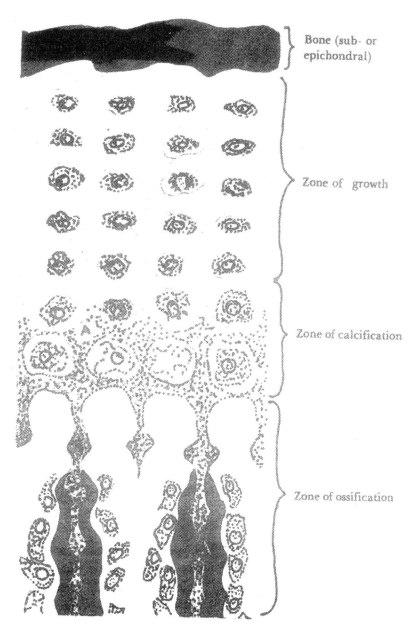

Bone (sub- or epichondral)

Zone of growth

Zone of calcification

Zone of ossification

Fig. 1.8. The structure of the growth plate

Zone of growth

The first layer of cells in this zone is that of chondrocytes in a 'resting' state. They are intimately associated with the epiphyseal vessels, which provide undifferentiated cells. Additional resting cells are also elaborated peripherally in a specialised area of the perichondrium called the zone of Ranvier. The next layer of cells is that of dividing cells. This division occurs in both longitudinal and transverse directions although mainly in the former. The next layer is that of columnating cells. In an active growth plate, these cell columns can comprise half the total height of the plate.

The randomly disposed collagen fibres in the resting and dividing layers take a more longitudinal orientation between the columnating cells.

Zone of cartilage formation
In this zone, the chondrocytes hypertrophy as a result of increased cellular activity. Increased amounts of intercellular matrix are formed and biochemical changes occur in it preparatory to its eventual ossification; it becomes metachromic and then calcifies. The fate of the chondrocytes is controversial. Some authors believe that they degenerate while others think that they become osteoblasts.

Zone of ossification
Following the calcification of the matrix in the zone of cartilage, metaphyseal vessels which bring in osteoblasts invade it. These osteoblasts form osteoid tissue on the preformed chondroid septi. The osteoid is quickly mineralised, forming the so-called primary spongiosa. With time this becomes replaced by a more mature variant, the secondary spongiosa which no longer contains remnants of its cartilaginous precursor.

Nutrition of Cartilage

Cartilage is largely avascular and acquired its nutrition by diffusion of nutrients from the surrounding tissue fluids. This is the mode of nutrition of articular cartilage, except during the growth period when the deeper layers of it receive a blood supply from the epiphyseal vessels. Mechanical activity acts as a pump, which aids diffusion of nutrients through the cartilage. In the epiphyseal growth plate, the major source of nutrition is the vascular plexus in the epiphyseal side of the plate next to the zone of growth, the rich metaphyseal blood supply being concerned mainly with endochondral ossification. This arrangement explains the clinical observation, fractures in childhood, which usually occur through the comparatively weak hypertrophied zone of cartilage formation, the nutrition of the growth plate (from the metaphyseal vessels) is undisturbed, whereas epiphyseal fractures frequently disturb cartilage growth (because of damage to the epiphyseal vessels).

Situations imposing non-use of joints or limbs (immobilisation following fractures or other injuries; paralytic conditions such as poliomyelitis) cause impairment of nutrition and both articular and growth plate cartilage may degenerate even to the point of total destruction. In poliomyelitis, for example, a severely affected limb is always shorter and smaller than an unaffected one.

Calcification of Cartilage

Cartilage may calcify (mineralise) at certain sites and under certain circumstances. We have already mentioned the calcification that occurs as a prelude to endochondral ossification in articular cartilage and in the epiphyseal growth plate. Another example is the calcification of cartilaginous bone tumours, e.g. the cartilaginous cap of an osteochondroma.

If mineralisation is impaired, as in rickets, the invasion of mineralised cartilage matrix by vascular tissue and, consequently, its ossification does not occur. As in bone, alkaline phosphates are essential for cartilage mineralisation and can be demonstrated at mineralisation sites. The mineral is a calcium apatite crystal similar to that of bone.

Epiphyseal Closure

At the end of the growing period (at 15-16 years in the female, 16-18 in the male), division of cartilage cells in the growth plate ceases and the plate becomes progressively ossified, beginning from the diaphyseal side of it. The epiphysis and diaphysis become one, the process of their union being called a synostosis. A thin horizontal and radiographically more opaque line is formed at the point of union and is called the epiphyseal scar.

In a typical long bone with two growth plates, one produces more total growth than the other, either because its cartilage cells multiply more rapidly, or because they grow for a longer period than those of the other plate. This 'more productive' end is called the growing end of the bone. Important examples include the proximal end of the humerus and lower end of the radius and ulna in the upper limb, and the distal end of the femur and proximal end of the tibia in the lower. These facts lie at the root of the memory aid phrase: "To the elbow I grow, from the knee I flee" which in effect, repeats the facts stated in the last sentence.

BASIC ANATOMY AND PHYSIOLOGY OF SKELETAL MUSCLE

The importance of skeletal muscle to the locomotor system cannot be over-emphasised: they move the joints and therefore the whole body. This they do by virtue of their ability to contract in response to nervous stimuli invoked by will, hence the alternative name, voluntary muscles. Knowledge of the gross anatomy and function of muscles is helpful in the understanding and management of congenital abnormalities, fractures and other abnormal conditions involving the musculoskeletal system.

The Gross Structure and Function of Skeletal Muscle

A whole skeletal muscle is a mass of muscle tissue, usually of a definite shape and size, enclosed in a connective tissue sheath called *epimysium*. It has at least one 'origin' and one 'insertion'. Some muscles e.g. the biceps, the triceps and the quadriceps as their names imply have two, three and four origins respectively. The origins and insertions of the muscles of the appendicular skeleton determine the displacements that occur when the major long bones are fractured.

It is important to bear in mind that no muscle acts alone and that very few muscles have only one action. Muscles always act in conjunction with several others as an integrated group. For example, a muscle which crosses a joint in such a way that its contraction produces adduction and internal rotation cannot produce either of these movements separately. However, when it acts in conjunction with other muscles as a group, some of them can be used to cancel out an unwanted action. For example, if pure adduction is required, the internal rotation component can be cancelled out by employing one or more of the external rotators. Similarly, if internal rotation alone is required, the adduction component can be cancelled out by the abductors.

The term, prime mover, is commonly used to describe muscle and their actions. A prime mover (muscle) is one whose contraction is largely responsible for bringing about a given movement. When a muscle acts in a subsidiary capacity to bring about a movement, it is called a synergist. Muscles which oppose prime movers are called antagonists. For example, flexor carpi radialis and ulnaris are the prime movers in wrist flexion, all the long flexors of the fingers are their synergists and the dorsiflexors (extensors) of the wrist are their antagonists.

The Muscle Cell (Fig.1.9)

Although a detailed knowledge of the finer structure and function of skeletal muscle will certainly help in the understanding of certain muscular diseases such as muscular dystrophy, it is of limited value in the management of most common orthopaedic

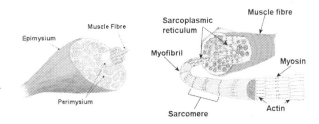

Fig.1.9a&b. Muscle fibre and muscle cell.

diseases, including injuries. Therefore only a brief summary of microanatomy and function will be given here.

The basic structure of a muscle cell is similar to that of other cells. Its basic peculiarity is its elongated shape and its possession of an excitable membrane called *sarcolemma*. In addition to the normal elements (organelles) found in all cytoplasm, the cytoplasm of the muscle cell, which is otherwise called *sarcoplasm*, possesses contractile protein filaments called *myofilaments*, which run along the long axis of the cell. A myofilament contains at least three proteins, *actin*, *myosin* and *tropomyosin*. A bundle of these filaments grouped together is visible in the light microscope and is called a *myofibril*. Mitochondria, the power-houses of any cell, are particularly large and numerous in the myofibrils. The smooth endoplasmic reticulum of a muscle cell is known as the *sacroplasmic reticulum* and is disposed along the myofibrils.

Each muscle cell is enclosed in a connective tissue tube called the *endomysium*. The so-called 'muscle fibres' are bundles of cells, each in its *endomysium*, enclosed in another connective tissue tube called the *perimysium*. The sheath around a whole muscle is called the *epimysium*.

The contractile unit of a skeletal muscle is called *a sarcomere*. It is a composite arrangement of thick myosin-containing and thin actin containing filaments. The architecture of a sarcomere imposes precise limits on the amount of shortening that can occur during contraction. A muscle fibre can shorten by more than 50% and a whole muscle can produce full movement in a joint from shortening to only 43% of its fully extended length.

Skeletal muscle is able to perform its special function of contraction because of its excitability. The excitation (impulse) comes from the motor nerve or nerves innervating it. Muscular contraction requires a lot of energy, the immediate source of which is believed to be *adenosine triphosphate (ATP)*. A lot of heat is produced by muscular contraction. Muscles are subject to fatigue (reversible exhaustion) and rigor (irreversible exhaustion).

BASIC ANATOMY AND PHYSIOLOGY OF JOINTS

A joint is the anatomical structure between two or more bones. This rather vague definition is given in order to avoid the temptation to think of a joint only in terms of a space or cavity between two or more bones, facilitating movement between them. Although the latter is the usual function, some joints are solid in nature, like the primary cartilaginous joint separating the epiphysis and metaphysis in the growing long bone, and do not allow movement.

Joints develop in the embryo from elements of the cartilaginous models of the skeleton and their mesenchymal precursor. In the more typical synovial joints, an interzone develops between two or more models. This zone consists of three layers - two parallel chondrogenic layers and an interposing and less dense intermediate layer. Complex processes occur in this zone, which result in the formation of a joint cavity (by cavitation) and development of a joint capsule, synovial membrane and intra-articular structures such as menisci and cruciate ligaments. The chondrogenic layers form the opposing joint surfaces (cartilage). Joint formation is firmly established by the 10th intrauterine week.

TYPES OF JOINTS

There are three main classes of permanent joints - *fibrous, secondary cartilaginous joint (or symphysis) and synovial joints.*

Fibrous Joints

Examples include the distal tibiofibular joint, also called a syndesmosis and the structures which separate the skull bones in the foetus and young child. Fibrous joints are characterised by the presence of fibrous tissue instead of a joint cavity between two bones and allow only limited movement.

Secondary cartilaginous joints (or symphysis)

The classical example is the symphysis pubis. The intervertebral disc is another example. In this type of joint, the bone ends are covered with hyaline cartilage (as in synovial joints) but a plate of fibrocartilage then unites these ends. This plate may become softened as in the intervertebral disc or may develop a cavity as in the symphysis pubis. Movement in individual joints is usually limited but can be considerable e.g. in the vertebral column.

Synovial Joints

These constitute the majority of the joints of the locomotor system. As their name implies, they are characterised by the presence of a synovial membrane. Their complex structure permits free movement to occur in them but these characteristics also make them subject to certain pathological conditions such as inflammatory joint disease (which is essentially a disease of the synovial membrane) and degenerative joint disease (which is in the main a result of the wear and tear of articular cartilage caused by movement at the joint).

Structure of a Synovial Joint (Fig.1.10.)

The moving bone ends are as a rule covered by hyaline cartilage. The few exceptions include the temporomandibular joint in which the articulating ends are covered by fibrocartilage. Starting from the outside and going inwards, other structures forming the joint are the joint capsule (a sleeve of collagen fibres surrounding the whole joint), the synovial membrane (a band of vascular tissue with a glistening inner surface) lining the inner surface of the capsule and intra-articular structures. Intra-articular structures may include cartilaginous discs which are typically found in the knee joint where they are called menisci (singular = meniscus).

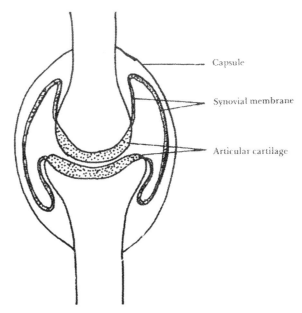

Fig. 1.10. The structure of a synovial joint. A synovial joint is characterised by its possession of a synovial membrane.

Also associated with synovial joints are ligaments, tendons and bursae. Ligaments are bands of fibrous connective tissue usually found on the outside of the joint capsule, on its medial and lateral aspects, as in the knee joints, but which could also be intra-articular, for example, the anterior or posterior cruciate ligaments of the knee. Tendons are the fibrous origins or insertions of muscles. They are usually related to the outside of the joint capsule but could also be intra-articular as in the case of the popliteus tendon in the knee.

A bursa is a pocket of synovial membrane that has protruded outside the joint through a defect in the joint capsule but, sometimes, there is no connection between a bursa and a related joint cavity. In the latter case, it develops in the connective tissue around muscles or tendons as a smooth-walled cavity containing a viscid lubricant closely resembling synovial fluid. Sometimes a bursa may wrap around a tendon so as to enclose it almost completely for much of its length; such elongated bursae are known as synovial sheaths.

Types of Synovial Joints

Synovial joints are usually classified according to the type of movements or movements that take place in them or according to the shape of their articular surfaces. The following types of joints are distinguished:

Hinge Joints allow movement only in one plane - the plane of flexion and extension. A classical example is the knee joint. The so-called condylar joints are actually hinge joints.

Pivot Joints resemble the hinges of a gate; they allow the movement of rotation. The superior radioulnar joint is of this variety. Hinged at this joint, the radius rotates around its axis in the movements of pronation and supination of the forearm.

The hip and shoulder joints typify *Ball-and-socket Joints*. They allow movement centred in the centre of the ball which, in the mentioned examples, are the heads of the femur and humerus respectively. The movements of flexion, extension, abduction, adduction, and internal and external rotation as well as a combination of all of them (called circumlocution) are all possible. The so-called ellipsoid joints, represented by the radiocarpal (or wrist) joint, is a variety of a ball-and-socket joint in which both the ball and the socket are ellipsoidal rather than spherical in shape.

The carpometacarpal joint of the thumb represents *saddle-shaped joints*. They have two saddled-shaped articular surfaces lying upside-down on each other. They allow rocking movements in other directions, including rotation.

It must be borne in mind that most movements of the body involve more than one joint whose actions must necessarily affect one another. Another point of practical significance about joints is the concept of stability. The most important factor determining the stability of a given joint is its anatomy. In this respect there are two factors - the bony anatomy and the soft-tissue (muscle and ligaments) anatomy. The shape of the articulating surfaces is important too, so also are the associated muscles and ligaments. It is therefore not surprising that the hip joint with its deep acetabular socket, congruently-shaped and well-covered femoral head, supported by powerful and well balanced muscles and ligaments, is the most stable joint in the human body. Its stability makes it difficult for it to dislocate except under the effect of enormous forces. On the other hand, the bony base of the shoulder joint is comparatively weak and so its stability depends to a large extent on the surrounding muscles (rotator cuff muscles). Consequently it dislocates much more easily that the hip joint.

Blood Supply and Innervation of Synovial Joints

The blood supply of joints is derived from a plexus of vessels lying outside the joint capsule. Its nerve supply comes from adjacent nerve trunks. The fibrous capsule and any fibrocartilagenous intraarticular structure such as intervertebral discs are freely supplied by sensory fibres. The synovial membrane also has sensory fibres but articular cartilage (as opposed to subchondral bone) has none.

Synovial Tissue

Synovial membrane is made up of synovial cells which derived from the embryonic mesenchyme of the skeletal blastema, like other connective tissue cells. They form a discontinuous layer, one to four cells thick, with the cells linked to one another by interlacing cytoplasmic processes.

A fibrocellular subsynovial layer of tissues richly supplied with blood vessels and lymphatics containing mast cells and macrophages supports the synovial membrane. In both structure and function the synovial membrane is similar to the peritoneum. Its scavenging role is very efficient. Its venous circulation absorbs crystalloid and similar very small particles. Larger particles are absorbed by the lymphatics, while very large particles are phagocytosed by the synovial lining cells.

Synovial membrane secretes the synovial fluid, which is a viscous, clear or slightly yellow fluid rich in protein. Chemically, it is a dialysate of plasma, with the addition of mucin, composed mainly of hyaluronic acid. It lubricates the joint, nourishes the articular cartilage and provides macrophages, which scavenge debris from the moving surfaces or other sources. In a normal joint, synovial fluid is present in very small quantities. For example, the knee joint, which has the largest amount of synovial tissue, normally contains less the 0.5ml of synovial fluid. However, in injury (ligamentous ruptures, fractures involving joints) and disease (rheumatoid arthritis, for example), a large quantity of fluid may form 'in sympathy' (sympathetic effusion).

BONE METABOLISM

Bone metabolism involves complex interactions involving bone, the endocrine and urinary systems, the nutritional status of the individual and genetic abnormality when present. Disturbances of these factors and their relationships can result in metabolic bone diseases, most of which have serious consequencies for the individual affected and for healthcare costs. For example, osteoporosis accounts for about 300,000 hip fractures a year in the U.S.A. and in 1995 alone, osteoporosis care was said to have cost that country the sum of $13m.

As mentioned earlier, the bone cells - osteoblasts, osteocytes and osteoclasts, contain receptors responsive to hormones, which control bone metabolism. Osteoblasts synthesise osteoid, the organic matrix of bone and also produce the enzyme, alkaline phosphatase, which can be measured in the serum as an indicator of bone formation. They have receptors responsive to parathyroid hormone (PTH), which is released when the body's ionised calcium level is falling.

Osteocytes also have receptors for parathyroid hormone (PTH). Stimulated osteocytes are said to mobilise poorly crystallised calcium salts surrounding them without affecting the organic matrix of bone. They do not actually resorb bone to release calcium.

Osteoclasts resorb bone by enzymatic degradation and are responsive to a variety of factors produced by the osteoblasts and osteocytes. One such factor produced by osteoblasts, *receptor activator of nuclear factor-kB ligand (RANKL)*, has recently been recognised as *a protein* essential for the control of bone metabolism.

It is postulated that there exists a signalling mechanism or pathway between osteoblasts and osteoclasts that regulates a balance between bone formation and bone resorption. A newly identified member of the tumour necrosis factor family is said to be a part of this pathway.

CALCIUM HOMEOSTASIS

Calcium is an important regulator of many cellular functions in the body, including muscle contraction, blood coagulation, intercellular signal transmission and the control of cell membrane potentials. Calcium homeostasis can be defined as a state of optimum calcium balance in the body. It is maintained by complex and co-ordinated interactions between the skeleton, intestines and kidneys. The skeleton serves as a calcium reservoir for maintaining calcium homeostasis.

The normal serum concentration of calcium ranges from 9 to 10.4 mg/dL. Approximately 45% is bound to proteins (primary albumin), a small fraction, about 5%, is bound to phosphate or citrate and the remaining 50% is in free ionised form. Ionised calcium levels are regulated within narrow limits and significant disturbances of these limits are the main trigger for the release of PTH.

All body calcium is derived from diet, its absorption from the intestines being regulated according to body needs. About 20% of calcium intake is absorbed by active transport in the duodenum by a calcium-binding protein, which is regulated by 1,25-dihydroxyvitamin D3. Passive transport of calcium also occurs in the jejunum.

Calcium is absorbed in the proximal tubules through a solvent gradient but active transport occurs in the distal portions by a sodium-calcium exchange pump. Some calcium absorption also takes place in the loop of Henle via an electrochemical gradient but the main regulation of calcium absorption is believed to take place in the distal convoluted tubules where active calcium transport occurs. Calbindin, a vitamin-dependent calcium-binding protein, is said to assist in this transport against chemical and electrical gradients.

Calcium is excreted by the kidneys at a rate of 150-200 mg/day, the same amount absorbed from the intestine.

The amount of dietary intake of calcium varies with age and the body's efficiency in absorbing it. Calcium needs are high during growth, pregnancy and lactation and dietary intake should be increased in old age to counter the calcium loss from increased bone resorption.

VITAMIN D METABOLISM

Vitamin D is a fat-soluble hormone, which plays a vital role in calcium homeostasis. The two main sources of this vitamin are:

- *The diet* – fatty fish, cod-liver oil, fortified cereals, bread and milk and
- *The skin.* – during exposure to ultraviolet light

The synthesis of vitamin D in the body follows exposure to sunlight and begins with 7-dehydrocholesterol (itself synthesised from steroids in the body) being converted to vitamin D3 (cholecalciferol), a biologically inert form of vitamin D. Carried in the bloodstream to the liver, cholecalciferol is hydroxylised to 25-hydroxyvitamin D3. This binds to alpha-globulin and becomes the principal circulating form of vitamin D. On getting to the kidney, a 2nd hydroxylation takes place in the proximal tubules and glomerulus to produce 1,25-dihydroxyvitamin D3, the biologically active form of vitamin D.

The main function of 1,25-dihydroxyvitamin D3 is the regulation of the production of the calcium-binding protein essential for calcium absorption and transport in the intestine. Its circulating level varies with age, decreasing in old age and with impaired renal function.

PARATHYROID HORMONE (PTH)

The parathyroid hormone is a peptide produced by the four parathyroid glands. The target organs are the kidneys, intestines and the skeleton. PTH synthesis and release are related to the level of extracellular ionised calcium, which is able to affect a receptor on the surface of parathyroid cells. The pathway for PTH release is said to involve cyclic adenosine monophosphate (cAMP). An increased serum calcium level inhibits cAMP formation and decreases PTH secretion and vice versa.

The functions of PTH can be summarised as follows:

- *stimulates the release of calcium from bone*
- *increases resorption of calcium in the distal tubule*
- *stimulates 1-alpha-hydroxylase activity in the kidney, increasing 1,25-dihydroxyvitamin D3 production, which leads to increased intestinal reabsorption of calcium*
- *decreases phosphorus reabsorption in the proximal tubule*
- *stimulates osteoblasts to form new bone*
- *stimulates the production of factors, such as interleukin-6, that stimulate osteoclasts to resorb bone.*

THYROID HORMONE

Thyroid hormones, T4 (*thyroxine*) and T3 (*3,5,3'-triiodothyronine*), circulate in the bloodstream bound to plasma proteins. Increased levels of thyroid hormones stimulate both bone formation and bone resorption but the latter effect is slightly greater, with eventual net bone loss. Consequently, thyroid hormonal replacement and chronic hyperthyroidism can contribute to osteoporosis.

OESROGENS

Decreased oestrogen levels are associated with increased rates of bone loss. In menopause and also following oophorectomy, oestrogen levels decrease by 80% and bone loss accelerates – from the normal 0.3%-0.5% per year to 2-3% per year, returning to normal only after 6-8 years. Oestrogen inhibits bone resorption by some unknown mechanism and oestrogen receptors are found on both osteoblasts and osteoclasts.

ANDROGENS

Androgens are known to play an important role in the maintenance of bone mass in men. Delayed puberty is associated with reduced bone mass and men with idiopathic hypogonadotropic hypogonadism also have reduced bone mass.

CORTICOSTEROIDS

Briefly, corticosteroids have the following effects on calcium metabolism (homeostasis):

- *they decrease protein synthesis, including that of calcium-binding proteins*
- *increase calcium excretion in the kidneys and through this mechanism can cause secondary hyperparathyroidism*
- *high doses inhibit both bone formation and bone resorption*

Further reading

Albright TA and Brand RA (ed). *The Scientific Basis of Orthopaedics.* New York. Appleton-Century-Crofts, 1987.

Passmore R and Robson JS, eds. *A Companion to Medical Studies, Vol.1,* 2nd ed. Blackwell Scientific Publications, 1976.

CHAPTER 2

PRINCIPLES OF CLASSIFICATION, DIAGNOSIS AND TREATMENT OF BONE DISEASES AND INJURIES

CLASSIFICATION OF ORTHOPAEDIC DISEASES

It is important that doctors who manage orthopaedic diseases speak "a common language", otherwise confusion will result, which may compromise treatment, comparison of results of various treatment options, clinical audit and the learning process. Classification means grouping of conditions according to specified criteria. Such criteria may be based on chronology, causative factors, characteristic features or a mixture of these.

Classifications of orthopaedic conditions are numerous and complex. However, the value of any given classification is directly proportional to the amount of help it provides in the understanding, diagnosis and treatment of a given condition. I think it is important not to spend too much time memorising classifications but to understand the principles behind them.

There is no classification so complete or clear as to earn universal acceptance. The following working classification can serve in most practical situations:

1. Traumatic conditions
2. Congenital abnormalities
3. Developmental abnormalities
4. Orthopaedic infections
5. Inflammatory joint diseases
6. Degenerative joint disease
7. Metabolic bone diseases
8. Bone tumours and tumour-like formations
9. Miscellaneous conditions

- **Traumatic conditions**
  These include fractures and all soft-tissue injuries of the musculo-skeletal system.

- **Congenital abnormalities**

  These are abnormalities existing at the time of birth. Congenital clubfoot is a good example: it is present and obvious at birth. Others, such as congenital dislocation of the hip, though present at birth, are less obvious.

- **Developmental abnormalities**

  Traditionally, abnormalities appearing in the first few months after birth are termed "developmental". These should also include all conditions occurring during the developmental period – e.g. bow legs and scoliosis.

- **Inflammatory joint diseases**

  These are characterised by inflammation, which can be loosely defined as pathological tissue metabolism producing swelling, redness, heat, pain and disturbed function. The inflammation is triggered by causative factors or agents, which are not infective.

- **Orthopaedic infections**

  These include bone, joint and soft-tissue infections. Here, symptoms and signs of inflammation are present and have been caused by one or more infective agent(s) e.g. bacteria. Tissue necrosis with the formation of pus is characteristic of an infective process. Acute haematogenous osteomyelitis and pyogenic myositis are classical examples.

- **Degenerative diseases**

  These are often conceptualised as "wear and tear" changes affecting the bones, joints and soft-tissues of the musculo-skeletal system. They are understandably common in the older age brackets. With regard to joints, they are typified by osteoarthritis, which is essentially wear of articular cartilage. A popular way of remembering this condition is that it can be abbreviated as "OA", which can also stand for Old Age.

- **Bone tumours and tumour-like formations**

  These are usually swellings or masses formed by abnormally fast-growing cells of the affected tissues. They may arise from either bony or soft-tissue elements of the MSS. They may be benign or malignant.

- **Metabolic bone diseases**

  These arise from abnormal bone metabolism. Such an abnormality may be in the bone cells, matrix or mineral and are often associated with defective hormonal control of bone metabolism. Examples include osteogenesis imperfect, osteoporosis, Paget's disease, rickets and osteomalacia.

- **Miscellaneous conditions**

  A few conditions, which do not clearly come under any of the above groups, can be discussed under this heading. Examples include Frozen shoulder, tennis elbow and golfer's elbow

PRINCIPLES OF DIAGNOSIS OF ORTHOPAEDIC DISEASES

INTRODUCTION

The diagnosis of orthopaedic diseases is slightly more difficult than that of fractures but the principles are the same. The symptoms and signs are also similar but whilst the symptoms and signs of fractures are usually obvious, those of orthopaedic diseases are not always so and their diagnosis requires considerable knowledge and experience. A systematic approach is imperative. This systematic approach should begin with good history-taking, physical examination, radiographic and laboratory investigations and end with a definitive diagnosis on which treatment can be based.

HISTORY

Like fractures, every disease has a story behind it. This story should be elucidated in a systematic manner. It usually begins with asking the patient what their complaint(s) is/are. A patient with bone disease will complain of one or a combination of the following:

- **Pain**. This could be mild, moderate or severe and may be present at rest, on palpation or with movement. Joint pain is usually made worse by movement or weight-bearing.

- **Swelling.** This may result from inflammation, infection or tumour. It may be accompanied by a *bruise* or *erythema (redness)*. Swelling is usually not obvious in diseases affecting deep-seated bones or joints e.g. the spine and hip.

- **Deformity.** This could be intrinsic in a given bone e.g. as in tibial bowing but most deformities occur at joints e.g. knock knee (genu valgum) or bowed knee (genu varum). Deformity could be angulatory, rotatory or both.

- **Loss of function.** Generally, movement is adversely affected by swelling, bone or cartilage defect or loss, deformity, weakness or pain. These abnormalities may make a joint *unstable*. In most cases, the patient is unable to use the affected bone or joint normally.

History of the complaints or symptoms

After sympathetically listening to the complaints, the doctor must now seek to know the history of the complaints. This includes elucidating all situations thought to be related to the patient's condition. The details sought should include the chronology, speed of development and severity of the individual symptoms as they may aid diagnosis and subsequent management. For example, in a 12-year-old young man presenting with a swelling in his proximal tibia, the speed of development of the swelling is important in thinking along the lines of acute osteomyelitis, osteosarcoma or osteochondroma. If a patient is unable to give an account of their symptoms, history can be obtained from parents, close relatives, carers or friends.

Past medical history (PMH)

The patient's past medical history must also be sought for they may have a medical condition such as asthma, psoriasis, chronic obstructive airways disease, hypertension or diabetes, which could influence the management of their condition. It is also important to find out if there is a *history of allergy* to drugs, food or other substances.

Medication

A *drugs history* is also important. The patient may be on drugs, which may adversely interact with the ones you may wish to prescribe for them. For example, many elderly patients are on anti-hypertensives, which may adversely interact with non-steroidal anti-inflammatory drugs commonly prescribed for orthopaedic conditions.

Social history (SH)

The social history is also important. If a child, what are the home circumstances? If an adult, does he/she live with a partner, family members or friends? A patient may be a hard drinker, a fact that may be important when anaesthetising them, if they require surgical treatment. Their cultural practices may influence their attitude to their hospitalisation, if this is considered necessary. Their social status, occupation, earning capacity, number of dependants and financial commitments to relatives are all factors that could influence their management, as are the requirements of their religion. The physician must patiently seek out and document these details.

PHYSICAL EXAMINATION

This part of disease management is very important and the temptation to cut ends must be resisted, no matter how obvious or simple a condition may appear at first sight. Physical examination must be systematic. First, a quick routine general examination of the body, system by system, is carried out. This is then followed by a more thorough examination of the affected region.

General examination

The aim here is to elicit any abnormal condition in the patient as a whole that may affect the management of their condition. Not infrequently, such a condition was in existence before the orthopaedic condition. For example, anaemia of various origins, cardiac, respiratory or other insufficiencies may be present. Any significant finding must be noted and recorded. Skin colour change, e.g. pallor or jaundice cannot be estimated in dark-skinned people, so, it may be necessary to examine the patient's eyes for possible conjunctival pallor or jaundice. The pulse, blood pressure, heart sounds, the pulmonary sounds and the state of the abdomen should also be noted.

Local examination

This elicits the *local status (status localis)*. In conditions involving a limb, comparison of the affected limb with the unaffected one is vital. In recording the findings of a physical examination, knowledge of the normal orientation of the human body for descriptive purposes and a uniform terminology are important (Fig.1.1).

The following steps in local examination are distinguished:

- **Inspection (LOOK)**. It is perhaps important to remind the young doctor that the word "inspection" means "looking". This synonym brings out better the role of the eyes of the examiner in the procedure. A careful look will reveal a *deformity, atrophy, swelling, and bruise,* if present. *Scars* or any other abnormality in the affected part should be sought; they may be pointers to the pathology in hand.

- **Palpation (FEEL)**. This is the procedure of examination with the hand. It includes touching, feeling and sometimes, exerting firm pressure with the fingers, thumb or clenched fist. It will define the bounds of a swelling, determine its texture or consistency and define points or areas of tenderness.

- **Movement (MOVE)**. Testing for the presence, restriction or absence of movement in a diseased part is fundamental to the physical examination of a patient with an orthopaedic complaint. *Active* and *passive movement* must be tested for. In testing for active movements, the patient is asked to move the diseased part. Usually, in the presence of disease, they will not be able to do so fully or comfortably. Passive movements are effected by the examiner and are liable to cause pain and so must be carried out with extra care. Except in neuromuscular diseases, the information obtained by testing for passive movements is generally more helpful than that obtained by testing active movements.

To recognise and interpret abnormal ranges of movement in a given joint, the examiner must know the movements and their normal ranges in a given joint.

TYPES OF MOVEMENT OCCURRING IN JOINTS

Flexion

Flexion occurs in the saggital plane. It is difficult to define in terms of the direction in which it takes place because the direction is different in different joints. For example, in the hip joint, it is a forward bend of the thigh, whereas, in the knee joint, it is a backward bend of the lower leg. Even the plane of movement is not always saggital: in the neck and lumbar spines, sideways movements are described as *lateral flexions* and elbow flexion can be effected in many planes. The best way to use the term is to individualise it for each joint.

Extension

Extension is the opposite of flexion and usually takes place in the saggital plane. It is also difficult to define in terms of the direction in which it occurs: in the hip, it is a backward bend of the thigh, whereas, in the knee, it is a forward bend of the lower leg.

Abduction

This is movement of a part e.g. the arm, away from the midline in the *coronal (frontal) plane.*

Adduction

This is movement of a part away from the abducted position to the midline in the *coronal (frontal) plane.*

Rotation

Rotational movements occur typically in *ball-and-socket* joints as represented by the shoulder and hip joints. These can take place in clockwise and anti-clockwise directions. *Internal and external rotations* occur in clockwise and anti-clockwise directions respectively. The term *circumduction* is used to describe a combination of flexion, extension, abduction, adduction and rotation in a joint and typically occurs in the shoulder joint.

NORMAL RANGES OF MOVEMENT IN VARIOUS JOINTS

- **The neck**
  The movements of the neck are the sum of the movements in the numerous joints located in the region. The normal ranges of flexion, extension, lateral flexions (left and right), and lateral rotations (left and right) occurring in the neck are summarised on Table 2.1.

  Table 2.1. Ranges of movement in the neck

Flexion:	0-45 degrees
Extension:	0-45 degrees
Left lateral flexion:	0-45 degrees
Right lateral flexion:	0-45 degrees
Left lateral rotation:	0-45 degrees
Right lateral rotation:	0-45 degrees

- **The shoulder joint**
  The movements of flexion, extension, abduction, adduction, internal rotation, external rotation and circumduction occur in the shoulder joint. In abduction/elevation, there is movement in the glenohumeral joint as well as in the scapulothoracic "joint" in the ratio of 2:1. That is, in full abduction/elevation of 180 degrees, 120 degrees occur at the glenohumeral joint whilst 60 degrees occur at the scapulothoracic joint. The ranges of shoulder joint movements are shown of Table 2.2.

Table 2.2. Ranges of movements in the shoulder joint

Flexion:	0-90 degrees
Extension:	0-45 degrees
Abduction:	0-90 degrees
Adduction:	90-0 degrees
Internal rotation:	50-60 degrees
External rotation:	40-45 degrees
Elevation	0-90-180 degrees
Circumduction:	360 degrees

- **The elbow joint**

The ranges of movements here are shown on Table 2.3.

Table 2.3. Ranges of movements in the elbow joint

Flexion:	0-150 degrees
Extension:	150-0 degrees
Hyperextension	5-15 degrees

- **The forearm**

The movements here are rotation and occur at three joints: the superior and inferior radioulnar and the radiohumeral joints. The ranges of movement are shown on Table 2.4.

Table 2.4. Ranges of movements in the forearm

Pronation	0-70-80 degrees
Supination	80-90-0 degrees

- **The wrist joint (Table 2.5)**

Table 2.5. Ranges of movements in the wrist joint

Flexion (Palmarflexion):	0-60 degrees
Extension (Dorsiflexion):	0-30 degrees
Abduction:	0-10 degrees
Adduction:	0-45 degrees

- **The finger joints (Table 2.6)**
  The main movements here are flexion and extension:

Table 2.6. Ranges of flexion/extension in the finger joints

Metacarpophalangeal joint:	0-70 degrees
Proximal interphalangeal joint:	0-90 degrees
Distal interphalangeal joint:	0-45 degrees

- **The spine(Table 2.7)**

Table 2.7. Ranges of movements in the thoracolumbar spine

Flexion:	0-110 degrees
Extension:	0-15 degrees
Left lateral flexion:	0-30 degrees
Right lateral flexion:	0-30 degrees
Left lateral rotation:	0-45 degrees
Right lateral rotation:	0-45 degrees

- **The hip joint (Table 2.8)**

Table 2.8. Ranges of movements in the hip joint

Flexion:	0-120 degrees
Extension:	0-30 degrees
Abduction:	0-45 degrees
Adduction:	0-30 degrees
Internal rotation:	0-45 degrees
External rotation:	0-45 degrees

- **The knee joint (Table 2.9)**

Table 2.9. Ranges of movements in the knee joint

Flexion:	0-135 degrees
Extension:	135-0 degrees

- **The ankle joint (Table 2.10)**

Table 2.10. Ranges of movements in the ankle joint

Flexion:	0-15 degrees
Extension:	0-15 degrees

- **The subtalar joint (Table 2.11)**

Table 2.11. Ranges of movements in the subtalar joint

Inversion:	0-15 degrees
Eversion:	0-10 degrees

MEASUREMENTS

- Atrophy or hypertrophy of part of a limb may be quantified by circumferential measurements with a tape-measure using marked identical points on the affected and unaffected limb.

- In suspected limb length inequality, limb lengths can be measured and compared. *Apparent limb length* is measured with the patient lying supine, from any point in the midline proximal to the hip joint level, usually the navel, to the medial malleolus. *Real limb length* is measured from the anterior superior iliac spine on each side to the corresponding medial malleolus.

NEUROLOGICAL EXAMINATION

Sensory loss, if present, can be graded as follows (Table 2.12):

Table 2.12. Grades of sensory loss

Grade 0	Total anaesthesia
Grade 1	Pain perception only
Grade 2	Pain and some touch perception
Grade 3	Pain and normal touch perception but no two-point discrimination
Grade 3+	Same as Grade 3 plus some two-point discrimination
Grade 4	Normal sensation

Muscle power should be determined, especially if muscular weakness is suspected. The grades of muscle power are shown on Table 2.13. The tendon reflexes as well as sensation should also be evaluated.

Table 2.13. Grades of muscle strength

Grade 0	Total paralysis
Grade 1	Muscle contraction insufficient to bring about movement in a joint
Grade 2	Contraction sufficient to bring about movement with gravity eliminated
Grade 3	Contraction sufficient to bring about movement against gravity
Grade 4	Contraction strong enough to bring about movement Against some external resistance
Grade 5	Contraction strong enough to bring about movement against full external resistance (Normal power)

INVESTIGATION OF THE ORTHOPAEDIC PATIENT

It is possible to make a diagnosis of an orthopaedic condition on the basis of the above examination alone but a more detailed knowledge of its characteristics and the differential diagnosis (which are essential for its management) can only be obtained with the help of radiological and other (laboratory) investigations.

RADIOGRAPHIC IMAGING

Radiographic imaging, very much in the forefront of Medicine as a whole today, acquires special significance in orthopaedics. Very few orthopaedic conditions could be fully managed without it. The following modalities are in frequent use:

Conventional X-rays

An X-ray picture of the suspected disease site is imperative. Usually, two views, an anteroposterior (AP) and a lateral view, are sufficient but oblique views may sometimes be necessary. In limb pathologies, it is usually necessary to insist on the inclusion on the X-ray of one joint above and one joint below the disease site.

An X-ray picture will show the disease site and some characteristics of the abnormal changes caused by the disease e.g. a bony swelling, a bend in a bone, a destructive process going on in a bone, periosteal reaction to a disease process such as a malignant tumour or "wear and tear" changes in a joint.

A chest X-ray may be indicated in the elderly, mainly for anaesthetic purposes.

Tomography is a conventional X-ray imaging in which the beams are concentrated on a small area of interest – *"cone view"*. This method has been largely overtaken by computed tomography.

Computerised Tomographic (CT) scan

This provides a cross-sectional image of a given bone and can be very useful in the diagnosis of diseases in deep parts of the body, especially the skull, spine and pelvis. A 3-dimensional reconstruction is particular useful in intra-articular pathologies (Fig.2.1).

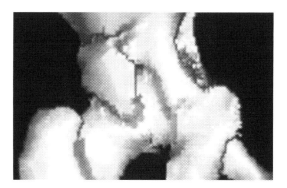

Fig.2.1. A 3-D reconstruction of a central dislocation of the right hip

Magnetic Resonance Imaging (MRI)

This investigation has progressed at a fast speed since Raymond Damadan produced a coarse MRI image of a rat tumour in 1974. It has revolutionised many aspects of the diagnosis and treatment of many orthopaedic diseases. The principle of the MRI is that when subjected to a magnetic field, different tissues react according to the number of protons in their nuclei. These reactions can be recorded on a film, providing pictures that are characteristic for the different tissues - bone, cartilage, muscle, tendon, nerve, fat, etc. These images or pictures are, so to say, tomographic maps of the distribution of protons in the tissue examined. They are obtained *without using ionising radiation*, which makes the method more desirable. Improvements of equipment and technique over the years have made it one of the most reliable of diagnostic tools available to the orthopaedic surgeon.

MRI is particularly useful in determining soft-tissue involvement in certain conditions such as spinal fractures, bone infections and malignant bone tumours (Fig.2.2).

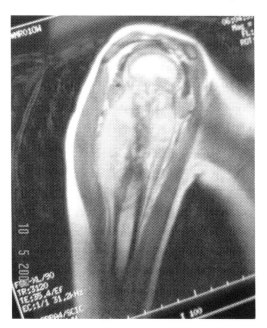

Fig.2.2. The massive soft-tissue involvement in this osteosarcoma of the proximal
humerus in a 12-year-old boy is best ap-
preciated on an MRI scan.

Ultrasonography (US)

Ultrasound is sound above the audible range, especially of frequency greater than 20 kilohertz (kHz). Diagnostic ultrasound operates in the frequency range of 1 – 20 megahertz (MHz). Equipment and technique are complex but the principle is that ultrasound, produced by piezoelectric effect using ceramic crystal elements and electric current, generates an electric pulse that is used to create an image. Subjected to ultrasound, different tissues, with differing acoustic and other properties, generate different characteristic images, which can be used for diagnostic purposes.

Like the MRI scan, *this investigation does not involve ionising radiation* and is particularly useful in the diagnosis of paediatric pathologies, rotator-cuff injuries and shoulder joint instability. A particularly important use of US in paediatric orthopaedics is in the assessment of congenital/developmental dysplasia of the hip for which it is clearly the imaging method of choice.

Ultrasound is used for therapeutic purposes in acute soft-tissue trauma.

Isotopic Bone Scan (Fig.2.3)

A radiolabelled phosphorus-based compound with affinity for bone tissue e.g. Technetium 99, Gallium 67 or Indium 111, is used as a physiological marker to detect abnormalities of bone metabolism. A 3-phase bone scan consists of the following:

- The first phase is an angiogram performed over the area of interest following the injection of the radionuclide. This is essentially a blood flow study.
- The 2nd phase consists of blood pool images taken after the injection. This phase detects superficial non-osseous pathology.
- The 3rd phase represents delayed images obtained 2-3 hours after the injection. These will show active osteoblastic activity and will be positive in various bone diseases.

Areas of increased uptake of marker are called "hot spots". Bone scan is indicated in the diagnosis and treatment of cellulitis, osteomyelitis, septic arthritis, avascular necrosis of bone and soft tissues and of bone tumours, especially metastatic tumours, which tend to be widespread. Its advantage over conventional X-rays is that it shows lesions much ealier. Unfortunately, it is non-specific, except if specific tracers are used e.g. Indium 111 and Gallium 67, in the investigation of suppurative diseases. In *acute osteomyelitis*, bone scan is positive within 24-48 hours of its onset in most cases.

Bone loss seen in a number of conditions e.g. avascular necrosis of the femoral head, is detected much earlier by bone scan. Up to 50% of bone loss has to be present before it is visible on an X-ray.

Single-Proton Emission Computed Tomography (SPECT) may be indicated in certain sites e.g. spine, femoral/humeral head and small bones of the hand and foot, where lesion detection may prove difficult with conventional bone scanning.

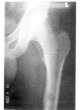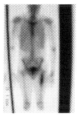

Fig.2.3. Osteosarcoma of the left femur on conventional XR and as a "hot spot" on a bone scan.

Arthrography

With the advent of MRI scanning, this investigation now has limited indications e.g. in the investigation of ligamentous lesions in the ankle.

Venography/Arteriography

A venogram is useful in the diagnosis of deep vein thrombosis, which may complicate disease management, especially post-surgery management. An arteriogram may also be indicated, though rarely.

LABORATORY TESTS

Blood and urine tests

Haemoglobin(Hb). Some bone diseases, e.g., rheumatoid arthritis; many bone tumour, e.g., osteopetrosis, cause anaemia. Furthermore, knowledge of the haemoglobin level is essential for the management of many orthopaedic diseases.

Full Blood Count (FBC). Elevated white cell count (leucocytosis) and thrombocytosis may be seen in many conditions, especially infections and the differential count may be helpful in the diagnosis of certain diseases, e.g., lymphomas.

Erythrocyte Sedimentation Rate (ESR) and C-reactive protein (CRP) are markers of acute inflammation; CRP is the more sensitive of the two. They are non-specific and are often raised in infections of bones, joints and soft tissues, including the internal organs; tumours of bones and soft tissues, etc. However, their being normal may exclude certain diagnoses.

Bone biochemistry.

- *Uric acid* is characteristically raised in gouty arthritis.

- *Alkaline phosphatase* is raised many times the normal level in Paget's disease. The *acid phosphatase* level is raised in prostatic carcinoma. *Abnormal proteins* are present both in the blood and urine in certain diseases.

- Abnormal proteins in the urine - Bence Jones protein – are characteristic of myelomas.

- *Vanillylmandelic acid* is present in the urine of patients with Ewing's tumour. There are other examples.

Joint fluid analysis

Naked eye appearance. The colour, viscosity and turpidity may indicate abnormality. Frank pus is recognisable. Acute synovial inflammation gives a thin turbid appearance.

Microscopy, biopsy and histology

The presence of large numbers of mononuclear cells on microscopy is consistent with a diagnosis of osteoarthritis. Polymorphonuclear cells predominate in RA, gouty arthritis and septic arthritis. In gout, urate crystals under polarised light are negatively birefringent whilst in pseudo-gout, calcium pyrophosphate dehydrate crystals are weakly positively birefringent.

Microscopy, culture and sensitivity studies are an essential part of day-to-day orthopaedic practice. The management of many orthopaedic infections, especially those involving Methicillin Resistant Staphylococcus Aureus (MRSA), require significant microbiological input. Many conditions, including inflammatory arthritis, metabolic diseases and bone tumours, require biopsy and histology for their definitive diagnosis. HLA tissue typing is useful in the diagnosis of ankylosing spondylitis.

Electrocardiography

An ECG may be indicated in the elderly or in patients with a history of heart disease.

PRINCIPLES OF TREATMENT OF ORTHOPAEDIC DISEASES

These can be divided into *non-surgical* and *surgical*.

NON-SURGICAL OPTIONS

- *Rest and Elevation*
  Rest and elevation of a diseased part are an essential part of management of most orthopaedic conditions. However, a balance has to be struck between the benefits of rest and the danger of deep vein thrombosis, which can be caused by immobility.

- **Splintage**
  In some cases, immobilisation of a diseased part facilitates its recovery. Dynamic splintage is also used e.g. walking calliper or the "lively" splint used in finger conditions.

- **Physiotherapy**
  Physiotherapy is quite inseparable from orthopaedic practice because it helps the surgeon to achieve one of the most important aims of orthopaedic disease management, namely, restoration of function. Several *physiotherapeutic modalities* are used to restore function to a diseased part:

  Active exercises help to mobilise joints, strengthen muscles and restore co-ordination and activities of daily living.

  Passive joint movements are used to activate weak or paralysed muscles.

  Local heat can be given by warm compress, short-wave diathermy, infra-red or radiant heat lamp.

Ice helps swollen or stiff joints to recover and is quite commonly used in the knee.

Wax baths are popular for mobilising arthritic feet and hands.

Ultrasound releases heat in tissues and also has a micro-massage effect, both of which are therapeutic.

Massage can be used to supplement active and passive exercises.

Electrical stimulation can reactivate muscles denervated by trauma or disease.

Hydrotherapy utilises the supportive effect of immersion of the body in water to facilitate the return of function in spinal and lower limb conditions.

Occupational Therapy

This encompasses measures designed to restore the patients ability to return to his usual occupation.

Drug Therapy

- *Analgesics* (Pain-killers) are commonly prescribed for orthopaedic diseases causing pain.

- *NSAIDs* (Non-Steroidal Anti-inflammatory Drugs) are frequently prescribed for degenerative and inflammatory bone and joint diseases

- *Antibiotics* are essential in the management of bone, joint and soft-tissue infections.

- *Steroids and other powerful drugs* are used in the management of inflammatory and metabolic bone diseases

- *Chemotherapy* uses powerful drugs to kill tumour cells and has contributed significantly to the on-going success of malignant bone and soft-tissue tumour management.

- *Radiotherapy*

  Radiotherapy is indicated in the management of certain bone and soft tissue tumours. It is usually used in combination with other treatment options such as surgical excision and chemotherapy.

- *Local injection of drugs*
  A drug can be delivered straight to the disease area by injection. In orthopaedics, local injections of a steroid and local anaesthetic are commonly carried out for knee joint diseases and for *tennis elbow, golfer's elbow* and *plantar fasciitis.*

- *Aspiration*
  This involves the use of a syringe and needle to suck up fluid from a joint, tissue or cavity

for the purpose of pain-relief, laboratory examination or both. Aspiration of the knee joint for these purposes is commonly done.

- *Manipulation of a joint*
  Forced manipulation is a last-resort measure used after physiotherapy has failed to restore movement in a joint. This is generally done under general anaesthesia for the purpose of increasing the range of movements in a joint e.g. in frozen shoulder (*adhesive capsulitis of the shoulder*) or in the treatment of knee stiffness following total knee replacement. Intensive physiotherapy must follow to ensure that the gained movement range is retained.

SURGICAL OPTIONS

- *Biopsy*
  Usually, this involves the removal of part of a tissue, suspected of being abnormal, for the purpose of histological examination but, sometimes, the whole tissue may be removed for the same purpose. If the later is the case, the procedure is called *excision-biopsy*.

- *Excision*
  This is removal of a part or the whole of a tissue or organ. Like biopsy, it is commonly done in tumour surgery but unlike biopsy, it is not always done for the purpose of histology. For example, in the procedure of total hip replacement for osteoarthritis, the femoral head is excised but not sent for histology, except if other pathology is suspected.

- *Debridement*
  Derived from French, this means excison or clearance. It is used mainly in relation to surgical clearance of dead tissues associated with open fractures or of necrotic tissues associated osteomyelitis or soft tissue infections.

- *Arthroplasty*
  This means reshaping or reconstruction of a joint. It encompasses the excision of the articular cartilage on one or more joint surfaces making up a joint. In the frequently performed operation of *total knee or hip arthroplasty* (also called *replacement*), the articular surfaces of these joints are excised and replaced with metallic and plastic implants moulded to articulate with one another. Artificial implants are sometimes not used to replace the cut surfaces, in which case the term *excision arthroplasty* is used. The classical example here is *the Girdlestone* operation in which only the proximal femur is excised and the acetabulum is left untouched. A *hemiarthroplasty* is one in which only one side/aspect of a joint is excised and replaced or reconstructed e.g. hip hemiarthroplasty with the Austin Moore or Thompson prostheses is frequently carried out for fractures of the neck of femur (Fig.2.4).

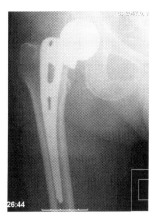

Fig.2.4. Hemiarthroplasty of the right hip using an Austin Moore prosthesis.

- *Arthrodesis*
This involves the excision of the articular cartilage of a joint and holding/fixation of the denuded bone ends to achieve fusion of the joint (*intra-articular arthrodesis or fusion*). However, fusion can also be achieved by placing a bone block across a joint capsule e.g. between the transverse processes of adjacent lumbar vertebrae – *extra-articular arthrodesis*. With the advent of arthroplasty, arthrodesis is no longer as popular as it used to be, especially with regard to the larger joints such as the knee and hip but it still retains a place in the treatment of hallux rigidus and infected knee joint replacement.

- *Bone grafting*
Bone grafting involves the harvesting and transfer of a piece of bone from one site to another and is usually carried out for the purpose of bridging a gap in a bone created by injury (fracture) or disease e.g. infection, tumour or congenital defect or for the purpose of stimulating new bone formation in the treatment of delayed or non-union.

  Three main basic types of bone grafts are recognised – *autograft* (graft from the patient themselves), *homograft* (graft from another person) and *heterograft* (graft from an animal). A graft could be of *cortical bone, cancellous bone or cortico-cancellous*. The iliac crest is the most common site/source of bone grafts.

- *Operations on the epiphyseal growth plate*
These operations are usually carried out in the management of limb deformities or leg-length discrepancies in children. Depending on the correction required, the growth plate may be wholly or partially:

  1. *destroyed* by excision or bone grafting to stop further growth
  2. *compressed* by stapling (*epiphysiodesis*) to slowdown growth or
  3. *stretched* with an external fixator (*epiphysiolysis*) to facilitate increased growth.

- *Decompression*
Decompression can be defined as "release/reduction of pressure in a tight tissue". The more common examples of surgical decompression include decompression of a tight carpal tunnel in the treatment of the carpal tunnel syndrome or the decompression of the ulnar nerve at the elbow in the treatment of peripheral ulnar neuritis at this point but we also have the so-called "core decompression" of the femoral head in the treatment of avascular necrosis of the femoral head.

- *Soft-tissue procedures*
These include operations on skin, muscles, tendons, nerves and other soft tissues.

PART II
ORTHOPAEDIC DISEASES

CHAPTER 3

ARTHRITIS

What is arthritis?

Arthritis is inflammation of one or more joints, characterised by pain, restricted movement, swelling and warmth of overlying skin. The involvement of one joint is termed **mono**-arthritis; **pauci**-arthritis is used to describe the involvement of a few joints and **poly**-arthritis describes the involvement of many joints. Let us remind ourselves of the structure of a synovial joint discussed in Chapter 1. The *joint cartilage* and *synovial membrane* are the structures initially affected by arthritis (synovial membrane in inflammatory arthritis and articular cartilage in osteoarthritis)

TYPES OF ARTHRITIS

1. **Inflammatory arthritis.** This is arthritis caused primarily by inflammation of the synovial membrane or entheses (the sites of insertion of tendons or ligaments into bone). Examples include **rheumatoid arthritis, ankylosing spondylitis, psoriatic arthritis, gout** and **pseudo-gout.**

2. **Degenerative arthritis**. This is arthritis caused primarily by wear and tear of the articular cartilage. The typical example is **osteoarthritis** and the terms "degenerative arthritis" and "osteoarthritis" are often used synonymously.

RHEUMATOID ARTHRITIS (RA)

Rheumatoid arthritis is an inflammatory disease of joints. In its acute stage, an affected joint is swollen and painful, especially on movement. The name "rheumatoid arthritis" is a bit misleading in that it may imply that the disease affects only joints. In fact, the disease is a multi-system one, affecting, in addition to joints, other systems, including the skin, the digestive system, heart, lungs, eyes and salivary glands. Involvement of joints does constitute a major part of the disease, hence the important role of the rheumatologist and orthopaedic surgeon in its management. Classically, a number of joints is affected simultaneously (*polyarthritis*) and usually in a symmetrical fashion, for example, both hands, both knees and both ankles.

Aetiology

The actual cause of rheumatoid arthritis is unknown. However, certain possible causative factors have been identified as follows:

Age. The disease affects both children and adults. The childhood variant is called *Still's disease.* The adult variant is seen mainly in the 25-50 age bracket.

Sex. It affects more women than men. A sex ratio of 3:1 is quoted.

Genetic considerations. There is a hereditary element in rheumatoid arthritis. Certain families appear to be more prone to the condition than others. Generally, those of African descent are less frequently affected than Caucasians.

Geographic considerations. Climate seems to be important: RA is more common in cold than in hot climates.

Possible role of infection. Infection with bacteria, viruses and mycoplasmas has been postulated. These agents have not yet been definitely identified.

Smoking has been shown to predispose to rheumatoid arthritis.

Pathogenesis

The main target organ in RA is synovial tissue and so any organ or structure possessing synovial tissue e.g. synovial joints, sheath and bursa, can be affected. In susceptible individuals, a yet-to-be-identified antigen is thought to trigger CD4 T lymphocytes in the synovium. These T lymphocytes are accompanied by neutrophils, mast cells, fibroblasts and macrophages, which induce an *acute inflammatory process.* The initial pathological lesion is highly vascularised through the activity of angiogenesis-stimulating factors released by the macrophages and fibroblasts. Macrophage-derived cytokines, interleukin (IL)-1, -6 and -8, tumour necrosis factor-alpha (TNF-alpha) and T cell-derived cytokines, IL-2, IL-4 and interferon-gamma, are all seen in the synovium.

The cumulative effect of the described processes taking place in the synovial membrane is that it not only hypertrophies but also undergoes hyperplasia, significantly increasing in size and forming a *pannus,* which is *a succulent band of "active" synovial membrane,* which "flows" on the articular cartilage, destroying it. There is comcomitant *enzymatic degradation of the matrix* of articular cartilage by proteolytic enzymes secreted by macrophages, neutrophils and fibroblasts. The pannus also destroys joint capsule, adjacent ligaments and tendon, with resulting instability.

As the disease process attains chronicity, *round cells, particularly lymphocytes and plasma cells,* become dominant, some organised as lymphoid follicles. Plasma cells in the synovium and the lymphoid system produce antibodies, known as *rheumatoid factors, RFs.* These are antibodies to autologous immunoglobulins, IgG, IgA and IgM. RFs are found in 70% of patients with RA and high titres (especially of IgG and IgA) are associated with severer forms of the disease. The remaining 30% are referred to as sero-negative.

Progressive destruction of joint structures results in a progressive appearance of joint deformity. In the hand, for example, there is typically a flexion deformity of the thumb at the metacarpophalangeal joint, ulnar deviation of the fingers at the metacarpophalangeal joints and flexion deformity at the proximal interphalangeal joints. These deformities constitute the so-called *rheumatoid hand* (Fig.3.1). In the knee, a valgus deformity is characteristic. Much later, a fibrous or bony ankylosis may develop.

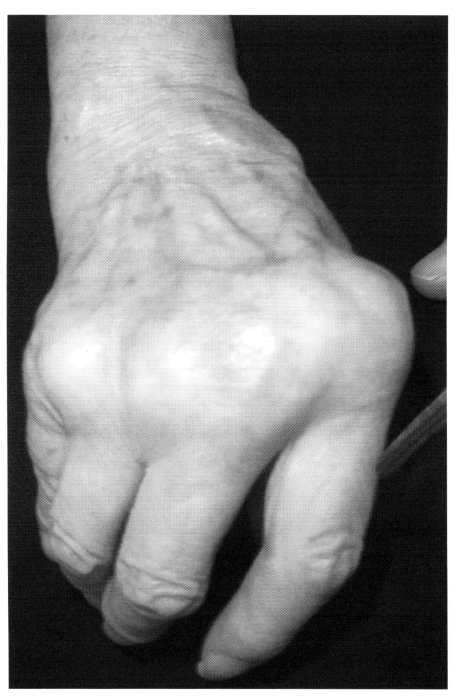

Fig.3.1. The rheumatoid hand. Note the generalised swelling and deformities of the fingers.

Extra-articular manifestations of RA include:

- *Tenosynovitis*

- *Rheumatoid nodules* are seen in about 20% of patients. They can be found (a) around tendons and tendon sheaths (b) lying subcutaneously in the posterior aspect of the elbow and forearm (c) in the gastrointestinal tract, lungs, heart, kidney and meninges. Histologically, a nodule is characterised by an irregular shape and a central zone of fibrinoid necrotic material surrounded by histiocytes and chronic inflammatory cells.

The primary involvement of the synovial membrane distinguishes RA from osteoarthritis, which is primarily targets the articular cartilage.

DIAGNOSIS

Symptoms of Rheumatoid Arthritis

General or systemic symptoms include:

- *malaise* (feeling generally unwell)
- *mild fever*
- *weight loss*
- *enlargement of lymph nodes* (lymphadenopathy), may be present at the onset or after
- *secondary anaemia* is common

Local symptoms are first seen in the joints of the hand or foot. Larger joints, especially the knee, may be affected on one or both sides. As a result of acute inflammation of the synovial membrane, the ***affected joints*** are:

- *swollen*
- *shiny*
- *warm to touch*
- *tender, painful and stiff.*

Muscle wasting around affected joints (peri-articular osteoporosis) is also a characteristic feature, especially in the larger joints such as the wrist and knee.

Deformities appear in the late stages of the disease following the involvement of other structures in and around the affected joint – tendons, capsules, ligaments and bone. These deformities can be quite characteristic e.g. hand deformities and knock-knee deformity of the knee joint.

Investigations

Blood tests.

Secondary anaemia is common. The white cell count is usually normal. The acute inflammatory markers – the Erythrocyte Sedimentation Rate (ESR) and C-Reactive Protein (CRP) are raised but they are non-specific for RA. The CRP is very sensitive to change and therefore is excellent for monitoring improvement or deterioration in the patient's condition.

The anti-body, *"Rheumatoid factor"*, is present in about 70% of patients, who are described as "sero-positive". Those in whom it is absent are termed "sero-negative). It must, however, be noted here that the rheumatoid factor is found in about 1% of the normal adult population.

Another antibody *Citrulline* (also referred to as anticitrulline antibody, anticyclic citrullinated peptide antibody, and anti-CCP) is present in most people with rheumatoid arthritis. Testing for citrulline antibodies is most helpful in looking for the cause of previously undiagnosed inflammatory arthritis in sero-negative patients. Yet another antibody called the <u>antinuclear antibody</u> *(ANA)* is also frequently found in people with rheumatoid arthritis.

A word of caution is appropriate here. The rheumatoid factor, ANA, ESR, and C-reactive protein tests can also be abnormal in other systemic autoimmune and inflammatory conditions. Therefore, abnormalities in these blood tests alone are not sufficient for a firm diagnosis of rheumatoid arthritis.

Regional distribution of rheumatoid arthritis in the body

Rheumatoid arthritis can affect any synovial joint of the body. The regional distribution and relative frequency are shown on Table 3.1.

Table 3.1. Regional Distribution of Rheumatoid Arthritis

Region	Part	Frequency
Spine	Cervical	Common
	Thoracic	Less common
	Lumbar	Less common
Upper Limb	Finger joints	Common
	Wrist joint	Common
	Elbow joint	Less common
	Shoulder joint	Less common
Lower Limb	Foot joints	Common
	Ankle joint	Common
	Knee joint	Common
	Hip joint	Common
Pelvis		Uncommon

Radiological features of RA

The radiographic changes in an affected joint depends on the stage of the disease. Characteristic features include:

- *Soft-tissue swelling around the affected joint* may be visible on X-ray.
- *Juxta-articular osteopenia* may be seen. This is caused by inflammation of the subchondral bone as well as by hyperaemia caused by inflammation of the synovium.

- *Loss of joint space* is progressive.
- *Bone erosions* and *Subchondral cysts* are seen in the later stages of the disease
- *Joint contracture and deformities* are seen in advanced disease

TREATMENT

Most RA patients are managed by Rheumatologists, who work closely with Physiotherapist and Occupational Therapists. The main objectives of management are the control of the inflammatory process and the resulting symptoms of joint swelling, pain and stiffness and to preserve joint function. A team approach is advocated for the best results. The orthopaedic surgeon is invited if surgical intervention is considered necessary.

Physiotherapy and Occupational therapy

The Physiotherapist and Occupational Therapist are early members of the management team. They help the patient to maintain good ranges of movements and strength in the joints, which together help to relieve pain. The occupational therapist has a role in teaching the patient how to cope with activities of daily living.

Drug treatment

- *Analgesics*
  Simple analgesics, such as Paracetamol, can be prescribed 4-6 hourly for pain relief. They have no anti-inflammatory effects.

- *Non-steroidal anti-inflammatory drugs (NSAIDs)*
  These drugs reduce joint swelling, stiffness and pain. Commonly used non-steroidals include Voltarol (Diclofenac sodium), Naproxen, Piroxicam, Indomethacin and Ibuprofen. Routes of administration include by mouth (oral), anal (as suppositories) and gels, liniments or creams applied to the skin. They vary in their potency and, even in right doses, are all plagued by varying degrees of gastrointestinal toxicity, manifesting as gastritis, peptic ulceration and bleeding. In some patients, there is also kidney toxicity. This is why it is so important that taking of these tablets is done under the doctor's supervision.

- *Corticosteroids*
  These are hormones secreted by the adrenal glands. They are potent anti-inflammatory and immunosuppressive drugs. The Cortisone analogues, Prednisone and Prednisolone, are commonly used to control the effects of active rheumatoid arthritis, especially joint swelling, pain and stiffness. Corticosteroids are toxic when used in high doses over a long period. Osteoporosis and hypertension are some of the possible complications. Corticosteroid therapy should be administered under the strict supervision of a Physician.

- *Disease-modifying anti-rheumatic drugs (DMARDs)*
  These are a group of drugs, which retard the development of joint erosions in RA. They include gold compounds, D-penicillamine, hydroxychloroqine and sulfasalazine.

- *Immunosuppressive drugs*
  Examples include Methotrexate, Azathioprine and Cyclophosphamide. Previously reserved for use in the later stages of the disease when joint erosion appears, these drugs are now recommended for use at the time of diagnosis. They are all potentially toxic and require careful and regular monitoring. Regular blood tests to monitor their toxic effects need to be carried out.

Surgical treatment

The place of surgery in the management of rheumatoid arthritis is relatively small but highly significant.

- *Synovectomy.* Excision of the synovial membrane of an affected joint can help to reduce joint swelling and pain. This is commonly carried out in the hand and knee

- *Repair of ruptured tendons* is commonly carried out in the hand

- *Joint replacement* is commonly carried out in the hand, knee (Fig.3.2) and hip. In knee or hip joint disease, joint replacement may provide the all-important relief of intolerable pain and restore mobility.

- *Arthrodesis.* This procedure joins together the bones forming affected joints so that there is no movement (and pain) in the joint. Though rarely performed these days, it remains a surgical option, especially in the wrist and cervical spine.

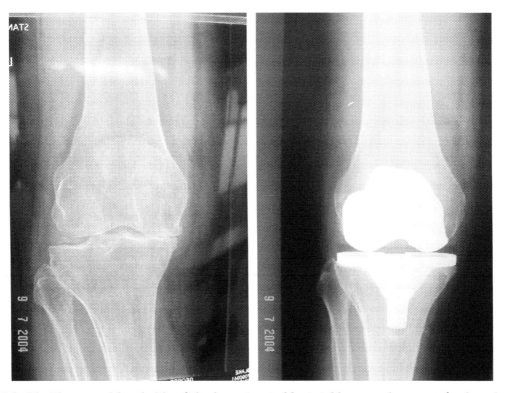

Fig.3.2a&b. Rheumatoid arthritis of the knee treated by total knee replacement (arthroplasty)

Juvenile rheumatoid arthritis (JRA)

This is also known as **Still's disease** and occurs in children aged less than 16 years. A number of sub-groups are distinguished on the basis of the course of the disease and the number of joints affected.

The *classic type* begins in early childhood (the child is often less than five), with marked generalised symptoms such as fever, enlargement of lymph nodes, liver and spleen and irritation of the eyes. The joints are affected but the systemic features overshadow the joint ones. Many of the children "outgrow" this variant of the disease. There are other varieties, including one in which joint involvement may start at an early age and predominate over the systemic symptoms, continue into adult life and cause progressive deformities

The diagnosis of Still's disease is made along lines similar to those used for adult RA. It should be suspected in a child with acute systemic symptoms and signs, even in the absence of joint swelling, pain and stiffness. Treatment is similar to that of adult rheumatoid arthritis but the approach has to be modified to accommodate the differences occasioned by age.

ANKYLOSING SPONDYLITIS

Ankylosing spondylitis is a disease characterised by progressive fusion (joining together) of the joints of the spine, causing back pain and stiffness. Ankylosing spondylitis, like rheumatoid arthritis, is a systemic disease, affecting not only joints but also other organs of the body. The disease is most common in white Caucasian men in the adolescent or adult age brackets. It tends to run in families.

Three patterns of affection can be distinguished as follows:

- *Spine and pelvic joints*
- *Large joints of the limbs e.g. hip and knee joints*
- *Systemic disease: fatigue, involvement of the eyes (iritis) and blood vessels*

The disease usually starts from one of the pelvic joints, the sacroiliac joints, and lumbar spine, causing low back pain and progressive stiffness. It gradually ascends to involve the chest and neck portions of the spine. The ribs may also be affected. Large joint involvement, especially the hip and knee joints, is seen in about 50% of patients. A variant of the disease has strong similarities with rheumatoid arthritis. However, unlike in rheumatoid arthritis, the small joints of the hand and feet are not commonly affected.

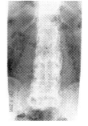

Fig.3.3. Ankylosing spondylitis in a 71-year-old man. Note the bamboo stem appearance.

Bridging bone formation between the vertebral bodies eventually results in the classical *bamboo spine (Fig.3.3).*

The diagnosis is made on the basis of the symptoms of pain and increasing stiffness of the spine, the characteristic deformity (Bamboo spine), a positive family history of the disease as well as characteristic findings in the blood of the patient. The latter deserves special mention: over 90% of patients with ankylosing spondylitis have the tissue antigen *HLA-B27* in their blood. However, this antigen is present in 7% of the general population, whereas only 1% develop ankylosing spondylitis. This means that most people with the antigen in their blood do not develop ankylosing spondylitis, so environmental and genetic factors are likely to play an important part in the development of the disease.

Treatment is mainly non-surgical.

- Constant exercises are essential in order to maintain as much suppleness of the spine and other affected joints as possible.
- Analgesics and non-steroidal anti-inflammatory drugs (NSAIDs) are usually helpful.
- Calcium and vitamin D supplements should be considered in an effort to reduce associated osteoporosis.
- Patients usually find the bent position of the spine comfortable but must be warned against this as it could lead to the spine fusing in the bent position.
- A programme of spine straightening exercises is instituted and brace support is sometimes indicated.
- Replacement of the hip is beneficial if hip disease is severe and there may be an indication for surgical cut (osteotomy) of the spine to straighten it.

GOUT

Gout is a particularly acute and painful form of inflammatory arthritis, caused by the deposition of *uric acid crystals* in a joint. Uric acid is the end-product of the breakdown in the body of a protein called *purine*. Uric acid crystals provoke an acute and painful inflammation in the affected joint.

Gout usually affects one joint at a time, usually in the **big toe,** which it attacks in 70% of patients. The reason for this preference for the big toe is not clear. Men are affected in 95% of cases and the first attack usually occurs in the 50s age bracket.

Two types of gout are distinguished as follows:

- *Primary gout,* which is caused by excess uric acid in the blood (*hyperuricamia*) due to defective workup of purine, a body protein, in the body.

- *Secondary gout,* which is due to disorders in which there is increased production of uric acid by cell breakdown as in leukaemia or cancers or other diseases which decrease the voiding of uric acid from the body, for example, chronic kidney disease. Certain drugs, e.g. those inducing urine formation (diuretics), can also cause gout.

Clinically, *Acute* and *Chronic gout* may also be distinguished. Briefly, acute gout is characterised by acute inflammatory arthritis, whereas chronic gout is characterised by diffuse deposits of chalky whitish material in skin and other tissues, especially in the hands, feet and earlobes (*chronic tophaceous gout*).

DIAGNOSIS

The diagnosis is made on the basis of characteristic clinical, laboratory and X-ray findings.

Symptoms

- Acute gout usually affects the big toe.

- An attack is characterised by a rapid onset of acute pain. It may be precipitated by local trauma, surgery, illness, alcoholic or dietary over-indulgence. The affected joint is swollen, red in light-skinned people, warm to touch and exquisitely tender and the patient walks with a limp. Low-grade fever may be present.

- Recurrent attacks lead to chronicity and joint destruction, especially in the fingers, where whitish chalk-like lumps of uric acid crystals can be seen or felt under the skin(*gouty tophi*.) Tophi may also be deposited in the earlobe, tendon sheath and bursae, especially at the point of the elbow and the knee cap. About 15% of gout patients develop uric acid stones in their kidneys.

Investigations

Examination of the joint fluid reveals the characteristic picture of uric acid crystals. Blood tests reveal a high level of uric acid. There is a need to differentiate it from pseudogout. X-rays may show typical well-demarcated rounded erosions close to the joint margins, usually in the hands. Joint destruction may be seen later.

Treatment

Diet

- As uric acid is formed from the breakdown of purines, adopting a low-purine diet will helpPlant purines have been shown by researchers to be safer than animal purines. Ideally, a low-purine diet needs to be worked out with the help of a Dietician.

Drug treatment

- It is important that treatment is prescribed and monitored by the doctor. High doses of anti-inflammatory drugs will normally control an acute attack. Amongst others, Indomethacin, Diclofenac sodium and Piroxicam are effective. Colchicine may be used instead of anti-inflammatories in patients with heart failure or who are on anti-coagulants as the latter may induce fluid retention or interfere with anti-coagulant therapy.

- Frequent attacks, the presence of chalky deposits (tophi) or signs of chronic gouty arthritis requires long-term control of uric acid levels in the blood with Allopurinol and other drugs.

Surgical treatment involves the excision of chalky deposits from the affected joint.

PSEUDOGOUT

This disease mimics gout but the crystals deposited in the affected joints are those of calcium pyrophosphate. (instead of uric acid as in gout). Men are again more frequently affected than women (ratio 3:2) and most patients are aged over 50 years. *The condition does not produce symptoms in some individuals.*

As with gout, there are also two forms:

- *Primary form*: this is due to a familial enzyme abnormality and

- *Secondary form:* this is due to some metabolic disorder such as an overactive parathyroid gland (hyperparathyroidism), an underactive thyroid gland (hypothyroidism), diabetes or gout.

In symptomatic cases, there is an acute onset of pain and swelling of the affected joint. The swelling is much less profuse than with gout and although one joint is initially affected as with gout, this is rapidly followed by involvement of other joints in the vicinity of the first. Large joints such as the knee, shoulder and wrists are frequently involved; the big toe is very rarely involved.

In common with gout, an attack may be provoked by local trauma, illness or surgery and although there are other similarities with gout, the doctor can distinguish between the two diseases using x-ray features, blood tests and examination of joint fluid under the polarised microscope.

Treatment. Indomethacin can take the edge off an acute attack. Injection of steroids into the affected joint may be used to control stubborn cases.

PSORIATIC ARTHRITIS

Like rheumatoid arthritis, **psoriasis** also affects a number of body systems, not only joints. It is characterised by patchy and itchy dermatitis (inflammation of the skin), damaged nails and inflammation of joints, the latter occurring in about 7% of patients. Three per cent (3%) of rheumatoid arthritis patients also have psoriaris. The skin problems usually appear before the joints become involved. Usually, outlying joints, especially the finger joints, are involved but large joints such as the knee and the spine are sometimes involved too.

Doctors distinguish five types of joint involvement in psoriasis, depending on the joints involved and on nail involvement.

Involvement of finger joints is common. In a typical case, involved fingers are sausage-shaped. The characteristic radiographic feature is best seen in the distal interphalangeal joints of the hand where severe erosions result in a "pencil-in-cup" appearance. Periostitis may be seen along the shafts of long bones. X-rays of affected larger joints, such as the knee joint, show features similar to osteoarthritis.

Treatment options include:

- the use of creams, ultraviolet light for skin problems and anti-inflammatories for joint problems.

- With regard to a possible role for diet, the initial hope that Omega-3 fish oils would bring relief to psoriasis patients was not fulfilled. However, a few recent studies have demonstrated improvement in general symptoms of psoriasis from adoption of a gluten-free diet (Gluten is a protein found in grasses such as wheat, rye and barley).

- Disease-modifying drugs such as Methotrexate, Azathioprine and gold may be used in severe cases. These are toxic drugs and their use requires constant monitoring by the doctor.

- *Surgical management* is indicated when joint destruction has resulted in severe pain and restricted movement. Severe affection of a large joint such as the knee can be treated by total joint replacement.

OSTEOARTHRITIS

Definition of Osteoarthritis

Osteoarthritis is a degenerative disease of one or more joints caused by wear and tear of the joint cartilage, with associated damage to neighbouring structures of the joint. It is, in effect, an age-related degenerative process in a joint.

AETIOLOGY

Primary and secondary OA are recognised:

Primary osteoarthritis is age-related wear and tear (degeneration) of articular cartilage with no known underlying cause i.e. it is **idiopathic**.

Secondary osteoarthritis is degenerative arthritis caused by previous injury or disease of the affected joint

Conditions predisposing to Secondary osteoarthritis

- previous injury to the affected joint (bony or cartilage)
- Previous infection
- Burnt-out inflammatory joint disease
- Congenital abnormality
- Abnormal weight (Obesity)
- Abnormal joint alignment and load sharing
- Joint instability

PATHOLOGY

The disease starts in the articular cartilage of the joint. There is softening and splitting of the cartilage (fibrillation). There is a breakdown of both the proteoglycan ground substance and the fibrous component of cartilage, collagen, mediated by enzymes. Mechanical, anatomical, physiological and biochemical factors are involved. There is evidence that mechanical factors precede the others: the earliest changes are found in areas of concentration of weight-bearing, load shearing and twisting stresses. Progressive cartilage wear results in the underlying bone rubbing against each other, resulting in abrasive wear, fatigue fractures and production of peripheral osteophytes, subchondral sclerosis and subchondral cysts.

REGIONAL DISTRIBUTION

Osteoarthritis has a broad distribution in the body (Figs.3.4-3.6):

- SPINE – Cervical (Cervical spondylosis) - common
  - Thoracic – less common
  - Lumbar (Lumbar spondylosis) - common
- UPPER LIMB – shoulder, elbow, wrist, finger joints
- LOWER LIMB – hip, knee, ankle, foot joints
- PELVIS – iliosacral joint OA

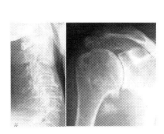

Fig.3.4. OA cervical spine and shoulder joint

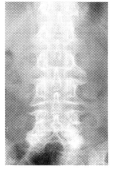

Fig.3.5. OA lumbar spine

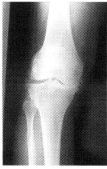

Fig.3.6a&b. OA of the knee joint treated by total knee replacement.

SYMPTOMS OF OA

- **Pain** – the most important single symptom. Varies in intensity. Exacerbated with use. More in weight-bearing joints of the lower limb than in the upper limb.
- **Stiffness** - usually associated with pain.
- **Swelling** - associated with joint fluid production plus/minus synovial hyperplasia
- **Deformity** - secondary to progressive joint damage and muscle pull imbalances

PHYSICAL SIGNS

- Abnormal posture and gait
- Deformity
- Tenderness – generalised/localised
- Limited movement
- Crepitus may be present

RADIOLOGICAL SIGNS

- Narrowing of joint space
- Peripheral osteophytes
- Subchondral sclerosis
- Subchondral cysts
- Deformity e.g. Genu varum/valgum

TREATMENT

Non-surgical treatment

- **Modification of activity.** The patient is advised to do less of those activities that put the affected joint under undue stress.

- **Drugs** – Analgesics and NSAIDs are prescribed as in rheumatoid arthritis.

Surgical treatment

Surgery has an important place in the management of osteoarthritis. Surgical options include:

- *Corrective osteotomy* can be carried out to correct mal-alignment. Particularly successful in the knee joint.

- *Joint replacement* is commonly carried out in the knee and hip joints (Fig.3.6 & 3.7), where it usually provides the all-important relief of intolerable pain and restores mobility. Other joints e.g. the shoulder and elbow, are also being replaced.

- *Arthrodesis.* This procedure joins together the bones forming an affected joint so that there is no movement (and pain) in the joint. Though rarely performed these days, it remains a surgical option, especially in the hand and toes.

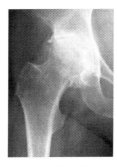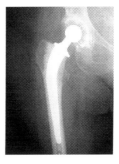

Fig.3.7a&b. OA of the hip joint treated with Total Hip Replacement

Further reading

Resnick D and Niwayama G. Diagnosis of Bone and Joint Disorders, 4th edition. Philadelphia, W B Saunders, 2002.

CHAPTER 4

METABOLIC BONE DISEASES

Metabolic bone diseases are diseases caused by disturbances in the normal formation, mineralization and remodelling of bone. They may result from familial, nutritional or hormonal abnormalities or a combination of them. Osteoporosis is the commonest and best-known of the metabolic bone diseases. Others include Paget's disease, rickets, osteomalacia and osteogenesis imperfecta.

OSTEOPOROSIS

What is osteoporosis?

Osteoporosis is thinning or shrinking of bone. The quality of the bone itself is normal but there is not enough of it because of decreased bone formation and increased destruction. It affects mainly the elderly, mostly women; it is widespread, affecting about 200 million women worldwide and 25 million people in the United States alone. Many affected individuals are unaware of it until they suffer a fracture because of it. Fractures resulting from osteoporosis are estimated at 1.5 million in the US and 250,000 in the UK. Figures for Africa are awaited.

Predisposing factors

- *Age* - it affects mainly people of the middle-age group or beyond
- *Sex* - it affects mainly oestrogen-deficient post-menopausal women
- *Heredity* appears to be important. People of African descent seem to be less prone to the disease than Caucasians. Also a positive family history is a factor.
- *Geography* - it is more common in temperate than in tropical climate.
- *Low body weight* - people weighing less than 120 lb or 85% of their ideal body weight are more prone to the condition.
- *Premature menopause* has also been identified as a cause of osteoporosis.
- *Environmental factors*, including poor nutrition and low dietary intake of calcium, have also been blamed.
- *Lifestyle* - smoking, inactivity, unfavourable medication, especially steroid intake, has been shown to have a negative effect on bone mineral density.

- *Various other diseases*. Diseases of the blood, thyroid gland, the kidneys and post-gastrectomy syndrome have also been blamed.

Types of osteoporosis

Type 1 - Occurs at menopause and is 6 times more common in women than men. It is more related to oestrogen deficiency than to calcium intake. This is a high turnover osteoporosis with net bone loss of bone at the rate of 2-3% per year for many years (6-10 years). This type is clearly associated with spinal fractures.

Type 2 – This is *senile osteoporosis* seen in people older than 75 years. Again, women are more frequently affected than men but in the lower ratio of 2:1. It is believed to arise from prolonged lack of calcium in the body. It is a low turnover osteoporosis associated with prolonged calcium deficiency.

SYMPTOMS AND SIGNS

Fractures (Figs 4.1)

Fractures are the commonest signs of osteoporosis. They are typically caused by trivial trauma and are described as "pathological" because it is thought that they would not have occurred had the bone not been weakened by disease. These fractures are most common in the spine (Fig.4.1), proximal femur, proximal humerus, wrist and ribs.

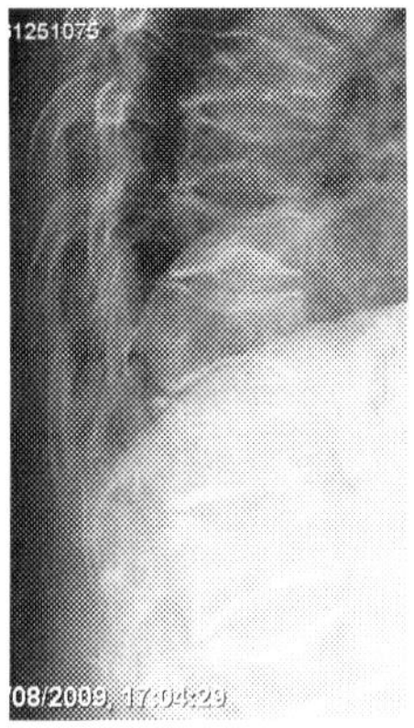

Pain

Pain is an important symptom of osteoporosis, especially of the spine, due to vertebral collapse.

Fig.4.1. Compression fracture in the lumbar spine secondary to osteoporosis

Round-back deformity (hunchback)

This is also a significant sign, which results from crushing of vertebral bones weakened by disease.

Diagnosis

In the non-emergency situation, the patient usually seeks help for back pain and spinal deformity (round back). In the emergency situation, they present with a wrist, hip or other fracture. X-rays will diagnose fractures but a **DEXA scan** (Dual-Energy X-ray Absorptiometry scan) and biochemical tests are essential for the confirmation of osteoporosis. It is important to emphasise that the most the important single diagnostic test for osteoporosis is the DEXA scan, which accurately measures **bone mineral density (BMD)** whilst emitting only low-dose radiation.

BMD is measured in the hip and/or spine and the figures obtained are compared to the peak bone mass in young adults. The difference is expressed as a T-score, which represents one standard deviation above or below the ideal bone mass. A BMD value less than 1 standard deviation below the young adult mean is considered normal. A value between -1 and -2.5 standard is defined as osteopenia, whilst a value lower than -2.5 standard deviations is defined as osteoporosis.

In summary,

T-scores: **Normal** 0-1   **Osteopenia** -1 to -2.5   **Osteoporosis** <2.5

Laboratory investigations include blood tests to measure the level of calcium (usually normal), phosphorus (usually normal), vitamin D, urea and minerals in the blood as well as thyroid and parathyroid gland function. For men, the serum testosterone level is measured as well.

Treatment

Drugs used to prevent and treat osteoporosis are very potent and can lead to serious complications. This is why it is important that all treatment and preventive procedures are prescribed and monitored closely.

Early prevention

This is the best policy but the opportunity to achieve this is largely lost by the time the condition is diagnosed. It should be started early along these lines:

- Children, adolescents and young adults should be encouraged to attain their peak bone mass in the 20-30 age bracket – by proper nutrition, adequate calcium and vitamin D intake and weight-bearing exercises.

- Females should be encouraged to maintain a normal menstrual cycle.

Late treatment

There are drugs that help to prevent fractures by strengthening the bones:

- *Hormone Replacement Therapy (HRT)* is suitable in healthy postmenopausal women but has been associated with a long-term risk of developing breast cancer, blood clots (deep-vein thrombosis) and stroke.

- *Bisphosphonate drugs:* Alendronate, risedronate, zoledronate reduce the rate of bone turnover and have been shown to decrease the occurrence of fractures of the spine, hip and other osteoporosis-related fractures in postmenopausal women.

- *Strontium ranelate (Protelos)* is a new anti-osteoporosis drug, which has the double action of promoting bone formation and reducing bone destruction. It has been shown to produce early and sustained reduction in vertebral (backbone), hip and other osteoporosis-related fractures.

- *Parathyroid hormone peptides* are promising new drugs. Positive effects have been reported after only four weeks of treatment!

- *Calcium and vitamin D supplementation* have been shown to reduce hip and other non-vertebral fractures in very elderly patients living in residential accommodation.

- *Lifestyle changes/advice and physiotherapy* can be of some benefit.

Treatment of fractures

Fractures of the spine, shoulder, wrist and hip are treated by the orthopaedic surgeon by casting or open surgery. Physiotherapy and rehabilitation are essential for a successful outcome. Preventive treatment as stipulated above should be instituted alongside fracture treatment.

The cost implication of osteoporosis

The cost implications of treating osteoporosis have been assessed mainly for the western world, where it has been estimated that 1 in 3 women and 1 in 5 men surviving to 80 years of age will suffer a hip fracture related to osteoporosis.

- In the United States, as long ago as 1996, the cost of treatment of osteoporosis-related hip fractures alone was put at between $13 and $18 billion yearly! Today, it is estimated at US$19 billion. If the cost of treatment of spinal, shoulder and wrist fractures is added, this figure may double.

- Cost figures for other western countries include 2.1 billion pounds for the UK and 25 billion Euros for Europe.

- Figures for the developing countries will come but with people living longer nowadays, the number of patients with osteoporosis worldwide is bound to increase and the cost of treatment will keep rising. Therefore, it goes without saying that prevention is the way forward.

RICKETS & OSTEOMALACIA

Decreased mineralisation of bone in children is called rickets whilst the adult variety is called osteomalacia. These conditions, though rare, are still seen in clinical practice. They are usually due to dietary deficiency in calcium or to defective absorption, synthesis or metabolism of vitamin D.

RICKETS

Pathology. Rickets can be caused by a number of disease conditions adversely affecting skeletal development. Classical rickets is caused by vitamin D deficiency due to decreased absorption of calcium and phosphorus, which causes a compensatory increase in the production of parathyroid hormone. Pseudo-vitamin D deficiency rickets is due to defective renal synthesis of vitamin D and vitamin D- resistant rickets is due to decreased renal reabsorption of phosphate.

Diagnosis. Rickets is characterised by widespread skeletal deformities affecting mainly the foci of rapid growth. It may be recognised in infants as young as 6 months of age. The diagnosis is based on the classical symptoms and signs of the condition, radiological and biochemical findings. The clinical features of rickets are summarized below and illustrated on Fig.4.2.

Skull: Protruding forehead(Frontal bossing) – from thinning and softening of the calvaria and bulging of the fontanelles

Chestwall: "Rachitic rosary" – from beading(enlargement) of the costochondral junctions of the ribs; "pidgeon chest" deformity; depression along the line of the rib-diaphragm attachment (Harrison's groove).

Protruding abdomen: this is a characteristic feature.

Wrists, knees, ankles: may be enlarged due to failure of mineralisation of metaphyseal primary spongiosa.

Long bones: a curvature may develop: anterior bowing of the tibia is characteristic.

Pathological fractures are common presenting features of rickets. They usually occur in the ends of the long bones.

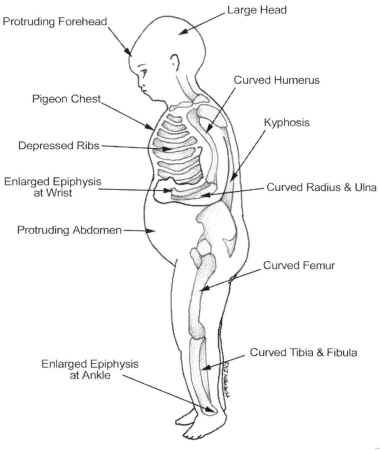

Fig.4.2. Clinical features of rickets

Radiological findings in active rickets include:

- *generalised osteoporosis* of bones
- *thickening and widening of the growth plate:* this may predispose to a slip.
- *cup-shaped concavity and flaring of the metaphyses ("cupping")*(Fig.4.3)
- *bowing of the diaphysis of long bones.*

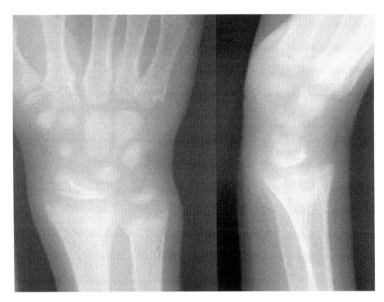

Fig.4.3. Widening and cupping of the metaphyses

Treatment.

- Classical rickets responds to small daily doses of Calciferol.

- Pseudo-vitamin D deficiency rickets is treated with high doses of vitamin D (Ergocalciferol).

- Vitamin D-resistant rickets (Familial hypophosphatemic rickets) requires large doses of vitamin D as well as neutral phosphate.

- Osteomalacia is also difficult to treat because it is invariably accompanied by osteoporosis as well. Larger doses of Calciferol and calcium are used.

- The treatment of pathological fractures in rickets and osteomalacia depends on their sites and the peculiarities of the fractured bone. In the long bones, treatment will likely follow lines of treatment similar to those used for non-pathological fractures. In the spine, some form of external support may be necessary. Concomitant systemic treatment is also advised.

Osteomalacia

Pathology. Failure of mineralisation in an adult results in the production of large quantities of unmineralised osteoid.

Diagnosis. The symptoms and signs of osteomalacia are more subtle than those of rickets, particularly in mild or moderate disease. Mildly affected patients may present with nonspecific bone pain and tenderness and possibly hypotonia. Severely affected patients may experience difficulty in walking and may have a waddling gait. Pathological fractures may occur at typical sites: vertebral bodies, long bones, axillary margin of the scapula, pubic rami, and ribs. Besides fractures, a classical radiological sign of osteomalacia is the presence of the so-called *looser's zone*, which is a thin transverse band of rarefaction in an otherwise normal-looking bone. This zone is due to healing of stress fractures with callus that lacks calcium and can be seen in long bones, the pelvis and the scapula.

Treatment. Osteomalacia is much more difficult to treat than rickets because it is invariably accompanied by osteoporosis. Larger doses of Calciferol and calcium are required. Pathological fractures are treated by the orthopaedic surgeon by bracing or operation.

HYPERPARATHYROIDISM

The parathyroid gland is a hormone-secreting organ lying next to the thyroid gland. It produces the parathyroid hormone (PTH), which mobilizes calcium from bone. Hyperparathyroidism is excessive functioning of the gland resulting in over-production of the hormone; this can weaken the bones, rendering them liable to deformity and pathological fractures.

Two types of hyperparathyroidism are recognized: primary and secondary. In *primary hyperparathyroidism*, a tumour (an adenoma) or overactivity of the gland is responsible for PTH over-production. In *secondary hyperparathyroidism*, the underlying condition is chronic renal failure, which produces acidic urine, which, in turn, requires a lot of calcium for its neutralisation. Removal of calcium from the blood for this purpose stimulates the parathyroid gland, causing it to produce more PTH in order to mobilise more calcium from the skeleton.

One of the main results of hyperparathyroidism is a general loss of bone substance due to increased breakdown of bone. The vertebrae, phalanges and long bones are commonly affected and could be the sites of pathological fractures. In severe cases, brownish tumour-like masses, the so-called *brown tumour of hyperparathyroidism,* may form. Such a site is particularly vulnerable to pathological fracture.

Symptoms of hyperparathyroidism include nausea, loss of appetite, abdominal pain, excessive passing of urine, kidney stones and bone pain. Laboratory investigation of the patient can confirm the diagnosis before a pathological fracture occurs. Treatment may involve the removal of a parathyroid tumour or part of an overactive gland. This is usually carried out by a specialist surgeon. Pathological fractures, if they occur, are treated by the orthopaedic surgeon.

SCURVY

This is a nutritional disease caused by lack of vitamin C (ascorbic acid) in the diet. Ascorbic acid is essential for the synthesis of collagen, the protein fibre found in bone, cartilage, muscle and other soft tissues of the musculo-skeletal system. Lack of adequate amounts of vitamin C in the diet results in inadequate production of normal collagen; this can result in the development of the disease.

The characteristic symptom of scurvy is an increased tendency to bleeding, especially beneath mucous membranes and the connective tissue sheaths covering bones (the periosteum). Wounds also heal poorly in scurvy. Bleeding of the gums on minimal trauma such as teeth-brushing is an early sign of vitamin C insufficiency.

From the orthopaedic view-point, bleeding under the periosteum and into joints, especially the knee and shoulder, are quite common and can be disabling. In children, the growth plate is usually affected, with resulting deformity. Bone formation (osteogenesis) is also impaired, and with resulting osteoporosis, pathological fractures may occur. Treatment is mainly by adding an increased amount of citrus fruits, fruit juices and ascorbic acid to the diet. Specific orthopaedic treatment is needed for fractures and deformities.

OSTEOGENESIS IMPERFECTA (OI)

Translated from Latin, osteogenesis imperfecta means imperfect or defective synthesis or manufacture of bone. It is the most common congenital (inherited) disease affecting the synthesis of collagen, the protein fibre found in bone, cartilage, muscle and other soft tissues of the musculo-skeletal system. The underlying abnormality is a failure of formation of normal bone ground substance (bone matrix).

Osteogenesis imperfecta is characterised by osteopenia (insufficient amount of bone), lax ligaments and thinning of the sclera. Fractures are common in this disease because of the bony deficiency. Six types of osteogenesis imperfect have been identified. They are all characterised by an increased liability of the affected bone to fracture.

Diagnosis

The symptoms and signs are diagnostic:

- General - The disease may be apparent at birth or may appear shortly afterwards. Many affected infants survive only a few weeks. Most of those who survive are short in stature and the most severely affected are dwarfed.

- Fractures - These are common and often multiple. Those with the more severe forms of the diseases sustain more fractures than those with the milder forms. Multiple fractures are more common in children than in adults. When repeated, they tend to occur at the same sites.

- A blue sclera is also a feature but not all aff ected individuals have it.

- Other features include lax ligaments, poorly formed teeth (dentinogenesis imperfecta) and deafness.

X-rays will show the characteristic bone changes, including fractures.

Treatment

This is necessarily multi-disciplinary, with a big role played by parents, carers, the Physiotherapist and the Occupational therapist. Orthopaedic management is mainly to do with the treatment of resulting fractures. Fortunately, the fractures heal well. Severe bowing of long bones can be corrected with multiple osteotomies and fixation.

MARFAN'S SYNDROME

First described by the French paediatrician, Marfan, in 1896, the distinguishing orthopaedic features of this syndrome are disproportionately long and thin limbs and digits, generalised joint laxity and scoliosis. Other features include dislocation of the lenses (of the eyes), heart defects and predisposition to developing hernias. Photographs of Abraham Lincoln are said to suggest that he was afflicted with this syndrome.

PAGET'S DISEASE (FIG.4.4)

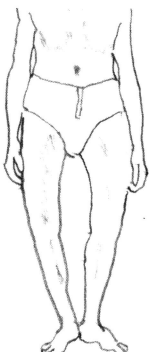

Paget's disease is characterised by excessive bone tissue formation and breakdown and the second most common metabolic disease - after osteoporosis. It was first described by Sir James Paget in 1877. The excessive bone tissue formation is greater than the bone breakdown, so, there is a net gain in bone tissue with resulting enlargement of the involved bone. The tibia and femur are classical sites of Paget's disease but virtually any bone in the body can be affected such as the skull, the lumbar spine and pelvis. However, before we go too far, let it be noted that many patients with the disease have no symptoms.

The cause of Paget's disease is ill-understood at the present time. However, a possible viral cause has been postulated. Heredity and geography are probably important too: its prevalence is comparatively high in northern Europeans, whilst it is very rare in black people and Asians. Age is also important: most affected individuals are aged over 40; so also is sex: the vast majority of patients are males.

Fig.4.4. Paget's disease. Note the shape of the lower legs.

Diagnosis

As noted earlier, most patients with the disease are symptomless, the disease being discovered by accident, usually by X-rays taken for some other complaint. Some patients may present with complications of the disease such as fracture, heart failure (from severe involvement of the bone marrow), arthritis and tumour. Local bone and joint pain and low back pain are common features. In lower limb involvement, thickening and deformity are common. The tibia usually bows forward ("sabre" tibia), whilst the femur bows forward and to the side. Despite progressive deformity, these bones remain strong enough for the patient to continue weightbearing for long.

In spinal involvement, kyphosis (round back), scoliosis (sideways bend) and spinal canal narrowing with nerve root or cord compression, are seen. Progressive thickening of the external cortex of the skull may result in enlargement of the head. The classical confirmatory laboratory test for Paget's disease is for serum alkaline phosphatase, which is found to be raised by up to 20-30 times the normal level.

Treatment

Patients with active disease are treated with a number of drugs, including Bisphosphonates and Calcitonin.

Complications

Apart from pathological fractures and the blood flow and heart complications mentioned above, Paget's disease can cause malignant bone tumours.

MARBLE BONE DISEASE

(Osteopetrosis) (Albers-Schonberg disease)

Osteopetrosis is a rare disease characterised by the formation of extremely hard, dense bones throughout the growing skeleton, which persists till the cessation of skeletal growth. The density and hardness of the formed bone is the reason for the alternative name of Marble bone disease. At the root of the disease lies decreased breakdown of bone and cartilage whilst bone formation is normal. The bone consists of cores of calcified cartilage, surrounded by areas of new bone, usually woven bone, which is fragile and so prone to fracture. Nine types of the disease have been identified.

Further reading

Favus MJ (editor). Primer on the Metabolic Bone diseases and Disorders of Mineral Metabolism, 4th edition. Philadelphia, PA, Lippincott-Williams & Wilkins, 1999.
Siris ES. Paget's disease of bone. *J Bone Miner Res 13: 1061, 1998.*
Mankin HJ. *Metabolic bone disease. Inst Course Lect 44:3, 1995.*

CHAPTER 5

BONE AND JOINT INFECTIONS

Introduction

For orthopaedic purposes an infection is a pus-producing disease caused by germs. It can affect any tissue of the musculo-skeletal system. Bone infection is termed osteomyelitis. Infection of a joint is termed septic arthritis, whilst that of muscle is termed pyomyositis. Bone infection can be a particularly dreadful disease, dreaded by patients because it is self-perpetuating and by doctors because it may take several months, even years to cure. Sometimes, it is incurable!

ACUTE HAEMATOGENOUS OSTEOMYELITIS

Causative organisms

The most frequently isolated organism is *Staphylococcus aureus,* which is involved in 70-80% of cases, singly or in combination with other microbes. The causative organisms may differ according to the age or other peculiarities of the patient:

Neonates: *Staphylococcus aureus; Streptococcus pyogenes; Gram-negative bacilli e.g. E. coli.*

Infants and children under 2-3 years: *Staphylococcus aureus; Streptococcus pyogenes; Haemophilus influenzae.*

Older children: *Staphylococcus aureus* is responsible in the vast majority of cases.

Sickle cell disease patients: *Salmonella* is the commonest causative organism in patients with sickle cell disease. Other commonly isolated organisms are *Staphylococcus aureus, Streptococcus pneumoniae* and *H. influenzae.*

Intravenous drug users: *Staphylococcus aureus; Streptococcus pyogenes; P. aeruginosa.*

Other organisms: *Pneumococcus, Pseudomonas aeruginosa, Proteus mirabilis, Escherichia coli (E. coli), Salmonella*

This list is not exhaustive.

Pathogenesis (Fig.5.1)

The causative organisms are known to originate from an infective focus in the body, such as boils, infected tonsils, tooth abscess, upper respiratory or lower urinary tract infection, from where they gain access to the bloodstream. Transported in the bloodstream, their deposition at the site of infection is determined and influenced by various factors. For example, *antecedent trauma* and *anatomical peculiarities of the affected sites* are thought to be important in children, in whom the most frequently affected sites are *areas of rapid growth and increased risk of trauma e.g.* the *metaphysis* of the proximal tibia, distal femur, proximal humerus and distal radius. It is postulated that trauma and the large calibre of the metaphyseal veins in these areas in children predispose to marked slowing of the blood flow in the veins, with resulting venous thrombosis, which, in turn, facilitates the deposition of blood-borne bacteria. Acute haematogenous osteomyelitis is uncommon in adults; cases seen are usually in intravenous drug abusers.

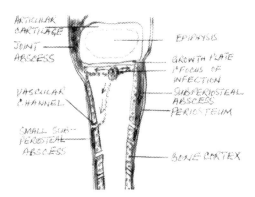

Fig.5.1. Acute haematogenous osteomyelitis: The pathological lesion and possible routes of local spread

Having been deposited at the infection sites, the causative organisms proceed to multiply. The result is *acute exudative inflammation,* with increased vasculiarity, oedema and polymorphonuclear leucocytes. Within 48 to 72 hours, thrombosis of more veins and increased medullary pressure result in bone ischaemia and necrosis. Bacteria, their toxins, an altered pH, local oedema and vascular occlusion all contribute to bone necrosis.

Formed abscess looks for a way out and may enter the joint, producing *a joint abscess* (septic arthritis) or tract under the periosteum, forming a *subperiosteal abscess,* which may perforate the periosteum to form soft-tissue abscess. If a subperiosteal abscess is circumferential in nature, part or the whole shaft may be cut off from its blood supply and undergo cell death, becoming a *sequestrum.* Usually, the elevated periosteum around this dead bone would produce an encircling new bone envelope - *involucrum* - around the dead bone. The involucrum may have holes, called *cloacae,* through which pus can escape. With time, a subperiosteal abscess may force its way to the outside; the passage thereby created is called *a sinus*.

In summary, acute pyogenic osteomyelitis is characterised by *bone destruction, new bone formation and the presence of dead bone (sequestrum).*

When does acute osteomyelitis become chronic osteomyelitis?

The commonly accepted view is that the time of formation of an established sequestrum marks the end of the acute and the beginning of the chronic stage. This is roughly two weeks from the onset of symptoms. Acute osteomyelitis becomes chronic in about 10% of cases despite early and appropriate treatment. *Sequestra, involucra, cloacae and sinuses are the characteristic features of chronic osteomyelitis.*

In children, the epiphyseal growth plate does not allow anastomoses across itself and so blocks the spread of infection from the metaphysis to the epiphysis. In adults, such anastomoses exist and so infection can spread from the metaphyseal to the epiphyseal region of a long bone.

Clinical features

The classical symptoms are general and local. ***General symptoms*** include malaise, fever, vomiting with resultant dehydration. The ***local symptoms*** are swelling, warmth and pain. Redness (erythema) is present in light-skinned patients. The adjacent joint is usually held in flexion in an effort to splint the painful part and minimise pain.

On examination, signs of a toxic illness – fever, weakness, dehydration – may be present. Locally, a swelling may be seen over the affected metaphyseal area, which is warm and tender on palpation. Movement of the adjacent joint causes pain.

Investigations

Blood tests are mandatory.

- A *blood culture* is done with blood aseptically taken from two sites for culture and sensitivity.

- A *full blood count and differential count* are carried out. The white cell count is usually significantly raised in about one-third of patients and the differential count shows neutrophila.

- *The erythrocyte sedimentation rate and C-reactive protei*n are usually raised in over 90% of patients. However, these acute inflammatory markers are non-specific and could also be raised in neoplasmata, recent surgery, other infections, rheumatoid arthritis and other inflammatory conditions.

- *Aspiration* aseptically carried out from the infection site is essential; the aspirate is sent for culture and sensitivity studies. A good yield suggests an abscess requiring incision and drainage.

X-rays do not clearly show the lesion in the first 10 days. However, a careful examination of the films may reveal soft-tissue swelling and some loss of clear definition of the trabeculae in the region. X-ray signs of bone destruction become apparent after this time in the form of irregular bone structure, with patchy translucencies intermingling with sclerotic bone. There are also signs of the periosteum being elevated from the cortex, with periosteal new bone formation.

If the history and physical findings are non-specific and blood test results and x-ray findings are non-diagnostic, additional imaging studies that may aid diagnosis include:

- *An MRI scan* is the most useful modality in early disease. It can detect medullary trabecular destruction and the resulting intramedullary and extramedullary oedema associated with early acute inflammation.

- *An ultrasound scan* is credited with showing periosteal elevation earlier than an x-ray and may demonstrate a subperioteal abscess.

- *A technetium bone scan* will also show early disease as an area of increased uptake of isotope. However, it lacks specificity but it may be useful if there are multiple sites, which is very rare.

- *A CT scan* may help in determining the extent of the lesion and help with biopsy or surgical planning.

Differential diagnosis

From Ewing's tumour. Moth-eaten type of bone destruction with associated layered periosteal new bone seen in acute haematogenous osteomyelitis in a child may be confused with Ewing's tumour in which there may also be general symptoms of fever and malaise. However, in acute osteomyelitis, the symptomatic period is short and there is a lack of a huge amount of soft-tissue swelling that is so characteristic of Ewing's tumour. Also, vanillylmandelic acid is characteristically present in the urine of patients with Ewing's tumour.

From acute rheumathic fever. Peri-articular and articular swelling and joint pain in rheumatic fever are polyarticular, acute osteomyelitis is usually localized to one bone.

From cellulitis. Cellulitis is inflammation confined to the skin and subcutaneous tissue. Bone involvement is rare and even without treatment will not occur for quite some time. There is swelling but this is much less than that associated with acute osteomyelitis. There is redness, which spreads faster than it does in acute osteomyelitis. The associated pain is much less and does not appear to be as deep-rooted as that seen in acute osteomyelitis.

From leukaemia. Leukaemia is symptomatically a more serious disease than acute osteomyelitis. The patient is more ill, local bone signs are multiple and haematological findings are characteristic.

Treatment

NON-SURGICAL

This constitutes the mainstay of management. Treatment begins after two very important investigative procedures – the taking of blood from two sites for culture and sensitivity and aspiration/attempted aspiration of material from the infection site, also for culture and sensitivity studies. The affected limb should be appropriately splinted to relieve pain emanating from movement.

Antibiotic treatment is then commenced on the basis of the patient's age and risk factors. The assumption almost always includes *S. aureus* as one of the organisms responsible. Anti-staphylococcal penicillin is initially given intravenously in appropriate doses based on the patient's weight. Cefuroxime is a suitable alternative. In case of allergy to penicillin or cefuroxime, other anti-staphylococcal antibiotics such as clindamycin or erythromycin can be used. Antibiotic therapy is reviewed as soon as the culture and sensitivity results are available; change is effected if necessary. If no pathogens are isolated, the empirically-chosen antibiotic regime should be continued.

The clinical picture is kept under constant review. Usually, there is noticeable improvement after 24-36 hours of i.v. antibiotics: the general condition improves and local symptoms and signs improve. If there is no improvement, further investigations, a change of the antibiotic and surgical intervention should be considered.

Assuming there has been a good response to treatment, what is the appropriate duration of antibiotic treatment? In general, the duration of therapy is dictated by the patient's response and the type of causative organism(s). For example, staphylococcal infections usually require longer therapy than Streptococcal infections. Historically, 4-6 weeks of i.v. antibiotics was recommended because failure was recorded with periods shorter than 3 weeks. However, subsequent experience showed that, if there has been a good response to i.v. antibiotic therapy, oral antibiotics can replace i.v. antibiotics after an initial period of 5-7 days; treatment is continued for another 5 weeks.

Treatment is monitored by the clinical response and by sequential laboratory studies. Of particular importance are the ESR and CRP levels, which should normalise before antibiotic therapy is discontinued.

SURGICAL

In early disease, surgical treatment takes the form of *incision and drainage*. It is indicated when any of the following situations exists:

- i.v. antibiotic therapy for 24-36 hours has not brought about significant improvement
- an abscess (pus) has formed subperiostally or intraosseously
- there are signs of spread of infection into an adjacent joint

At operation carried out under general anaesthesia, pus is evacuated, dead bone and other tissues are cleared away (debridement) and the infection site is copiously lavaged and irrigated. Material obtained is sent for further culture and sensitivity studies. This is particularly important because some malignant bone tumours not only have similar sites as osteomyelitis but also similar symptoms and signs. Ewing's tumour is a good example. For the same reason, if there are doubts regarding the diagnosis, material should also be taken from the "growing edge" of the lesion and sent for histology as well.

Pre-existing conditions can adversely alter the clinical course and the response to treatment as summarised above. Examples of such conditions include the following: **malnutrition, immune deficiency, extremes of age, malignant tumours, diabetes mellitus, kidney failure, liver failure, steroid therapy, alcoholism and smoking**.

Prognosis

The prognosis for untreated acute haematogenous osteomyelitis is poor. It can be fatal in a neonate and life-threatening in a child under two years of age. In the older child and adult, it will almost certainly progress to chronic osteomyelitis.

Acute implantation osteomyelitis

Two main types may be distinguished as follows:

- *secondary to accidental injuries*
- *secondary to surgical wounds*

Implantation osteomyelitis secondary to accidental injuries

In adults, the sources of bacteria are puncture wounds and open fractures. Road traffic accidents produce most of the patients. The wounds are usually contaminated by a lot of foreign bodies, including metallic debris, pieces of clothing and soil, which can be seen in the medullary canal and around the ends of broken bones. Staphylococci, Streptococci and Gram-negative organisms (Pseudomonas; E. coli) abound in these wounds. The potential for development of acute osteomyelitis in these circumstances is high.

Management begins with stabilising the patient. Associated life-threatening conditions must be attended to first. Local treatment consists of the following:

- Covering the wound with swabs soaked with an antiseptic agent such as Bethadine
- Bandaging the wound and splinting the limb
- Booking the theatre for *debridement and stabilisation of fractures*(in appropriate cases)
- Commencement of prophylactic antibiotic cover; this should reflect local susceptibility patterns. An example could be: I.V. Flucloxacillin 500 mg 6 hourly plus Metronidazole 500 mg 8 hourly given for 72 hours, followed by oral antibiotics, given according to culture and sensitivity studies and the patient's response. In severely contaminated open fractures, this treatment should be continued for 6 weeks.

The surgery itself consists of *wound extension, debridement, brushing, (pulsed) irrigation and fracture stabilisation if necessary.* The irrigation aspect is really very important and cannot be over-emphasised.

It does not have to be "pulsed" but it really needs to be copious. The saying that "Dilution is the solution to pollution" is very true here. With regard to fixation, recent reports suggest that even Gustillo Type IIIB open fractures can be stabilised by internal fixation with good results. External fixation is recommended for Type IIIC fractures.

Implantation osteomyelitis secondary to surgical wounds

This is also an important category of implantation osteomyelitis. It is iatrogenic, resulting from implantation of microorganisms in the wound at the time of surgery. Procedures commonly associated with this type of infection are:

- Open reduction and internal fixation of closed and open fractures
- Joint replacements e.g. total hip or knee replacement

Staphylococcus aureus, Pseudomonas aeroginosa, Proteus mirabilis and Escherichia coli have been isolated from implantation lesions.

Treatment may require:

- *In the case of an infected ORIF:* Removal of all metalwork, debridement and institution of a new fixation.
- *In the case of an infected joint replacement:* Two methods are used:
  a. removal of all metallic or plastic implant, debridement and insertion of new implants, all in one seating
  b. removal of all metallic or plastic implant, debridement and insertion of bone cement impregnated with antibiotics (usually Gentamycin) for 2-4 weeks, then coming back to insert new implants

Prognosis

This depends on the causative injury, the amount of contamination and the virulence of implanted microbes. In general, it can be good if treatment is prompt and adequate but a significant fraction of lesions proceed to chronicity.

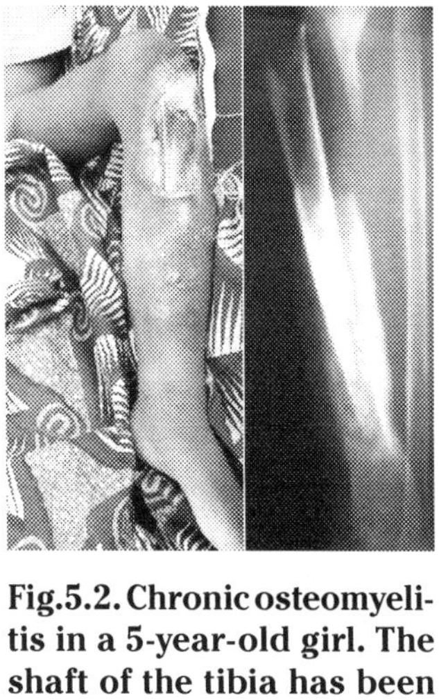

CHRONIC OSTEOMYELITIS

Between 15% and 30% of patients with acute haematogenous osteomyelitis go on to develop the chronic disease. The most common cause is either inadequate antibiotic therapy or inadequate surgical debridement of a lesion. At the centre of the pathology of chronic osteomyelitis is *dead bone – sequestrum* (Fig.5.2).

Dead bone is beloved of bacteria because it provides them with a cozy dwelling place in which they can multiply and proliferate and,

Fig.5.2. Chronic osteomyelitis in a 5-year-old girl. The shaft of the tibia has been sequestrated and an involucrum has been formed (Courtesy of Dr Suleiman Giwa, Chief Consultant Orthopaedic Surgeon, Lagos University Teaching Hospital, Nigeria)

together with associated scarring, protects them from the full effect of antibiotics. They produce the so-called bacterial bio films, housing colonies of bacteria, which give rise to mobile colonies that multiply and disperse rapidly.

A classification of chronic osteomyelitis may be based on the anatomical features of the lesion, the host response to it or both.

Clinical features

Chronic osteomyelitis is characterised clinically by *suppuration, discharging sinus, sequestra* and *cloacae.* Two main clinical courses of the disease may be distinguished as follows:

Type 1. The infection remains persistent and active, with recurrent sequestration of bone and continuous drainage from sinuses.

Type 2. Active infection may cease and the sinuses may close up but residual infection persists inside, only to flare up intermittently. When this happens, the affected part is swollen, inflamed and painful. The closed sinuses re-open, pus discharge resumes and dead pieces of bone may be extruded from the lesion.

Radiological features

The affected bone is irregular in shape, enlarged and dense (sclerotic), with visible cavities, sequestra and an involucrum (Figs.5.3).

Treatment

The principles of treatment can be outlined as follows:

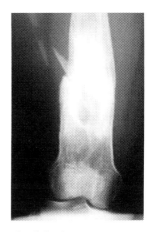

- all dead bone and infected associated tissue should be removed/ excised by radical surgical debridement

- any resulting defects – bony and soft tissue – should be made good by an appropriate method. This may involve the use of bone grafts, muscle flaps and skin grafts

Fig.5.3. A sequestrum sticking out of a chronic osteomyelitic cavity in the distal femur.

- appropriate antibiotics should be given throughout the treatment period in an effort to prevent re-infection

Antibiotic cover
This is mandatory. The choice of antibiotic(s) should be dictated by culture and sensitivity studies. If these are not available, an appriopriate broad-spectrum antibiotic should be used intravenously. Local instillation of 3 grams of Vancomycin and 3.6 grams of Tobramycin powder has been used with success by some authors.

Complications of chronic osteomyelitis

Pathological fractures through bone compromised by the osteomyelitic process or its treatment are not uncommon. Chronic drainage of pus over a long period of time may lead to *nephritis, amyloid disease or squamous cell carcinoma* in sinus tracts.

SEPTIC ARTHRITIS

Septic arthritis is an acute infection of a joint caused by bacteria. It is common in neonates and infants, affecting most commonly the hip joint. Hip joint infection is relatively so common because the proximal femoral metaphysis, in which the infection is initially located, is intracapsular, so that spread into the joint is easy. Less commonly affected are the knee and ankle, followed by other joints. The other group of patients particularly susceptible to septic arthritis are adults immunologically compromised by chronic disease such as rheumatoid arthritis, diabetes, malignancy, renal failure, immunosuppressive states or parenteral drug abuse.

Apart from arising from contiguous osteomyelitis, joint infection may arise from haematogenous infection of the synovium or direct inoculation of organisms into the joint following trauma.

Causative organisms

- *In all age group:* the most common organism isolated is Staphylococcus aureus.
- *In the neonate:* Staphylcoccus aureus and Group B Streptococci are the most common, followed by Gram-negative organisms such as Neisseria gonorrhoeae, which account for 10-15% of infections.
- *In young children aged 2 months to 2 years:* S. aureus, Streptococci and Haemophilus influenzae.
- *In young adult:* S. aureus and N. gonorrhoeae
- *In the elderly:* S. aureus and Gram-negative bacilli.
- *In drug abuse patients:* S. aureus, Pseudomonas aeroginosa, Serratia marcescens

A *clinical classification* of septic arthritis is based on the number of joints affected and on the chronicity as follows:

- *Acute monoarticular septic arthritis*

) 90% of patients
- *Chronic monoarticular septic arthritis*)

- *Polyarticular septic arthritis* *) 10% of patients*

Clinically, in neonates, acute symptoms and signs are minimal, due to yet-poorly developed immune response to inflammation. In toddlers and adults, the typical symptoms and signs of fever, local swelling and pain, as well as limitation of motion in the affected joint, are present. The pyrexia varies from low-grade to "boiling hot".

The diagnosis is best confirmed by joint aspiration carried out under aseptic conditions. It is recommended that the aspirate be expeditiously sent to the laboratory for direct smear, aerobic and anaerobic cultures and antibiotic sensitivity studies.

The treatment of septic arthritis is one of the few true orthopaedic emergencies because articular cartilage is quickly destroyed by the enzymes released by the causative bacteria and inflammatory cells. Unless prompt and effective intravenous antibiotic therapy, based on lab studies, can be instituted within 24-48 hours of the start of the infection, a washout of the joint, preferably by arthroscopy, is the only effective treatment.

The clinical course of chronic monoarticular septic arthritis is different from that of acute monoarticular septic arthritis. Basically, the symptoms and signs in the chronic form are indolent and the course is subdued. The disease is usually chronic by the time of clinical presentation and diagnosis. The typical causative organisms are mycobacteria, fungi and saprophytic bacteria (Brucella species).

Polyarticular septic arthritis is seen mainly in gonococcal arthritis. Five to eight per cent of cases involve children whilst in adults only 10-19% are nongonococcal. There are acute and chronic forms.

Complications of acute septic arthritis of the hip include pathological dislocation, osteomyelitis of the proximal femur and pelvic abscess.

PYOMYOSITIS

Pyomyositis is an infective pathology characterised by the formation of abscesses in muscles. Collection of pus in muscles may be seen in septicaemia but the discussion here is mainly about the "classical pyomyositis" in which the infection of the muscle(s) is the main event and constitutional/systemic illness occurs as a secondary event. In septicaemia the patient is firstly very ill with a swinging fever, weakness and prostration. There may be a history of a skin laceration, blister or boil. The condition is rapidly progressive. Muscle involvement is secondary and manifests with tenderness over and abscess formation in a number of muscles.

In *classical pyomyositis*, one or more of the patient's muscles becomes exquisitely painful, swollen and tender. The overlying skin becomes smooth and shiny. A single muscle or a muscle group may be involved or there may be several abscesses in different parts of the body. The affected muscles are indurated and hard to feel. Movement in neighbouring joints is painful. Later, the signs of acute inflammation subside as the infected muscle literally liquefies and becomes fluctuant with pus. If formed abscess is large, the patient may have systemic symptoms, such as malaise, fever and rigor. Commonly affected muscles include those of the thigh, calf, buttock, back and abdominal wall.

The main causative organisms are staphylococci. If suspected early before pus is formed and treated with a broad-spectrum antibiotic, cure may be achieved. After pus has formed, treatment is by incision and drainage, with antibiotics given before and after the procedure.

CHRONIC GRANULOMATOUS INFECTIONS

TUBERCULOSIS OF BONE AND JOINT

Tuberculosis is a systemic infection caused by *Mycobacterium tuberculosis*, resulting in focal lesions in the respiratory and digestive systems, with involvement of regional lymph nodes. Through lymphatic spread and arteriolar infarction, the infection gives rise to secondary lesions in other organs, notably the urogenital and skeletal systems. Up until the discovery of Steptomycin in 1944, infection with tuberculosis was seen virtually as a death sentence. Skeletal tuberculosis was the most important single cause of childhood crippling. Although there is evidence of recent resurgence, TB has, by and large, been eradicated in Europe, North America and Australia.

Tuberculosis remains a problem in the developing countries of Asia and Africa, where millions of people are still infected. The recent increase in the number of affected patients has been linked to an increase in the number of immunocompromised patients, especially those with acquired immune deficiency syndrome (AIDS). The situation has been compounded by poverty, as effective treatment, though available, is outside the reach of the most vulnerable – the poor. Skeletal TB, though only a small part of the whole problem, still poses considerable strain on the healthcare system of many developing countries.

Skeletal TB is thought to constitute about 10% of all TB infections. It is believed that most bone and joint infections occur within two years of the primary infection. Most of the patients are children, the peak age at infection being 5. Reduced immunity compared with adults is said to account for this predilection. The hip and knee are the most frequently affected joints and together with infection of the spine account for about 95% of all skeletal lesions. Infection of joints of the upper limbs are relatively rare and occurs more frequently in adults than in children

Pathogenesis of skeletal tuberculosis

It is important to emphasise that involvement of the skeleton in the tuberculosis process is a secondary process. Therefore, in a given case, the primary disease focus must be sought and identified, if possible. If such a focus is found, it must be decided if it is active, quiescent or healed.

Bone tuberculosis. The pathological response of bone tissue to *Mycobacterium tuberculosis* is quite characteristic. The organisms cause local necrosis of bone, with the production of caseous material and destruction of bone structure. Endarteritis of local vessels is an important part of the pathology, with the effect of causing further bone and tissue necrosis. Necrotic caseous material may burst through joint capsule and follow tissue planes to present under the skin as an abscess, classically described as "cold abscess", in contrast to the "hot abscess" from pyogenic pus. Unlike the situation seen when bone is infected by pyogenic organisms, bone infected with tuberculosis appears unable to offer any resistance to the invaders. Accordingly, new bone formation is absent on x-rays. *The typical x-ray picture of bone tuberculosis is, therefore, the presence of bone destruction and absence of signs of bone repair.*

Joint tuberculosis. Tuberculous infection of joint begins with the involvement of the synovial membrane, which becomes sprinkled with tubercles. It hypertrophies (thickens) and secretes excessive synovial fluid, giving rise to considerable swelling. It forms a *pannus* of tuberculous granulation tissue, which gradually covers the articular hyaline cartilage of the joint, gradually destroying it and the underlying subchondral bone, as in rheumatoid arthritis. X-rays show bone destruction and no evidence of repair. Joint narrowing gradually occurs and continued weight-bearing results in the collapse of the joint.

Macroscopic specimen and histology. Gross examination of bone or joint affected by tuberculosis reveals thickened oedematous tissue, frequently loaded with grayish small nodules, with occasional white opaque centres (granulomas). These granulomas sometimes coalesce to form larger areas of white necrotic material – *caseous material.* The process is called *caseation necrosis.* This is characteristic of tuberculous infection. In bone infection, this caseous material occupies the created defect in the bone. In joint infection, it often separates the articular cartilage from the subchondral bone.

Microscopically, a typical granuloma consists of a central necrotic area surrounded by pale histiocytes, also called epitheloid cells. Giant cells, with nuclei arranged at the margin of the cell – Langerhan's giant cells – are seen scattered among them. At the periphery of the granuloma or tubercle is a rim of chronic inflammatory cells, such as plasma cells. Often, the granulomas merge to form extensive central caseation necrosis. Acid-fast bacilli (AFB) can be demonstrated in the giant cells and at the margin of the caseous area with Ziehl-Neelsen stain.

Principles of diagnosis

The symptoms of musculoskeletal tuberculosis may be general or local. A history of malaise, loss of appetite, loss of weight and low grade pyrexia is usually present. Local symptoms include pain, swelling, limitation of movements and possible deformity of the affected part. If the characteristic x-ray picture (described above) is also present, a tentative diagnosis of tuberculous infection can be made. However, this needs to be confirmed by laboratory studies, as dependence on clinical and x-ray features can lead to a wrong diagnosis in up to 25% of cases.

Apart from routine blood tests – Hb, FBC, ESR and CRP, the findings of which are non-specific – important tests include:

- *Tuberculin test.* This gives no specific information if positive but is of value if negative. In the *Mantoux test,* a diagnostic dose of Tuberculin Purified Protein Derivative (PPD) is given by intradermal injection. In the *Heaf test,* a solution containing Tuberculin PPD (100,000 units/mL) is injected by multiple puncture. In a positive test, within 2-6 weeks, a small swelling appears at the injection site, which progresses to a papule or to a benign ulcer about 10 mm in diameter and heals in 6-12 weeks. This reaction is absent in a negative test.

- *Ziehl-Neelsen (ZN) stain.* A Ziehl-Neelsen (ZN) stain of tissue, joint aspirate or exudate may yield AFB.

- *Culture and sensitivity studies.* Culture and guinea pig innoculation of tissue, joint fluid or exudates can yield AFB but the results will not be available for weeks and may be negative.

- *Synovial biopsy and histology.* This is an important diagnostic test but will confirm the diagnosis in only 50% of cases. Biopsy of a regional lymph node is preferable to that of synovial tissue. Biopsy of the spine is difficult but can be made easier by CT guidance. Biopsies are fallible and a negative result should be taken with caution. About 50% of cases of tuberculous synovitis are reported as "non-specific chronic inflammation".

- *Interferon-gamma (IFN-g) assays.* These measure cell-mediated immune response by quantifying IFN-gamma released by T cells in response to stimulation by Mycobacterium tuberculosis antigens. Current evidence on the value of IFN-gamma assays as compared with the tuberculin skin test suggests that both tests have advantages and disadvantages and further studies are needed to establish the association between IFN-gamma values and subsequent risk of active disease.

Principles of treatment

These principles are:

- *Rest of the affected part.* Options range from bedrest to the use of various splints.

- *Use of chemotherapeutic agents.* The usual drugs currently used in combination are Isoniazid, Rifampicin, Pyrazinamide and Ethambutol; Streptomycin is still sometimes used. Rifampicin is bactericidal and active against rapid metabolising mycobacteria and should be included in all regimens. It is expensive, however. These drugs have significant side effects. Detailed treatment protocol is not given here. Drug treatment of primary tuberculosis should be prescribed and supervised by an experienced Physician.

Surgical treatment in appropriate cases. Despite their known effectiveness, chemotherapeutic drugs have not eliminated the need for surgical intervention, especially in advanced lesions with caseation, fibrosis and destruction of bone and joint. Surgical options include:

- *Evacuation or debridement of soft tissue abscesses*
- *Synovectomy, including biopsy*
- *Curettage and bone grafting of extra-articular skeletal lesions*
- *Arthrodesis of joints*
- *Resection of joints*
- *Amputation*

Surgery is mandatorily carried out under antibiotic cover to prevent bacterial spread. The choice of drug(s) used and the duration of administration is made in consultation with an experienced Physician.

TUBERCULOSIS OF INDIVIDUAL BONES/JOINTS

Tuberculosis of the spine (Pott's disease)

The spine is the most frequently affected part of the skeleton, accounting for about 50% of all skeletal affections. The thoraco-lumbar junction is the most frequently affected part, followed by the rest of the lumbar spine and then the thoracic spine. Spinal tuberculosis was first described by Sir Percival Pott in 1779, hence the alternative name "Pott's disease".

Pathology. Infection may begin in the intervertebral disc space or in the vertebral body, in the anterior part in both locations, which is fortunate because the neural elements are posteriorly situated. In the disc infection type, the lesion spreads to involve the adjacent vertebral bodies. In the case of initial vertebral body involvement, the disease destroys the bone directly. In both cases, collapse of the vertebral body results. Multi-level affection can occur, especially in the thoracic spine. As the vertebra collapses, caseous necrotic material is squeezed out into the soft tissues to form *paravertebral abscesses,* which can track down along fascial planes or within muscle sheaths. A typical example is the tracking down of such an abscess along the psoas muscle sheath to present in the groin as a *psoas abscess.* An abscess of the same origin may spread backward through the lumbar triangle to form a *lumbar abscess.*

Another effect of vertebral collapse is the formation of deformity – *gibbus,* which is a sharp kyphosis, centred at the level of the involved disc. A more serious effect is neural compression from caseous material, granulation tissue or bone, with resulting *paraplegia.* This later complication is more likely to happen in the thoracic spine, where the spinal canal is narrow and the spinal cord occupies most of the space. Abscess rupture into the dura may facilitate proximal spread of disease, resulting in *tuberculous meningitis*.

Clinically, the main complaints are of back pain and restricted spinal movements. The patient reflexly guards spinal movements and walks with a "stiff back" gait. In the early period, palpation is painful and restricted movements are a common feature. If vertebral collapse has occurred, a gibbus (hunchback) is present. The clinical picture may include those of complications, - abscess, sinus and paraplegia.

X-rays in the early period show rarefaction/osteoporosis of affected vertebral bodies and narrowing of the intervening disc space(s). As the disease progresses, bone destruction leads to progressive anterior wedging of the vertebra(e), culminating in their collapse.

There is often a need to differentiate spinal tuberculosis from a few other spinal conditions, such as *congenital hemivertebra, idiopathic kyphoscoliosis, spinal metastases* and *Burkitt's lymphoma.* The diagnosis of hemivertebrae can be made with the help of x-rays, which show characteristic missing half of a vertebra. In idiopathic kyphoscoliosis, a child slowly develops a progressive curve, starting from the age of 3 or so. The characteristic symptoms of tuberculosis are absent. In spinal metastases, the vertebral bodies are involved whilst the discs are spared. Furthermore, the serum alkaline phosphatase is raised and if the metastases are of prostatic origin, the serum acid phosphatase will also be raised.

The treatment of spinal tuberculosis is mainly with antibacterial drugs. There may be indication for surgical intervention in the form of biopsy, incision and drainage via a costotransversectomy and debridement with internal fixation.

Note on tuberculous paraplegia. Paraplegia is the major complication of spinal TB. It is seen in about 10% of patients. If a patient with spinal TB complains of clumsiness and weakness and incoordination of their legs, he/she is becoming paraplegic. The clinical picture may range from a slightly spastic gait to complete paralysis.

Two forms may be distinguished as follows:

- *Early type*: Paraplegia is due to inflammatory oedema around a paraspinal abscess. Responds well to antibacterial therapy or surgery, if necessary.

- *Late type*: This is due to pressure and stretching from a bony deformity and is seen when there has been no treatment or treatment has been late or incomplete. Prognosis is poor with antibiotics alone and even with surgical fixation.

Tuberculosis of the hip joint

The patient is usually a child, who presents with a painful hip and limp. The symptoms usually start slowly but the affected child ultimately becomes ill and fretful. There is wasting of the thigh muscles and a painful restriction of movements in the affected hip. Initially, the leg is held in flexion and abduction, then in flexion and adduction, all due to soft tissue involvement. Abscesses may form in the buttock or groin. X-ray features depend on the stage of the disease. Initially, there is loss of joint space and severe osteoporosis of the bones around the hip joint is characteristic. There may also be evidence of local bone destruction. In late disease, there is gross destruction of bone, with collapse of the joint.

In the differential diagnosis in a child, septic arthritis, slipped upper femoral epiphysis and Perthes disease should be excluded using their characteristic features.

Initial general treatment is chemotherapy. Specific treatment initially aims to prevent the development of flexion contracture. Traction usually achieves this. If the disease has been diagnosed early (within 6 weeks), joint destruction may be minimal or at least incomplete and immobilisation and chemotherapy may produce healing and preserve joint mobility. If total joint destruction has occurred, only surgical fusion can provide early and adequate control of the infection and relieve pain. The operation involves debridement of all tuberculous tissue and articular cartilage, then apposition of the cancellous bone of the femoral head and acetabulum, followed by cancellous bone grafting from the iliac crest and immobilisation in a hip spica.

Tuberculosis of the knee joint

The knee joint is the 3rd most common site for skeletal tuberculosis. The patient, who is usually a child, usually presents with a swollen and painful knee and a limp. The symptoms also start slowly and the affected child may become ill and toxic. There is wasting of the thigh muscles and a painful restriction of movements in the joint, especially extension. The leg is held in flexion and a flexion deformity may develop. X-ray may show some loss of joint space and osteoporosis of the bones around the joint.

As in the hip, general treatment consists of chemotherapy and initial local treatment is directed at preventing a flexion contracture. A Thomas splint or extension skin traction over a 3-month period can achieve this. The patient is then mobilised on crutches. Alternatively, a long-leg cast cylinder may be applied.

Further reading

Saul N Faust, Julia Clark, Ann Pallett, Nicholas M P Clarke. Managing bone and joint infection in children. *Arch Dis Child*, March, 2012.

Watts H G and Lifeso R M. Current Concepts Review - Tuberculosis of Bones and Joints. *JBJS* 78(2):288-299,1996.

Li J Y W Lo S T H Ng C S. Molecular Detection of Mycobacterium tuberculosis in Tissues Showing Granulomatous Inflammation Without Demonstrable Acid-Fast Bacilli *Diagnostic Molecular Pathology:* Vol.9 (2); 67-74, 2000.

CHAPTER 6

CONGENITAL AND DEVELOPMENTAL ABNORMALITIES

Congenital abnormalities are abnormalities a child is born with. Developmental abnormalities become apparent as the child grows.

Congenital torticollis (Wry neck)

Introduction

Wry neck is a neck abnormality in which the head is tilted to one side and the chin points toward the opposite shoulder, as shown on the illustration below. Congenital wry neck is caused by injury to the sternomastoid muscle during birth. As a result, a visible or palpable lump forms inside the muscle.

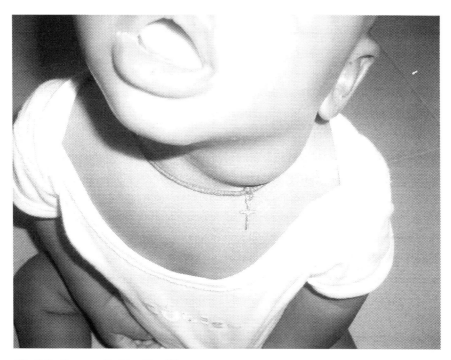

Fig.6.1. Congenital torticollis:

Symptoms & Signs

A lump appears in the muscle on one side of the neck at birth or soon after, reaching its maximum size in the first two months of life. The condition is easily diagnosed on the basis of the history, inspection and palpation. An MRI scan will show finer details of the disease. The doctor will also search for other congenital abnormalities known to be associated with wry neck - such as spinal deformity, congenital dislocation of the hip, clubfoot and other foot abnormalities, as well as eye problems. Differential diagnosis: wry neck may arise from infection in the neck region but this can easily distinguished from congenital wry neck by the presence of other signs of infection such as malaise, pyrexia and local warmth.

Treatment & Outlook

- If diagnosed shortly after birth and the deformity is mild, it can be corrected by gentle stretching of the neck. This is done several times a day by the parents after instruction by the Physiotherapist.

- If the deformity has been left untreated for a long period of time, e.g. two years, the chances are that the resulting contracture would have matured gradually and become more established. Then, physiotherapeutic measures alone may not suffice and surgery may have to be resorted to.

- After treatment, the deformity may recur to a greater or lesser extent and further surgery may be necessary.

SPRENGEL SHOULDER

Sprengel's shoulder is characterised by an elevated and internally rotated scapula. The baby is unable to bend the neck forward or sideways. Non-surgical treatment by physiotherapy is hardly effective. Functional or cosmetic problems can be treated by surgery.

KLIPPEL- FEIL SYNDROME

This abnormality is characterised by a short and stiff neck, low posterior hairline and bony abnormalities in the cervical spine. Associated abnormalities are common and a Sprengel shoulder, congenital scoliosis, congenital heart disease, renal disease and impaired hearing may be present as well.

A full physical examination must be carried out and must include an assessment of the child's nervous system, heart, kidney and hearing functions. An X-ray examination should include the whole spine. MRI studies of the spine may be required too.

Treatment & Outlook

The parents and carers of the child may be under the impression that the disease is only a neck problem. A full explanation of its complex nature should be given to them. Advice on exercises and abnormal positions of the neck to avoid is provided. Problems arising from the involvement of other organ systems of the body are attended to as they arise.

CERVICAL RIB

Introduction

We know that ribs are normally found in the chest and that there are twelve of them on each side. However, due to errors of tissue formation in the unborn child, a rib may form on one or both sides of the lowermost vertebra of the neck, the 7th. This is a "cervical rib". Both sides are frequently affected but, generally, the right side is more frequently affected than the left.

Symptoms & Signs

An extra rib causes symptoms because it presses on blood vessels and nerves in the area. It is rare for the symptoms of an extra rib to be seen in childhood. People who have symptoms complain of pain, numbness, "pins and needles", coldness and discolouration in the arm and hand on the affected side. There may also be weakness and wasting of the muscles of the hand. Gangrene of the finger-tips may occur in an extreme case. Symptoms improve or worsen depending on the position of the arm. The condition can be confirmed with x-rays and an MRI scan. Many people with extra ribs do not have symptoms.

Treatment & Outlook

A neck collar may relieve acute symptoms. Physiotherapy is generally helpful. If symptoms persist, surgical options may be considered. This may include removing the offending rib. I have seen only a few patients with wry neck in my surgical practice. Residual deformity persists in untreated or incompletely treated cases.

CONGENITAL DISLOCATION OF THE HIP - CDH (DEVELOPMENTAL DYSPLASIA OF THE HIP - DDH)

Introduction

This is a serious disease affecting one or both hips of a newborn child. There is a partial or complete displacement of the head of the femur out of the acetabulum, as shown on the X-ray picture below. The term "Developmental Dysplasia of the Hip (DDH)" is now preferred because it is considered to reflect the pathology better than the term "Congenital dislocation of the hip". It is rare in African countries where the baby is carried straddled on the back or side of their mother, which stabilizes a congenitally unstable hip, but objective studies are awaited to confirm this rarity.

Aetiological factors

- *Geographic considerations* - The frequency with which it is seen in the world varies from region to region and race appears to be important. Some areas of the world are known to have a high occurrence rate e.g. Manitoba in Canada, with an occurrence rate of 188.5 in

1,000 births and in parts of the former Yugoslavia, with an occurrence rate of 75 in 1,000 births. By comparison, the disease is virtually unknown in Bantu Africans.

- *Genetic considerations* – familial joint laxity accounts for the condition running in families

- *Sex* -The sex of the child is also important and girls are more likely to have the condition than boys - in the ratio of 6:1.

- *The position of the baby in utero:* CDH is more common in *breech presentation* than in head-first presentation.

- *How the baby is carried after birth* - The traditional way Bantu African women carry their babies – on the carrier's back or side, with the hips bent forward and spread out appears to be an important factor in the low occurrence rate of DDH in this region. On the other hand, the America Indians' way of carrying their babies with their hip joints extended has been shown to lead to a higher occurrence rate of the condition.

Pathology

A combination of aetiological factors enumerated above results in instability of the femoral head in the acetabulum. As a result, the femoral head may be dislocated at birth. The presence of the femoral head in the acetabulum acts as a stimulus for the development of both the head and the acetabulum. Therefore, absence of the femoral head in the acetabulum results in poor development of both structures, as well as abnormal development of other structures, such as the labrum acetabulare and the ligamentum teres, which hypertrophy with time and obstruct reduction of the head.

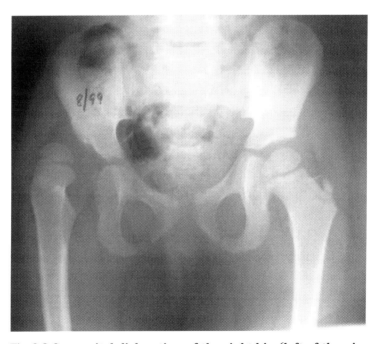

Fig.6.2.Congenital dislocation of the right hip (left of the picture). The pelvic socket is also shallow in comparison with the other hip.

DIAGNOSIS

Tell-tale signs of congenital dislocation of the hip

There are tell-tale signs a mother or carer may be able to notice in the baby:

- *Clicky hip* -Clicking of the affected hip during nappy change. This is popularly known as the clicky hip and may be felt or heard.

- *Shortening of a limb* - Sometimes, shortening of the limb on the affected side is obvious.

- *Unequal groin and thigh skin creases (Fig.6.3)* -Because the thigh is foreshortened, there is an increased number of skin creases on the affected side and resulting asymmetry. However, the value of this sign is diminished by the observation that groin and skin creases could also be unequal and asymmetrical in some unaffected individuals.

- *Limited ability to spread the baby's legs (Fig.6.3)* - The affected hip does not spread out normally like the unaffected one. If both hips are affected, then the limitation is seen on both sides.

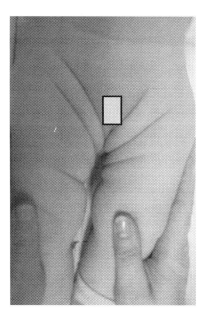
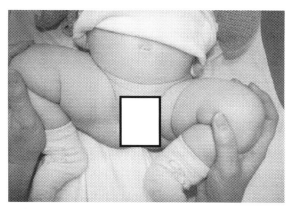

Fig.6.3. There are more creases and limited abduction on the left, signifying dislocation of the left hip.

In making a diagnosis, the doctor looks for any information in the history of the pregnancy that may point to the diagnosis. For example congenital dislocation is known to be more common in breech presentation than in head presentation. There may also be a family history of the condition, which may raise the chances of the child having it. Physical examination of the child includes a search for the above-mentioned tell-tale signs and carrying out of specific tests for the condition, *followed by confirmation of the diagnosis with an ultrasound scan.*

Specific tests for CDH in the neonate

The Galeazzi test (Fig.6.4)

The child is laid on the examination couch, the knees are bent to 90 degrees and the feet are placed flat on the couch so that both heels are touching. On looking at the level/height of the knees, an apparent shortening of the femur on the affected side is seen.

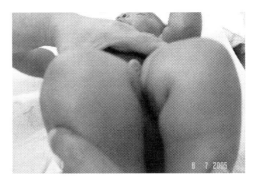

Fig.6.4.The Galeazzi test

The Ortolani test

This test confirms that *the femoral head is dislocated*. The baby is laid on its back. The examiner holds both bent knees together and gently abducts the hips while lifting up the greater trochanter with two fingers. As the hip is further abducted, if the femoral head is lying outside the acetabulum, it will re-enter it, giving a palpable "clunk" in the process. If this happens, the test is said to be positive.

The Barlow test

Unlike the Ortolani test, this test confirms that *the femoral head is dislocatable*. In performing the test, the examiner attempts to sublux or dislocate the femoral head from within the acetabulum with their thumb. The suspected hip is adducted and a gentle push is applied to the inner thigh with the thumb in an attempt to slide the hip posteriorly. Success at doing this denotes a positive test, whilst failure denotes a negative test.

Comment. The Barlow and Ortolani tests become difficult to carry out and less clear as the patient gets older, whereas the classic finding of limitation of abduction becomes more prominent. The greatest diagnostic problem lies in identifying the anatomically dysplastic but clinically asymptomatic and stable hip, which may become symptomatic in adolescence or early adulthood.

Treatment

Treatment is led by the doctor but active participation of the parents and carers is essential to success. Treatment options include the following:

In the first 6 months of life

- **"Double or triple nappies"**
  The use of two or three nappies instead of one enhances getting the legs into abduction. This is a temporary treatment whilst waiting for the result of the ultrasound scan of the hips. If CDH is confirmed, the nappies are exchanged for a splint e.g. Pavlik harness.

- **Hip splints -Pavlik harness & others**
  Some named splints have been used to treat DDH in the first 6 months of life. Examples are the von Rosen splint, Craig splint and Pavlik harness. They all aim to place and keep the dislocated or subluxed femoral head in the acetabulum. The Pavlik harness is perhaps the most commonly used splint in the treatment of DDH in the first six months of life (Fig.6.5).

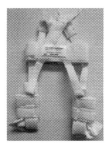 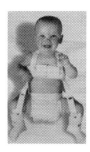

Fig.6.5. The Pavlik harness, like other hip splints keeps the head of femur in its normal position in the pelvic socket (acetabulum). 2ⁿᵈ picture shows a Pavlik harness in use. The young man's happy expression is proof that he is wearing a comfortable device.

- **6 months to 2 years**

1. **Resetting the hip and casting**
   The hip is repositioned in the pelvic socket under a general anaesthetic and held in the corrected position in a special plaster cast.

2. **Surgical treatment**
   Repositioning may have to be achieved by open surgery and there are many methods of doing this. One method is shown on the Fig.6.6:

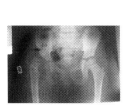 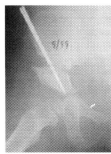 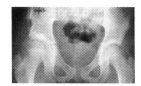

Fig.6.6. This picture shows a dislocated right hip (left picture) in a 3-year-old girl
The dislocated hip was repositioned by the author by appropriate osteotomies (bone cuts) in September 1999 (middle picture). The bone cuts had healed in less than 2 months and by October 2003, both the head of the femur and its socket in the pelvic bone had remodelled well (right picture).

Prevention is better than cure: carrying the baby right may avoid all the trouble! (Fig.6.7)

In most African countries (and in China too), infants are carried on their mother's/carer's backs from their first few weeks of life as shown on the above photograph. The child's chest and tommy lie in the depth of the lower spine of the carrier, with the legs bent forwards at the hips and spread out, straddling the carrier. Babies tolerate being carried in this manner intermittently for hours each day. In this position, the head of the femur is nicely positioned in its pelvic socket. Little wonder CDH is rare in these countries. Having grown up in such an environment, I can vouch that rare is the occasion in which this method of carrying babies does not succeed in calming down a crying baby. To realise that we may be successfully treating a baby with an unstable hip at the same time is a big bonus.

Happily, in Europe and America, the benefits of carrying the baby with their legs spread out have now been realized. The pictures below show not only happy children but also happy mothers!

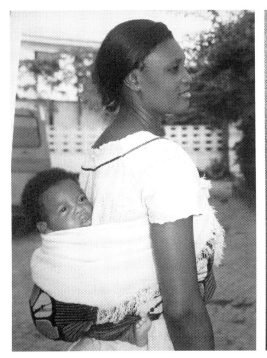 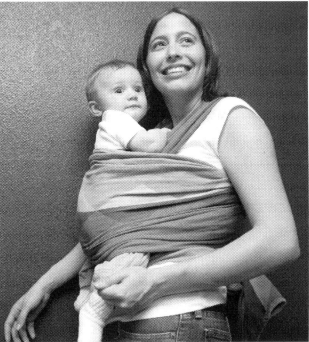

Fig.6.7. An African mother carrying her baby on her back. The legs are abducted and flexed at the hips, which ensures that the heads of the femurs are positioned well in the acetabulum. A European mother carrying her baby on her tommy exerts the same stabilizing effect on the baby's hips.

Outlook for CDH

The outlook is good for a CDH diagnosed early and treated promptly. Again, we should practice prevention.

CONGENITAL TALIPES EQUINOVARUS (CTEV) (CONGENITAL CLUBFOOT)

Introduction

In this abnormality, the baby's hindfoot is plantar-flexed and inverted at the ankle, the forefoot is plantar-flexed and adducted and the lower leg is thinner than it should be. There is a superficial resemblance of the affected foot to a club, hence the term "clubfoot" (Fig.6.8).

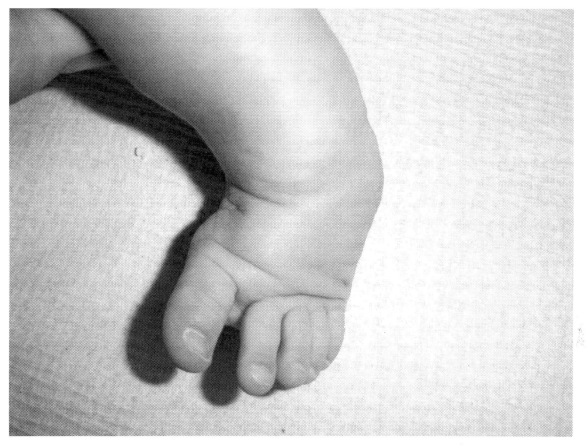

Fig.6.8. Congenital clubfoot affecting the left foot in a newborn child.

Types of clubfoot

Three types of clubfoot may be distinguished as follows:

- **Postural clubfoot** - due to bad position of the foot in the womb
- **Teratologic clubfoot** - the clubfoot is a part of other birth defects in the body
- **Idiopathic clubfoot** - "idiopathic" means that we do not know the cause. This is the "true" clubfoot and the subject of the following discussion.

Pathogenesis

The real causes of clubfoot are unknown but they are thought to include genetic/familial and environmental factors. It is quoted as occurring in about 1 in 1,000 births. Bilateral involvement is seen in about 50% of cases. Boys are more frequently affected than girls in the ratio of 2:1. Although popularly thought to be only a foot and ankle abnormality, the whole of the lower leg is in fact affected, with under-development of the calf and distal leg as well as the ankle and foot.

Aetiological factors cause abnormal development of muscles and other soft tissues on the posterior and medial aspects of the ankle, resulting in shortening of the Achilles' tendon and the inverters of the foot, which, in turn cause the foot to go into plantar flexion and inversion. If left untreated

(Fig.6.9), the bones of the foot, especially of the hindfoot, will adapt to the deforming forces of the muscles and soft tissues, perpetuating and worsening the deformities and making treatment more difficult.

Symptoms & Signs

- The foot does not look normal: the hindfoot is plantar-flexed and inverted at the ankle
- The forefoot is plantar-flexed and adducted
- There are skinfolds on the inner aspect of the ankle
- The affected leg looks thinner than the normal side
- The ankle joint is stiff, resisting movement of the foot

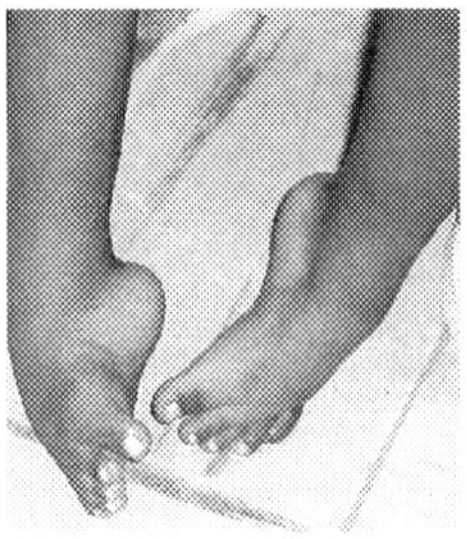

Fig.6.9. Late untreated clubfoot in 10 year old boy.

The diagnosis of clubfoot in the newborn is easy: the shape and stiffness of movement is characteristic. There is a frequent association of clubfoot with other congenital abnormalities e.g. CDH or spina bifida and these must be looked out for. X-rays are of limited value in the infant because most of the bones are yet to ossify and so do not show up. Ultrasound and MRI scans can be used to assess clubfoot but in practice are rarely used, as they are not considered essential for diagnosis or treatment.

Treatment

Successful treatment is based on the principle of first obtaining a complete correction of the various elements of the deformity and then maintaining the correction until all danger of recurrence has receded, sometimes up to five years later. Complete correction of all deformities is virtually impossible, except in the mild forms.

Non-operative methods include massage, stretchings, strapping and POP casting.

Operative methods. Operative intervention is indicated for correction of deformities persisting after three months of active non-operative treatment.

They include:

- *Early clubfoot*: soft tissue procedures: lengthening of Achilles' and tibialis posterior tendons and incision of the posterior capsule of the subtalar joint

- *Late, untreated or relapsed clubfoot* needs bony procedures for correction of resulting deformities e.g. a wedge excision of the calcaneo-cuboid joint (Dilwyn Evans' procedure) will shorten the lateral curvature of the foot and correct the inversion deformity.

The Physiotherapist and the parents have an important role to play in the overall management of clubfoot.

LATE-PRESENTED OR UNTREATED CONGENITAL CLUBFOOT

Late presentation is common in parts of the developing world, including Nigeria. The reasons for late presentation include fatalistic cultural beliefs, poverty and lack of access to good medical care. Late presentation is encumbered with all the negative effects of the evolution and development of congenital clubfoot. Initially correctable soft-tissue deformities become incorrectable and bones of the foot undergo adaptive changes. The only effective treatment option then is surgical, the result of which is almost always less satisfactory than that obtainable with early and combined treatment.

CONGENITAL TALIPES CALCANEOVALGUS (CTCV)

Introduction

Fig.6.10 below shows what a congenital talipes cacaneo-valgus looks like: the dorsum of the foot appears to be gummed to the front of the lower leg.

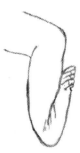

Fig.6.10. The CTCV foot: "It is as if the upper surface of the foot has become gummed to the front of the leg".

Characteristics include:

*   The occurrence rate is quoted as 1 in 1,000 live births.
*   Girls are more frequently affected than boys.
*   First-borns are more frequently affected than subsequent children.
*   The cause is unknown but it is thought to arise as a result of wrong positioning of the foot in the womb.
*   It is frequently associated with other congenital abnormalities, e.g. congenital dislocation of the hip.
*   There is sometimes an associated bowing of the tibia.
*   There are mild, moderate and severe forms.

Symptoms & Signs

*   The foot is lying in an abnormal position: the heel bone is tilted upwards in such a way that the foot comes to lie against the front of the leg.
*   It is not painful.
*   In the mild form, the foot is mobile and can be brought down to the normal position

- In the moderate form, the foot also mobile but cannot be brought down to the normal (plantigrade) position
- In the severe form, it is even more difficult to bring the foot down.

Diagnosis is not difficult and the distinction between it and other foot abnormalities can be made from the appearance and signs.

Treatment

Treatment is non-operative and successful in all patients correctly diagnosed. The mild form does not require formal treatment. The moderate form is treated with gentle stretching exercises whilst the severe form may require plaster of Paris casting, in addition to stretching exercises. An ankle-foot orthosis (AFO) is sometimes required to ensure satisfactory foot position when the child begins to stand and walk.

CONGENITAL METATARSUS ADDUCTUS (HOOK OR SERPENTINE FOOT)

Introduction

Fig.6.11. illustrates a hookfoot: the metatarsals are adducted at the midtarsal joint, giving a picture resembling a hook or a snake. It is noticed from the age of six months or so, when the child begins to pull itself upright. The hindfoot is normal. The deformity is reported as occurring in 1 out of 1,000 births. There is a familial propensity e.g. if one child in the family is affected, the risk of a second child also having it is said to be 1 in 20. A possible cause of the deformity is compression of the foot in the womb. A number of patients with hookfoot also have congenital torticollis, so, this should be looked out for.

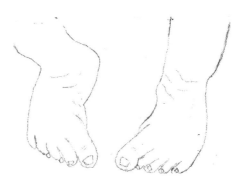

Fig.6.11. The hookfoot - Congenital meta-tarsus adducto-varus.

Symptoms & Signs

The baby's foot is turned inwards on the ankle and there is a superficial resemblance to a hook or snake. There are three degrees of severity:

- Mild – the foot can be stretched with the hands and made to assume a normal shape

- Moderate - the deformity is slightly fixed and making the foot to assume a normal shape is more difficult compared to the mild form
- Severe – the deformity is more rigid and surgical correction may be required.

Treatment

- Mild – the deformity corrects spontaneously and no formal treatment is required beyond massaging and simple stretching.
- Moderate - the deformity may resolve on its own in most patients or massage and simple stretching may be required. Shoe modification or serial casting is sometimes needed in some patients in this group.
- Severe – the deformity is more rigid. Serial casting is tried to begin with but surgical correction is often required.

Outlook

The outlook is good for most children with hookfoot. However, deformity does persist in a few, which may require surgical correction with bone cuts.

IN-TOEING

The baby's toes are turned inwards as s/he walks. It is one of the commonest cause of parental concern necessitating a paediatric orthopaedic consultation. It is usually first noticed in the second year, when the child begins to walk.

Causes of in-toeing

- Anteversion of the femoral neck. Most cases are due to internal torsion of the femur or tibia or both.
- Congenital metatarsus adductus
- The occasional less-benign causes include:

    1. *neurological disorders such as static encephalopathy*
    2. *infantile Blount's disease*
    3. *metabolic bone diseases*
    4. *skeletal dysplasias*

The diagnosis is easy but an examination of the nervous system must be carried out to exclude more serious diseases of the nervous system, as outlined above.

Treatment

- **Mild to moderate in-toeing**
  Most children have mild to moderate in-toeing and do not require treatment. Parents should be reassured that the condition usually resolves on its own in most cases. Regular follow up is arranged to ensure that the deformity is correcting itself.

It is doubtful that treatment in the form of splintage confers long-term benefit but most parents would prefer splintage to "doing nothing". If considered necessary, night splintage should be favoured as day-time treatment modalities interfere with the child's sitting, walking and running and may lower their self-esteem and cause conflict between them and their carers.

- **Severe in-toeing**
  Severe deformities may require treatment with casting, bracing or surgical correction of specific deformities.

Out-toeing

In this condition, the foot is turned outwards. The cause is usually in the hip joint, femur or tibia. In the womb, the hips are rotated outwards, so it is normal for the foot to turn outwards when the child is stood on their feet. Often, only one foot out-toes, usually the right. The deformity usually corrects itself and no treatment is required.

FLATFOOT

As the name implies, the foot is flat in this condition. On looking at the foot from the inner aspect, the in-step is flat or lower than usual and the heel is turned out. Broadly, two types of flatfeet can be distinguished – mobile (physiological) and rigid (pathological).

Physical examination distinguishes between the two types:

- **Mobile (Physiological)**. Most flatfeet in the infant and young children as well as in about 15% of adults with flat feet come under this group. To establish this in a child, ask or help the child to stand on their toes and you will notice that the medial longitudinal arch reforms perfectly. The feet are flexible and cause no symptoms.

- **Rigid (Pathological)**. This type is seen in certain congenital foot and ankle abnormalities e.g. congenital vertical talus, in which the talus assumes a vertical position. To establish this in a child, ask or help the child to stand on their toes and you will notice that the medial longitudinal arch DOES NOT reform. Abnormal flatfeet generally cause pain and stiffness.

X-rays do not add to diagnostic accuracy but an MRI scan can be useful in showing the relationship between the bones and the soft tissues in the abnormal variety.

Treatment

- Physiological flatfoot - Parental pressure accounts for treatment by some surgeons with medial longitudinal arch supports (insoles), heel cups and special shoes but none of these has proven benefits.

- Pathological flatfoot - the treatment here is more complex: muscle transfers and bony surgery may be required and can be done successfully.

- **The cavus of High-arched foot (Fig.6.12)**
  A high-arched or cavus foot is characterized by an abnormally high arch of the foot . It is a complex deformity, which should always be taken seriously as it is often the tip of the iceberg, being a manifestation of a more serious underlying nerve disease, such as diastematomyelia, in which a bony spur in the spinal canal splits the spinal cord, causing neurological symptoms. The usual cause is a neurological disease causing muscle imbalance, although it can also result from (a) tumours of the sciatic nerve (b) as a complication of the treatment of congenital clubfoot or (c) from injuries to the foot or leg, including the compartment syndrome

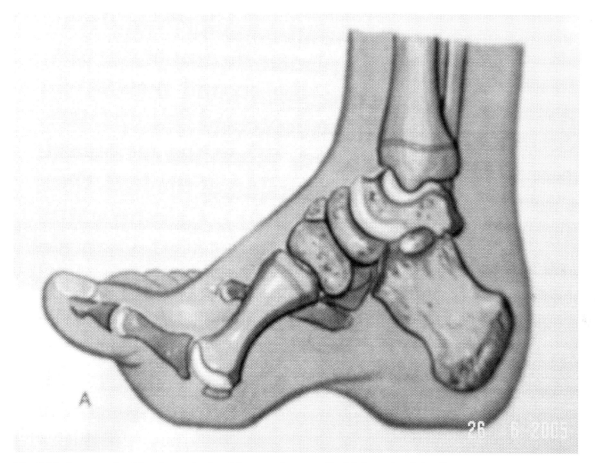

Fig.6.12. A cavus foot is characterised by an abnormally high arch of the foot

The presenting complaints are *frequent ankle sprains, foot pain and callosities* (thickened skin due to excessive pressure) on the toes and sole of the foot. Clawing of the toes results in callosities from footwear over the joints. Diagnosis includes an assessment of the state of the nervous system.

Treatment

The treatment of the high-arched foot is complex and depends a lot on the cause. Non-surgical treatment includes stretching of contracted plantar soft tissues and the use of various shoe inserts. AFOs (Ankle Foot Orthoses) can be used to improve the gait (walking posture) in children with peripheral nerve disease but, on the whole, these measures are not very successful. Surgical treatment options require specific indications and include soft tissue procedures e.g. Achilles' tendon elongation; soft-tissue releases; tendon transfers; corrective bone cuts and joint fusions.

TOE WALKING

Toe walking is seen in children with

- neuromuscular disorders (neurologic toe-walking) e.g. cerebral palsy
- in otherwise normal children (idiopathic toe-walking) and
- in untreated or inadequately treated clubfoot

Clinically, the child walks on its toes, with a characteristic forward stoop and cannot squat with the heels on the ground. S/he falls over backwards on attempting to stand upright. Dorsiflexion of the ankle is limited or absent.

Treatment

Physiotherapy and stretching exercises are ineffective. Serial casting may effect correction in the early stages but recurrence is common. Failure of initial conservative management is indication for surgery. Surgical treatment consists of Achilles tendon elongation.

Tibial bowing

The medical term for bowing of the legs is genu varum. Bow legs are usually a normal finding in the infant, when they are referred to as physiological. But there are other types of bow leg, which are the result of other abnormal conditions. These are described as pathological and it is important to distinguish between them. The bone mainly involved in bowing is the tibia but, in fact, the lower part of the femur and the knee joint are also involved.

Types and their Treatment

Altogether, five different types of bowing of the tibia bone are described, according to where the apex of the curvature is pointing:

- *Lateral tibial bowing* is normal in the infant and young child and is referred to as physiologic bowing. The condition is usually mild, symmetrical and unassociated with any skeletal disease. It usually resolves spontaneously.

- *Anterior tibial bowing* is associated with fibular hemimelia and considerable limb shortening usually results from it.

- *Posteromedial bowing* is a rare condition associated with dorsi-flexion deformity of the foot and mild limb shortening. The dorsi-flexion deformity usually resolves with time, the bowing also improves with time but the shortening tends to get worse, necessitating operative intervention, which may take the form of epiphysiodesis or leg lengthening.

- *Anterolateral bowing* is perhaps the most serious form of tibial bowing. It is usually associated with *pseudoarthrosis of the tibia* resulting from an unhealed fracture. Pseudoarthrosis of the tibia is very difficult to manage. Intramedullary nailing, plating and bone grafting may be required.

- *Focal fibrocartilagenous dysplasia of the tibia.* This condition is rare. A focal defect is seen in the proximal tibia with an associated area of sclerosis. The defect tends to heal with growth.

Prognosis

The prognosis for physiological bow leg is excellent. The prognosis for the other variants are guarded.

COMPLEX BOW LEGS

BLOUNT'S DISEASE

This is a serious form of bowing, which may affect one or both legs. It has come to be known as Blount's disease after Blount, who described it in 1937, although Erlacher had described it earlier in 1922. The medical term for Blount's disease is *infantile tibia vara*. The pictures below show a child and an adult with Blount's disease. There is a thin line between physiological bowing and Blount's disease (Fig.6.13). Physiological bowing should correct by the time the child reaches 18-24 months and most authors consider that for the diagnosis of Blount's disease to be made, the child should be 2 years old or older.

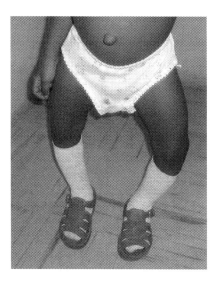

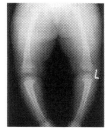

Fig.6.13. There is a thin line between physiological bowing and Blount's disease. This X-ray of a 21-month old child probably shows physiological bowing progressing to Blount's disease.

The actual cause is unknown but early walking and obesity appear to contribute to this condition.

At the root of the pathology is avascular necrosis of cartilage in the inner part of the growth plate of the tibia due to excessive pressure or mechanical stress in the course of walking on a physiological bow leg.

- It is more common in black children than in children of other racial groups.
- The child is usually in the 12-36 months age bracket.
- Females are more frequently affected than males.
- Tends to worsen with age. If left untreated, it would persist into adulthood (Fig.6.14).

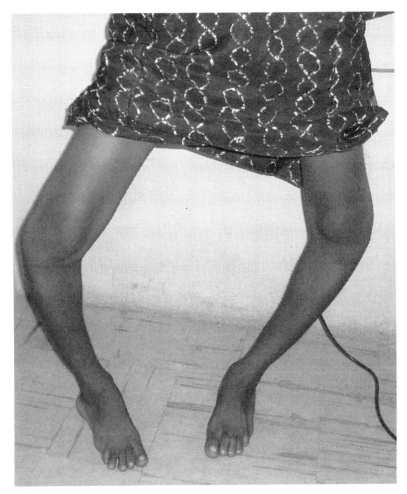

Fig.6.14. Untreated Blount's disease in an adolescent

Symptoms & Signs

- One or both legs are bowed and it can be seen that the bowing is more severe than physiological bowing.
- In severe forms of the disease, there is pain on the outer aspect of the affected knee

The diagnosis is based on the history and physical findings as noted above. Differential diagnosis considers other leg conditions with similar features, such as physiologic bowing, congenital bowing, rickets, osteomyelitis affecting the growth plate, epiphyseal growth plate injury, multiple enchondromatosis (Ollier disease) and metaphyseal chondrodysplasia.

In differentiating infantile tibia vara from physiologic bowing of the legs, in physiologic bowing, angular deformity results from a gradual curve involving both the tibia and the femur whereas, in

Blount's disease, the proximal tibial angulation is acute, occurring immediately below the medial metaphyseal beak (Fig.6.15).

The severity is determined using the Langenskiold's six-stage classification (Figs.6.15) and other parameters, such as the metaphyseal-diaphyseal angle, which is greater than 11º in Blount's disease.

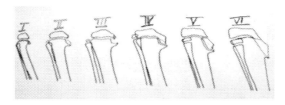 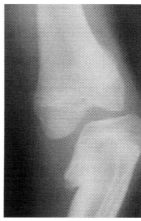

Fig.6.15. Langenskiold's six-stage classification of Blount's disease and a Stage 6 Blount's disease in a 22 year old man

Treatment

This depends on the age of the child, the stage of the disease and racial considerations. Broadly, treatment options include non-operative and operative methods.

Non-surgical treatment consists mainly of bracing. Some surgeons treat the milder forms with a long-leg brace e.g. the knee-ankle-foot orthosis. It is worn during play and at night. If brace management is chosen, definitive treatment should be completed before the age of 4 years. Some surgeons do not think that bracing works, given that the milder forms are known to resolve spontaneously.

Surgical treatment is carried out for the more severe forms of the disease. It consists of bone cuts (osteotomies) by the surgeon aimed at correcting the slope of the knee joint surface as well as the bowing of the tibia.

Outlook

The outlook for Blount's disease depends on the age of the child, the stage of the disease as well as racial considerations. Significant differences in results of treatment have been noted between Caucasian and black patients. The disease course has been shown to be more stubborn in black than in white children. A late complication of the disease is the development early osteoarthritis of the knee in adult life.

Knock-knee deformity

This is *genu valgum*. Popularly known as knock-knee in the UK, it is popularly called K-leg in Nigeria. It is the opposite of bow leg. The leg or legs angle out at the knee joint, giving an awkward standing and walking posture. This is noticed after the child has started to walk. Most cases are of benign cause and will resolve with growth without treatment. Deformity persisting into adolescence can be corrected with surgical stapling of the medial growth plate or corrective osteotomies in the proximal tibia.

PERTHES' DISEASE (FIGS 6.16)

This is idiopathic avascular necrosis (AVN) of the femoral head in a child.

Aetiological factors

Possible aetiological factors have noted as follows:

- *Sex* - Boys are more frequently affected than girls in the ratio of 4:1.

- *Age* - The most susceptible age bracket is 3-10 years. It is very rare before 3 and after 12.

- *Familial factors* - There is a significant familial incidence of the disease. It is rare in black children.

- *Environmental factors* - A high occurrence rate of the disease was seen in a study of an inner city area in a British town, prompting the suggestion that low socioeconomic factors e.g. poor nutrition, may be significant. This role remains unclear.

- *Trauma* - Trauma has been repeatedly blamed. Hyperactive children, being more prone to injury than other children, have a higher occurrence rate of the disease than non-hyperactive children.

- *Blood clotting problems* - These have been identified in some cases. An interesting example is sickle-cell disease but the cause of AVN of the femoral head in a sickle-cell disease child (SCD) is known and so should not be described as Perthes' disease. Furthermore, the radiological features in classical Perthes' are quite different from those of AVN in SCD.

Pathological features

A series of pathological processes follows the cutting off of the blood supply to the femoral head: increased density of the femoral head on X-ray, fragmentation of the affected segment, flattening of the femoral head and subsequent healing. The overlying articular cartilage survives. Healing may be excellent, with no residual deformity or there may be residual deformity in the form of coxa magna (big head) or metaphyseal widening.

Symptoms & Signs

The classical symptoms of the disease depend on the disease stage - from those of the initial inflammation to those of severe bone changes:

- Hip/thigh pain - the pain is located in the groin and hip area, as well as the front of the thigh.

- Knee pain is quite common. The knee pain is thought to be referred pain via a nerve, called the obturator nerve, which provides nerve supply to both the hip and knee joints.

- Limp - The limp is the result of an automatic mechanism acting to reduce pain when walking.

- Stiffness - This occurs because soft tissues around the hip joint are inflamed as part of the disease, especially in the early stages.

- Some muscle wasting occur in the thigh and buttock, due to reduced use because of pain.

Treatment

The final aim of treatment is to obtain a round femoral head and a full range of movements in the hip joint at the end of healing.

- *Initial bedrest by putting traction on the legs to immobilize them and control of pain with pain-killers*

- *Treatment is based on the concept of "containing" the femoral head in the pelvic socket.* Containment, which means "Holding or keeping in", becomes necessary when more and more of the femoral head becomes exposed laterally as a result of progressive flattening. It can be achieved by both non-surgical and surgical methods.

- *Non-surgical containment of the femoral head*
  The femoral head can be contained in the pelvic socket by bracing. However, bracing is cumbersome and prone to non-compliance and surgical containment may be preferred.

- *Surgical containment of the femoral head*
  There are many ways the surgeon can contain the femoral head in the acetabulum. They can cut the femur or the pelvic bone or both to achieve this, depending on specific indications. Treatment options are based on the age of the child. One method favoured by the author is illustrated below (Figs.6.16)

Prognosis

- Because the course of the disease is unpredictable, the prognosis is also unpredictable.
- The younger the child at the onset of symptoms, the better the chances of getting complete healing with the attainment a spherical femoral head.

Certain factors make for less-than-good outcome

- The presence of the so-called physeal bridge (a bony bridge between the epiphysis and the metaphysis) is a bad prognostic sign because it is known to impede remodelling.

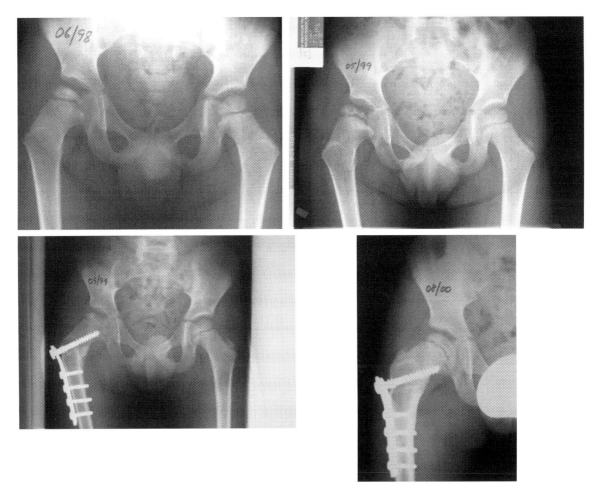

Fig.6.16.
(Top row): Whole-head Perthes' disease of the right hip in the pre-collapse stage in a 5 year-old boy. Eleven months later, the femoral head had fragmented and flattened out and the head is no longer fully contained in the acetabulum
(Bottom row): Same case: A varus subtrochanteric containment osteotomy was carried out by the author in July, 1999. Eleven months later – good containment, healing and remodelling have been achieved.

- Late onset disease e.g. after the age of 7-8 years, is more likely to be associated with a physeal bridge and considerable residual deformities, which result in symptoms in later childhood, adolescence and adult life. Pain with vigorous physical activity is common.

- Degenerative arthritis develops during middle to late adult life, necessitating hip joint replacement.

SCHEUERMANN'S DISEASE (FIG.6.17)

Scheuermann's disease is a disease of the spine, involving mainly the rib cage area (thoracic spine) in young people, aged 13-16 years, and causing the upper spine to bend forward. A segment of the spine, consisting of three or more consecutive vertebral bodies is involved. The alternative name for the disease is *round back deformity.* The upper part of the lumbar spine may also be involved. It is slightly more common in boys than girls.

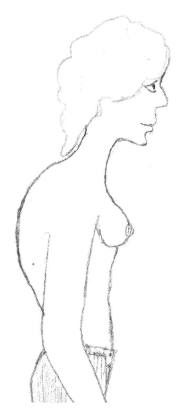

**Fig.6.17. Round back deformity –
Scheuermann's disease**

The cause of Scheuermann's disease remains unknown but hereditary factors are thought to play a part. The actual sites of the disease are the cartilage rings of the upper and lower ends of the vertebrae where growth of the vertebrae takes place and the problem is an abnormality of bone formation in these cartilage rings. Simply put, this abnormality softens the affected parts of the vertebrae and this allows the spine to bend forward from the pressure of weight-bearing, with a resulting hunchback.

Symptoms & Signs

The characteristic symptoms are *kyphosis (forward bend of the spine), poor posture* and *back pain*. A severe bend may cause problems with heart and lung function. Apart from the symptoms and physical signs, characteristic X-ray signs include wedge-shaped vertebrae and defects in the end-plates of a few vertebrae or the entire thoracolumbar spine. The severity of the hump in degrees determines the best treatment option for a given patient. MRI and CT scans may also be requested but are not essential for diagnosis.

Treatment

The treatment is controversial. Some doctors do not recommend formal treatment because they believe that the disease is benign, with few adverse effects. Others believe that treatment is necessary, especially in children who are still growing, because they believe treatment will prevent progression of the kyphosis, with development of pain and possible compression of spinal nerves, the heart and the lungs. Treatment depends on the degree of the kyphosis and the age of the patient.

- Non-operative management is satisfactory in most children who are still growing. Mild cases may do well with only pain-killers and physiotherapy in the form of backward bending exercises, which counteract the forward wedging of the vertebral bodies and the rib cage.

- Patients with significant deformity (kyphosis greater than 40 degrees) may require bracing or casting.

One such brace, called the *Milwaukee brace*, is recommended for kyphosis predominantly in the chest region and there are braces for more extensive deformities involving other regions of the spine e.g. the thoraco-lumbo-sacral orthosis (TLSO).

- Some patients with severe curves may need operative management. Operative options should only be carried out by orthopaedic surgeons specially trained in spinal surgery.

Outlook

- The kyphosis can progress, especially in those still growing, with increasing back pain and possible compression of spinal nerves, the heart and the lungs.
- In those treated by bracing, a gradual loss of correction can occur after the brace is removed.
- The outlook for those treated by surgery varies from patient to patient.

Scoliosis

Scoliosis is defined as a sideways bend of the spine greater than 10 degrees (Figs.6.18). In reality, however, the deformity is much more complex than that because there is usually a rotational component, which converts it into a three-dimensional deformity:

- there is an intervertebral extension in the saggital plane, resulting in lordosis of the scoliotic segment
- lateral intervertebral tilting in the frontal plane and
- a rotatory component in the axial plane

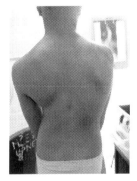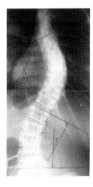

Fig.6.18. Scoliosis is defined as a sideways bend of the spine greater than 10 degrees. This 14- year-old girl has a primary thoracic curve, convex to the right and a compensatory lumbar curve, convex to the left. X-ray of the spine of the same patient shows lines drawn to determine the Cobb angles.

Classification

Mild bends of the spine to the side less than 10 degrees are quite common, affecting as much as 10% of the general population. They do not progress and are not considered to be pathological.

In general, scoliosis can be classified into two main groups (Table 6.1):

- Idiopathic scoliosis and
- Non-idiopathic scoliosis i.e. scoliosis of known aetiology

Table 6.1. A classification of scoliosis

Idiopathic scoliosis – classified on the basis of time of onset:

- *Infantile* – patients less than 3 years old
- *Juvenile* – patients aged 3-10 years
- *Adolescent* – patients aged between 10 years and skeletal maturity
- *Adult scoliosis* – scoliosis recognised after skeletal maturity

Adolescent idiopathic scoliosis is the most common form of idiopathic scoliosis.

Non-idiopathic scoliosis

- *Congenital* (Failure of formation or segmentation; neural tissue disorders)
- *Neuromuscular* (Upper motor neurone e.g. cerebral palsy; Lower motor neurone e.g. poliomyelitis; Myopathic e.g. muscular dystrophy)
- *Functional* (Secondary to spinal muscle spasm, leg-length discrepancies or some functional disorder)
- *Constitutional* (Associated with known syndromes e.g. neurofibromatosis; secondary to metabolic diseases or arthritis)
- *Miscellaneous* (Secondary to trauma, neoplasmata or contractures; iatrogenic e.g. radiotherapy or chest cage surgery)

Curve severity

Two grades of curve severity are generally recognised:

- *Established (structural) curve.* A segment of the spine has a fixed lateral curvature.

- *Not-established (non-structural) curve.* The curvature is not fixed. It may be due to poor posture, muscle spasm, leg length discrepancy or some other cause and can resolve with the resolution of the underlying cause.

Principles of management of scoliosis

Diagnosis

The *history* of the development of deformity is important. The age at onset and course/progression should be ascertained. Is there a family history of spinal deformity? Is pain a feature? Painful scoliosis in a child suggests an inflammatory or neoplastic cause.

Physical examination should aim to find or exclude features known to be associated with scoliosis. In a general survey, features of Marfan's syndrome, neurofibromatosis, limb length discrepancy, injury, infection and neoplasm are sought.

In local examination, the following features are specifically sought: **truncal asymmetry, differencies in left and right shoulder height, scapular prominence, flank crease and pelvic symmetry or asymmetry.**

Symmetry and balance of the spine is assessed with a plumb line. The presence or absence of vertebral rotation is assessed using *Adams forward-bending test:* the child is asked to bend the spine forward at the waist until the spine is horizontal and the examiner observes from behind. The patient's feet should be together, the knees straight and the arms dependent on the sides. If vertebral rotation is present, one side of the back will be higher than the other: there will be a rib hump in the thoracic region or paraspinal fullness in the lumbar region. This assymetry can be measured with a scoliometer. Forward spinal flexion is also recorded e.g. *"In forward spinal flexion, the tips of the middle fingers reach the mid-tibial level".*

X-ray assessment is mandatory. A baseline picture is necessary for assessment of possible progression of a curve. The scoliotic angle (Cobb angle) is the angle between the right angles to horizontal lines drawn along the endplates of the uppermost and lowermost vertebrae of a given curve. Curves greater than 10 degrees are considered significant. The rib-vertebral angle difference is also an important diagnostic and management feature.

Treatment

- *Observation and reassurance.*
  The diagnosis of "scoliosis" provokes anxiety in parents and a lot of explanation of the different courses and prognosis of the disease is required. Reassuring them is always helpful. Regular follow-up is instituted. Mild curves (Cobb angles less than 20 degrees) should be observed. Curve progression, i.e. an increase of 5 degrees or more, is noted and may necessitate a change to brace treatment.

- *Brace treatment.*
  This is indicated in skeletally immature patients with curves between 25 and 40 degrees. Some surgeons do not believe that braces work.

- *Operative treatment*
Operative treatment is usually indicated in immature patients with curves greater than 40 degrees. A number of operative options are available, including using rods to straighten out the curves and local bone fusions plus instrumentation. Operative treatment is the most definitive and effective method of treating scoliosis. However, it is a highly specialised area of orthopaedics. The indications are strictly defined and the operative techniques and instrumentation are highly specialised. High costs are involved.

CEREBRAL PALSY

The disease

This condition is also known as Little's disease or Static encephalopathy. It is a non-progressive central nervous system disorder characterised by malfunction of the voluntary muscles. The main malfunction is that of movement and/or posture but there are non-muscular problems such as mental impairment, epileptic fits (seizures), speech problems, hearing and visual deficits and perceptual difficulties.

The cause of cerebral palsy is brain damage, which may be the result of inadequate supply of oxygen, low blood levels of glucose or infection occurring before, during or immediately after the delivery of the baby but the symptoms and signs appear in infancy or early childhood. The incidence or prevalence of cerebral palsy is variously quoted as between 6 and 60 cases per 1,000 births.

Types of cerebral palsy, their Symptoms and Signs

There are five types:

- **Spastic type:** this is the best known type. It is characterized by a lot of muscle spasm, especially of the limbs, which results in deformity, contracture and dislocations of joints; the hip joint is especially prone to dislocation. The spine may also develop scoliosis.

- **Athetoid type**: this is characterized by the presence of apparently purposeless movements in various parts of the body. It used to be caused by transfusion of incompatible blood; it is now rare.

- **Ataxic type** is rare too. It is characterized by poor balance and loss of deep sensation, such as sensation to temperature changes.

- **Rigid type** is characterized by marked rigidity. The joints tend to bend like a lead pipe. Also rare.

- **Mixed type** has elements of spasticity and purposeless movements.

Treatment

The main problems requiring treatment are (a) spastic muscles (b) joint deformity (c) joint dislocations (d) joint contracture. Making treatment more difficult than it could be is the additional presence of mental, speech, visual and hearing impairment in most patients. There are surgical and non-surgical options.

Non-Surgical options include:

- *Physical therapy*: this is the mainstay of management. Modalities needed include passive stretching, techniques for relaxation, teaching of coordination, use of mobility aids and equipment and of the therapeutic pool. The physiotherapist, parents and/or carers have to be very patient because associated mental retardation tends to slow down progress. Management efforts need to be sustained over a long period of time.

- *Mobility aids*: wheelchairs; casting (corrective casting; night splints); orthotic devices and adaptive equipment are almost always needed.

- *Speech therapy* and *Educational assistance* are essential.

- *Drugs* may be required too.

Surgical options

These include relocation of a dislocated hip, soft-tissue release of contractures, tendon transfers, fusing affected joints in order to stabilize them and rhizotomy in which selected nerve roots in the spine are cut in order to reduce muscle spasm.

POLIOMYELITIS (INFANTILE PARALYSIS)

The disease

Poliomyelitis (polio) is a highly infectious disease caused by the *polio virus*. The virus enters the body through the mouth and multiplies in the intestines from where they invade and attack cells of the spinal cord and brain stem, responsible for moving our muscles. Total flaccid paralysis of or weakness of the limb or trunk muscles can occur in a matter of hours and the resulting deficit is usually permanent in nature.

Now virtually unknown in the developed world, anterior poliomyelitis is still seen in parts of the developing world where immunisation programmes remain incomplete.

Polio can strike at any age, but affects mainly children under the age of three (over 50% of all cases). Initial symptoms include fever, fatigue, headache, vomiting, stiffness in the neck and pain in the limbs. One in 200 infections leads to irreversible paralysis. The distribution of paralysis is random and deformities usually result.

Stages of polio

Three stages of poliomyelitis are distinguished: *acute, convalescent* and *chronic.*

Acute stage

This manifests as a flu-like illness, which comes after an incubation period of about 2 weeks. A progressively increasing paralysis without sensory involvement then develops over the next 2 weeks. Most affected muscles become weak; few are totally paralysed.

Convalescent stage

This stage lasts up to 2 years after infection and encompasses the recovery of many affected muscles as well as the development of contractures. Most of the recovery occurs in the first few months. Contracture affects muscle, tendon, joint capsule, fascia and neurovascular structures.

Chronic stage

This stage is deemed to start after about two years. The features include muscle imbalance, soft-tissue contractures and deformity. Limb atrophy and shortening, and bending of the spine are characteristic features.

Treatment

The management of patients with anterior poliomyelitis is complex but the results and prognosis are better than with those obtained with cerebral palsy patients. The most important reasons for this are that the patients have normal IQ as well as normal sensation, features which are lacking in most CP patients.

Non-operative management includes stretching exercises and splintage. Operative management includes a careful pre-operative assessment, soft-tissue release of contractures, tendon transfers, fusing affected joints in order to stabilize them and leg length equalization procedures.

Outlook

A lot depends on how many nerve cells have been destroyed by the disease. Paralysis of the muscles supplied by the destroyed nerves is usually permanent, the muscles shrink and the limbs are thin.

Further reading

Michael Benson John Fixsen Malcolm Macnicol Klaus Parsch. *General Principles of Children's Orthopaedic Disease [Paperback] Springer, 2011*

CHAPTER 7

BONE TUMOURS

INTRODUCTION and CLASSIFICATION

Bone tumours are abnormal swellings, lumps or masses, which have arisen from bone or associated tissues or have been brought to the skeletal system from elsewhere in the body. They are characterised by their ability to grow fast and outside of the control of the body, conferring no apparent benefit to it. A bone tumour which has arisen from elements of the skeletal system is classified as *primary*, whilst one which has come from another organ is classified as *secondary*.

Primary bone tumours are classified as *benign* or *malignant*. A benign tumour is one which does not spread to other organs; a malignant tumour is one which does. A malignant tumour is a cancer arising from bone and related soft tissues and is given a special name - *sarcoma*. Thus, we have **osteo**-*sarcomas*, if they originate from bone, **chondro**-*sarcomas*, if they originate from cartilage and **fibro**-*sarcomas*, if they originate from fibrous connective tissues.

Secondary bone tumours or metastatic bone tumours are carcinomata transported to bone from their organs of origin, such as the breast, lung, kidney, prostate or the intestines. Carcinomas spread to bone and other organs by a process known as *metastasis*. Secondary bone tumours are more common than primary bone tumours for the simple reason that they represent tumours that have spread to bone from quite a few different organs (Table 7.1).

Classification of bone tumours

Table 7.1

Name	Subtype	Origin
Primary	1. Benign 2. Malignant	Elements/tissues of the MSS
Secondary	Always Malignant	Metastasis from carcinoma of another organ

The *causes* of primary bone tumours are unknown but age is certainly a factor as most affected patients are children and young adults. On the other hand, secondary or metastatic bone tumours are much more common in adults and the elderly than in young people. Genes are important causative factors in some tumours.

Sites of bone tumours

The different bone tumours have characteristic sites, knowledge of which is helpful in their diagnosis and differential diagnosis.

BENIGN BONE TUMOURS ARISING FROM BONE

Osteoid osteoma

This is a benign tumour known to originate from the cortex of long bones, especially the tibial shaft. However, no bone is exempt and atypical locations have been noted in the head of the femur (Fig.7.1) and the posterior elements of a vertebra, where it may cause scoliosis as a result of muscle spasm (Fig.7.2).

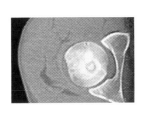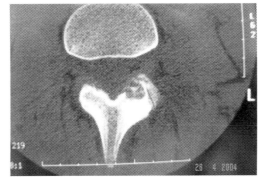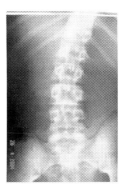

Fig.7.1. & Fig.7.2. CT scan showing an osteoid osteoma in the femoral head of an 11-year-old boy (left) and of the left pedicle of L3 (middle). The latter has caused lumbar scoliosis (right) (The middle and right pictures are by courtesy of Mr. Steve Cannon, FRCS, Royal National Orthopaedic Hospital, Stanmore, England).

Clinically, most of the patients are children and young adults and males are more often affected than females. The characteristic symptom is pain, which is often relieved by Aspirin and other NSAIDs. The tumour hardly attains a large size; there is little or no swelling. The radiographic picture is that of a lucent lesion, called a *nidus*, which is surrounded by densely sclerotic bone.

The nidus measures under 1.5 cm and is usually located in the cortex, although it can also occupy a subperiosteal or intramedullary position. A bone scan shows the nidus as the active part of the tumour. CT is very effective in identifying the tumour. Histologically, the lesion consists of a vascular fibrous stroma with varying proportions of osteoid tissue and fine new bone trabeculae.

The traditional treatment is en bloc excision of the nidus with surrounding sclerotic bone but, recently, simple excision and curettage of the nidus has been advocated. Radiofrequency ablation and CT-guided percutaneous core needle excision have also been reported to be effective. Recurrence rates are low.

Osteoblastoma

Characterised by the production of immature bone (osteoid), this tumour is commonly sited in the posterior elements of the spine, where it may be confused with an osteoid osteoma but it is larger than an osteoid osteoma (more than 2cm in length). A CT scan will locate the tumour. Treatment is by curettage but has a higher recurrence rate than an osteoid osteoma.

MALIGNANT BONE TUMOURS ARISING FROM BONE

Osteosarcoma (Fig.7.3)

Osteosarcoma is a malignant primary bone tumour consisting of a malignant stroma in which malignant osteoid, bone, and/or cartilage are formed. With the exception of bone marrow tumours, osteosarcoma is the commonest and most fatal, accounting for 20% of all primary malignant bone tumours. The peak incidence is the 10-20 age bracket and males are again more frequently affected than females. Until recently, the prognosis for this tumour was appalling and affliction with it was seen as a death sentence. Most victims succumbed to the effects of pulmonary metastases within one year of diagnosis. Fortunately, with the introduction of more effective treatment modalities and protocols, the five-year survival rates have improved from 10-20% twenty years ago to about 80% or more now.

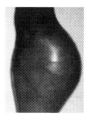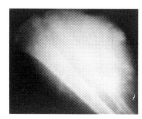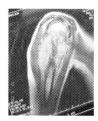

Fig.7.3. Osteosarcoma of the proximal fibula (left and middle pictures). The "sun-burst" appearance on x-ray is illustrated here. Right picture: MRI scan of osteosarcoma of the proximal humerus in an 11 year old boy (right picture) (Left and middle pictures are by courtesy of Dr. S.U. Eyesan, Consultant Orthopaedic Surgeon, National Orthopaedic Hospital, Igbobi, Lagos, Nigeria)

Diagnosis. The classical site for osteosarcoma is the metaphysis of a long bone; about 80% of them occur around the knee and shoulder joints. Flat bones such as the scapula, ribs and ilium are only occasionally affected. Local tumour growth results in local bony mass. Soon, the cortex is penetrated and surrounding soft tissues are invaded, resulting in considerable soft-tissue swelling. At the same time, spread along the medullary canal, with the formation of skip lesions, and to the lungs occurs.

Clinically, the patient complains of a painful swelling, arising from bony enlargement and soft-tissue induration. The pain is excruciating and persistent and the patient cannot find a position of comfort. Movement in the adjacent joint is severely restricted and painful. There may also be systemic symptoms of ill-health, such as pyrexia and malaise.

X-rays of the affected bone show an irregular and poorly-defined area of bone destruction and bone formation and destruction of the cortex. A number of classical radiographic features have been described:

Codman triangle: this is formed by the elevated periosteum at the proximal and distal borders of the tumour as well as tumour new bone. When complete, the vertical arm of the triangle is formed by the cortex of the bone, the short (horizontal) arm is formed by spicules of tumour bone and the hypothenus is formed by periosteal new bone. However, it is hardly a complete triangle: one of the three sides, usually the horizontal arm, is imaginary.

Sun-burst appearance: this arises from reactive and tumour bone deposited along blood vessels running through the tumour in a radial fashion (Fig.10b).

Onion-skin appearance: this is produced by successive layers of reactive periosteal new bone. However, it is more characteristic of Ewing's sarcoma than of osteosarcoma.

MRI scan and a bone scan are required for staging, treatment monitoring and prognostication. A CT scan of the lungs is carried out to identify possible metastatic lesions.

Differential diagnosis. The conditions needing to be distinguished from osteosarcoma include infection, fracture callus, pathological fracture through a benign tumour, aggressive osteoblastoma, non-ossifying fibroma and fibrous dysplasia and eosinophilic granuloma.

Treatment. Classical treatment used to take the form of amputation or disarticulation of the part bearing the tumour. Modern treatment comprises open biopsy, tumour staging, chemotherapy and then local tumour resection.

Typically, high-dose methotrexate in conjunction with adriamycin and cis-platinum, is given pre-operatively, often by intra-arterial perfusion of the affected limb. The tumour is then reviewed and re-staged and then locally resected with wide margins. With this regime, limb salvage is possible in up to 90% of patients. Local recurrence rates correlate with the completeness or otherwise of local resection and the patient's response to chemotherapy.

It has been recommended that patients with insufficient surgical safe margins should undergo immediate amputation, especially if they also have a poor response to chemotherapy.

Prognosis. Prognostic factors include:

Large tumour size and *vascular invasion* are poor prognostic signs

Tumour stage at the time of presentation. Patients presenting with lung metastases fare much worse than those without metastases.

Poor response to chemotherapy is a bad prognostic sign

Tumour site. The prognosis is better for tumours arising from appendicular skeleton than for those arising from the pelvis or spine.

BENIGN BONE TUMOURS ARISING FROM CARTILAGE

Solitary osteochondroma (Fig.7.4)

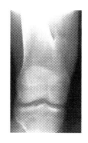

Also called *cancellous exostosis,* solitary osteochondroma is the most common of all benign bone tumours. Thought to arise from a defect in perichondral cartilage, it consists of a sessile or stemmed bony spur, capped by cartilage and covered by periosteum. It usually arises from the metaphyseal portion of a long bone and characteristically grows and points away from the nearest joint. Frequently, a bursa develops over the projecting bony mass. They account for 35% of all benign bone tumours and 9% of all bone tumours. Most are found around the knee and shoulder joints but location in flat bones is not uncommon.

Fig.7.4. Solitary osteochondroma of the distal femur. Note that the apex is pointing away from the knee joint.

The lesion begins during the growth period. The cartilage cap is most prominent in young patients and involutes with age. Growth of the tumour ceases with closure of the epiphyseal growth plate at the end of skeletal growth.

Generally, the patient complains of a painless mass but pain may become a feature if adjacent tendons or associated bursa become inflamed from trauma. Other possible causes of pain include neural compression, fracture, avascular necrosis of the cartilaginous cap and malignant transformation. Malignant transformation is very rare and does not occur before skeletal maturity. If it occurs, it is a chondrosarcoma, which arises from the cartilaginous cap; proximal appendicular and axial lesions seem to be at a greater risk of this complication than distally-situated ones.

The management is by initial observation. The development of pain or location in areas in which trauma by knocking against objects is common, e.g., proximal tibia or fibula, may be an indication for total excision, in which the tumour mass, cap and bursa are removed together with some healthy bone at the base. In growing children, excision should avoid injuring the growth plate.

Hereditary multiple osteochondromatosis (or Diaphyseal eclasia)(Fig.7.5)

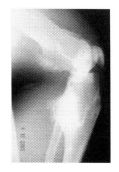

This is an autosomal dominant condition said to be associated with mutations of gene loci EXT1 and EXT2, which are tumour suppressor genes. The distal femur, proximal tibia and proximal humerus are frequent sites and the growth plates may be involved, which can result in considerable deformity. Generally, they are more fast-growing than solitary osteochondromas and malignant transformation is much more common in them than in solitary lesions. Surgery is indicated in symptomatic lesions.

Fig.7.5. Hereditary multiple osteochondromatosis

Enchondroma (Fig.7.6)

Enchondroma is a common benign tumour composed of facets of mature hyaline cartilage. It is said to develop when growth plate cartilage fails to undergo ossification and becomes trapped in bone, ultimately locating in the metaphysis or diaphysis. *It is the most common benign bone tumour seen in the hand,* although affection of other bones, e.g., ribs, humerus, pelvis, femur and tibia, is not uncommon. Simultaneous involvement of many bones is known as *enchondromatosis or Ollier's disease.* It may be associated with skin haemangiomas in *Maffucci's syndrome).*

The tumour is believed to develop during the growth period but it lies unmanifested for many years, presenting clinically in adult life. It is asymptomatic for a long time and often presents with a pathological fracture after trivial trauma.

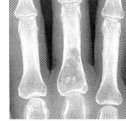

X-rays reveal a well-circumscribed lytic area in the end of the affected bone. There may be calcification within the tumour. Differential diagnosis includes a bone cyst, fibrous dysplasia and small inclusion cysts lined by squamous epithelium. There is some danger of malignant transformation, which is significantly increased in enchondromatosis. Endosteal scalloping on x-rays or CT is considered to be a feature of malignant transformation.

Fig.7.6. Enchondroma of base of the proximal phalanx of the middle finger

Treatment for a solitary enchondroma is meticulous curettage followed by filling of the resulting cavity with bone chips from the iliac crest.

Benign chondroblastoma

Benign chondroblastoma is a relatively rare tumour believed to arise from cartilage cells or cartilage-forming connective tissue. It is characteristically located in the epiphyseal portion of a long bone, especially the femur, tibia and humerus but, with growth, it may come to lie in the metaphyseal region. It is associated with genetic abnormalities in chromosomes 5 and 8. Affection of bones of the ankle and foot is also well known. In the foot, the talus is most frequently affected and cystic changes from the lesion are often confused with features of a simple bone cyst.

Chondroblastoma is often painful and, because of its epiphyseal location, may cause effusion in the adjacent joint. X-rays show a round or ovoid rarefied lesion, which may be mottled due to calcification within the tumour, surrounded by well-defined sclerotic bone. An aggressive one may be destructive and have poorly defined borders.

Treatment of the non-aggressive variant consists of curettage plus bone-grafting. Recurrence has been reported in 15 – 25%. Some authors recommend applying phenol after curettage but this should be done with caution because of the proximity of the lesions to the growth plate and the joint.

Chondromyxoid fibroma (Fig.7.7)

This benign tumour is relatively rare. It is believed to arise from cartilage-forming connective tissue exhibiting certain chondroid and myxoid properties. It has a characteristic rearrangement on chromosome 6 at position q13 but it is not clear if this genetic alteration is important in the formation and development of the tumour.

It is usually seen in adults in the 30–40 age bracket. The most commonly affected sites are the distal femoral metaphysis, the proximal tibial metaphysis, the distal fibula, the metatarsals and the calcaneum; the bones of the hand are less frequently involved. Local pain is an important feature.

X-rays show a radiolucent rounded or oval lesion eccentrically located in the metaphysis of the involved bone. This is usually surrounded by a shell of thinned cortex, which may be scalloped. Histologically, a mixed pattern of cellularity is seen, with hypercellular spindled areas lying in a hypocellular loose fibromyxoid stroma.

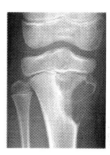

Treatment is by aggressive curettage followed by bone grafting from the iliac crest. Local excision may be indicated. The tumour may recur. Malignant transformation to chondrosarcoma has been reported.

Fig.7.7. Chondro-myxoid fibroma

MALIGNANT BONE TUMOURS ARISING FROM CARTILAGE

Chondrosarcoma

This is a malignant cartilaginous tumour, which produces hyaline cartilage. It is the second most common primary malignant bone tumour (osteosarcoma is the first). It is seen mostly after the age of 40; it is unusual under the age of 30. It is more common in males than females. The most common site is the pelvis; other sites include the rib, femur, tibia, humerus, spine and scapula. The tumour may arise as a *primary chondrosarcoma* or as a *secondary chondrosarcoma* in a pre-existing benign tumour such as osteochondroma, enchondroma or in a previously irradiated tissue. It is characteristic of a chondrosarcoma to attain a large size.

Three main histological variants are distinguished: *well-differentiated, poorly-differentiated* and *dedifferentiated*. Clinically, a well-differentiated tumour grows slowly, with only about 50% metastasising. The clinical course is worse with a poorly-differentiated tumour and worst with a dedifferentiated tumour, which is a high-grade poorly-differentiated tumour arising in a previously low-grade tumour.

Treatment consists of a large block excision or amputation of the part containing the tumour. The use of chemotherapy in high-grade chondrosarcoma is controversial. Survival of patients depends on tumour size, grade, location and adequacy of surgical extirpation.

BENIGN BONE TUMOURS ARISING FROM FIBROUS TISSUE

Fibrous cortical defect

This is a subperiosteal cortical defect, usually small and eccentrically located cortical bone craters filled with fibrous tissue. They are thought to be quite common in normal children, affecting as many as 35% of them at some stage during skeletal growth. Sometimes referred to as "bone islands", they are completely asymptomatic, being discovered by accident. Many are said to regress spontaneously. They require no treatment.

Non-ossifying fibroma (Fig.7.8.)

Although histologically similar to a fibrous cortical defect, non-ossifying fibroma is generally larger in size and many authors consider them to be different entities. Patients are usually under 20 years of age.

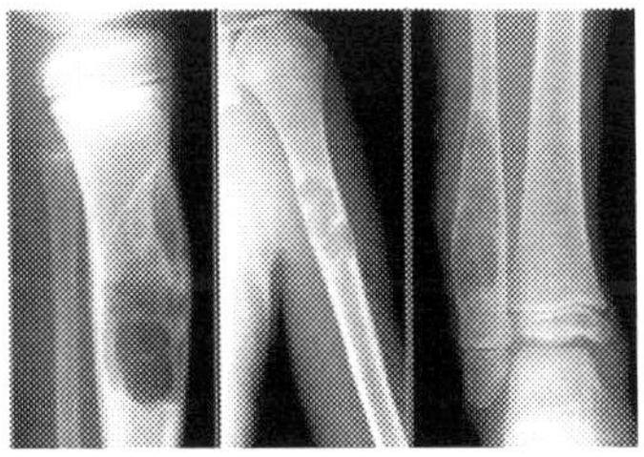

Non-ossifying fibroma is frequently seen in the proximal tibia, just distal to the metaphysis, but other bones may also be affected. Because of its large size, it can cause pain or pathological fracture or both. It has quite a distinctive x-ray appearance: an irregular translucent area with a scalloped border of sclerotic bone. Surgery may be indicated to relieve pain or to prevent or treat a pathological fracture.

Fig.7.8. Non-ossifying fibroma of the tibia, humerus and fibula

Simple bone cyst

This is considered to arise from a developmental anomaly of the growth plate caused by a transient failure of ossification of its cartilage, with subsequent cyst formation. The most frequently affected age bracket is 3-14 years; there is no distinct sex predilection. The most common site is the proximal humerus, followed by the proximal femur. It is not uncommon in the calcaneum. In the long bones, it is known to migrate distally with time.

The tumour is quite often symptomless, being quite often discovered by accident or following a pathological fracture. X-rays reveal a round or oval defect in the metaphysis, with its long axis parallel to the long axis of the host bone. There is cortical thinning. Evidence of recent fracture, e.g., periosteal new bone, may be present.

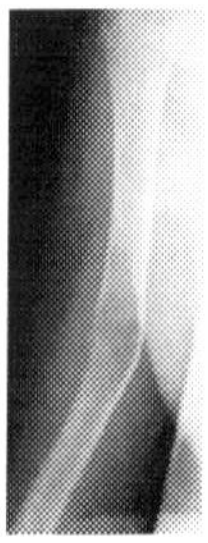

A solitary cyst should be differentiated from an aneurysmal bone cyst, eosinophilic granuloma, enchondroma, giant-cell tumour and solitary foci of fibrous dysplasia. The presence of multiple bone cysts suggest *hyperparathyroidism*.

Spontaneous resolution of a solitary cyst is common in late adolescence. Pathological fracture through a cyst is common (Fig.7.9.), following which healing usually occurs. A pathological fracture is treated by appropriate

Fig.7.9. Pathological fracture through a solitary bone cyst.

immobilisation. Curettage, followed by bone grafting may be indicated. Recurrence following this treatment is not uncommon.

Aneurysmal bone cyst (Fig.7.10)

This is a benign, usually solitary and expansile lesion seen most frequently in the metaphysis of long bones, the vertebrae and flat bones. It is a highly vascular tumour, eccentrically located and cortically-based. It forms bubble-like cavities, partially demarcated by bony septi, filled with blood. Some grow outwardly whilst others are more centrally located. With erosion of the cortex, the periosteum is stimulated, making it to form reactive new bone, which forms a shell around the tumour, contributing to the bubble-like appearance.

Patients are usually aged between 20 and 30 years. Pain is the presenting complaint and a mass is palpable if the tumour arises from a superficial bone. Occasionally, a pathological fracture is the

presenting feature, in which case severe bleeding results. Tumour growth may be rapid or slow and may involve a neighbouring bone. This is particularly true in vertebral lesions. X-rays show a honey-comb appearance and fluid levels can be demonstrated on MRI and CT scans.

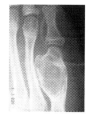

The treatment of cortically-based lesions is curettage and excision. Thermal or chemical therapy is advocated for central lesions. Radiotherapy is another option, although still under study.

Fig.7.10. Aneurysmal bone cyst in the 5th metatarsal bone

Giant-cell tumour

This is a benign but potentially aggressive and destructive tumour. It is thought to arise from the mesenchymal cells of connective tissue and starts after skeletal maturity, the incidence peaking in the 3rd decade. Females are more frequently affected than males in the ratio of 3:2. It is typically located in the epiphysis of long bones, abutting on the articular cartilage and moving into the metaphysis with continuing growth. The distal femur, proximal tibia and distal radius (Figs 7.12 and 7.13) are particularly favoured sites but almost all bones have been involved.

Judged by their rates of growth and aggressiveness, variants of this tumour range from slow-growing to fast-growing, with inclination to malignant change. Clinically, it presents as a growing and painful swelling, with resulting stiffness in the neighbouring joint. The x-ray picture is characteristic: there is an epiphyseal, juxta-articular lytic lesion, which may also involve the metaphysis. The cortex is thinned and expanded but there is no evidence of new bone formation. Quite often, it presents a multilocular cystic picture resembling a conglomeration of soap bubbles (Fig.7.11).

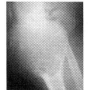
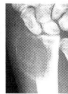

Fig.7.11. Giant-cell tumour of the proximal tibia and Giant-cell tumour of the distal radius (The left picture is by courtesy of Dr. S.U. Eyesan, Consultant Orthopaedic Surgeon, National Orthopaedic Hospital, Igbobi, Lagos, Nigeria)

The treatment of giant-cell tumour depends on the stage of the disease and the bone involved. With early disease, the option of choice is curettage with filling of the resulting defect with bone chips from the iliac crest or with allografts. However, tumour recurrence of up to 60% has been reported with this treatment. Long-standing and extensive lesions present management problems. Excision, followed by replacement with a vascularised or free graft, may be required. If a joint is compromised by the excision, joint replacement with customised components may be indicated. A tumour located in a surgically inaccessible site, may require radiotherapy. About 10% of giant cell tumours undergo malignant transformation, mainly to fibrosarcomas but also to osteosarcomas.

MALIGNANT BONE TUMOURS ARISING FROM FIBROUS TISSUE

Fibrosarcoma

This is a rare tumour of bone, which arises from fibrous tissue. It affects mainly the femur, tibia and humerus in adults. Presentation is with pain or a slow-growing mass. A biopsy is essential for diagnosis. High-grade and low-grade variants are distinguished. Treatment is by wide resection for a low-grade lesion and radical margins resection or amputation for a high-grade lesion. Adjuvant chemotherapy or radiotherapy is usually used.

BONE TUMOURS OF BONE MARROW ORIGIN

Myeloma

This tumour derives from plasma cells and is associated with abnormalities of protein synthesis. It is the most common of malignant bone tumours. Alternative names are *Multiple myeloma, Plasma cell myeloma and Plasmacytoma*. It is rare before the age of 40 and males are more frequently affected than females. Usually, the bone marrow of most or all of the skeleton becomes involved. Solitary involvement is more common in the axial than appendicular skeleton.

Clinically, pain is the usual presenting symptom; back pain is common. Pathological compression fracture of vertebrae is common; other bones may also suffer this complication. X-rays show lytic "punched-out" defects in the affected bones, without surrounding sclerosis. Cortical expansion may be present. Biopsy is necessary for establishing the diagnosis in a solitary lesion but multiple myeloma can be diagnosed with confidence by blood tests. The ESR, CRP, serum calcium and serum proteins are all elevated and Bence Jones and other abnormal proteins are found in the urine. Serum and urine protein electrophoresis are usually abnormal.

The place of surgery in the management of myeloma is limited to biopsy and treatment of pathological fractures. The mainstay of management is chemotherapy, radiotherapy and general supportive therapy under the supervision of a Haematologist and Oncologist. Survival is linked to the development severe anemia, debility, infection, renal failure, mylopathy and amyloid disease.

Lymphoma of bone

Lymphoma usually represents disseminated disease and rarely represents a primary tumour. It is seen in people in the 3rd to fifth decades of life. X-ray show a moth-eaten bony lesion. Treatment is with chemotherapy and radiotherapy.

BONE TUMOURS OF UNKNOWN ORIGIN

Ewing's tumour (Fig.7.12)

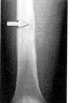

Fig.7.12. Ewing's tumour of the femur and calcaneum

Ewing's tumour is an uncommon primary malignant tumour of bone affecting mainly children and young adults in the second decade of life. Males are more frequently affected than female. The long bones – femur, tibia, humerus and radius - are frequently affected but no bone, including the flat bones, are exempt. It is said to be rare in black people. Recent studies (genetic, biochemical and electron microscopic) suggest that it may represent a mixture of tumours. It starts in the medullary region and destroys bone from within, gradually eroding the cortex to present in the surrounding soft tissue.

Clinically, there is a mass and the associated extensive bone necrosis causes severe pain. There is palpable local warmth and with blood tests showing anaemia, leucocytosis, high ESR and CRP, the stage is set for confusion of this tumour with acute osteomyelitis. At diagnosis, 25% of patients have metastasis to the lungs and other bones.

The onion-skin appearance on conventional x-rays is characteristic of Ewing's tumour but a biopsy is essential to confirm the diagnosis. It is difficult to distinguish from lymphoma, oat-cell carcinoma and neuroblastoma and special studies, such as urine vanillylmandelic acid determination, tissue glycogen stain, immunohistochemical tests and electron microscopy are needed to make the distinction. Cytogenetic testing show that the small, round cells of the tumour have a common karyotypic translocation between chromosome 11 and 22.

The recommended treatment over the years has been a combination of chemotherapy and local radiotherapy but because of increasing reports of high recurrence rates (20%-30%) with this treatment, surgery is now being given a bigger place in the treatment. Preliminary chemotherapy, followed by wide resection and then radiotherapy are being used for lesions of inexpendable bones. Mortality in patients with Ewing's tumour used to be high mainly because of metastasis to the lungs and viscera but survival is improving with modern management.

SOFT TISSUE TUMOURS

Soft tissue tumours do affect the musculoskeletal system. Broadly, these could be *benign, locally aggressive* or *malignant*. Benign tumours include lipomas, angiolipomas, haemangiomas, myxomas, synovial cysts and neurofibromas. The most common locally aggressive tumour is fibromatosis, also called extra-abdominal desmoid tumour. Malignant tumours pose the greatest management problems because they tend to metastasise early to the lungs and other organs.

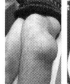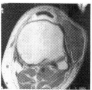

Fig.7.13. Pleomorphic spindle-cell soft-tissue sarcoma in a 60-year-old man

Soft-tissue sarcomata (Fig.7.13) form the main type treated by the Orthopaedic Surgeon. Irrespective of their histological grade, malignant soft-tissue tumours should be treated with either a radical surgical margin and no radiation or a marginal or wide surgical margin plus radiation therapy. Most limb salvage procedures are marginal resections followed by radiation therapy. Radiation therapy can be internal or external. Radiation administered after biopsy but before surgical resection can interfere with wound healing.

LIMB SALVAGE AND AMPUTATION IN PRIMARY MALIGNANT BONE TUMOURS

Patients with malignant bone tumours naturally prefer limb salvage to amputation. Doctors treating them want the best for them but the issue is much more complex than that. At the root of the complexity is the issue of tumour recurrence, which is closely tied to patient survival, and the question of function after treatment. If a limb salvage procedure can guarantee total tumour excision, good function and no recurrence, it is definitely the only desirable procedure. However, if it cannot guarantee these outcomes, then the option of amputation comes in. Recent studies comparing limb salvage with amputation for distal femoral osteosarcoma suggest equal overall survival but a slightly higher risk of recurrence in the limb salvage group. Both groups received adjuvant chemotherapy.

There are no absolute contra-indications to limb salvage. After tumour resection, reconstruction can be effected with autografts, allografts and metal implants and prostheses. However, limb salvage may be associated with large limb length discrepancy, resection of major nerves, especially the sciatic nerve, and pathological fracture, all of which are associated with poor function and decreased survival. Accordingly, amputation should be considered when these circumstances and others, e.g., distant metastases, especially extrapleural lesions and skip metastases, exist. In general, amputations are classified as *intralesional, marginal, wide* or *radical,* depending on the margins achieved. Amputation techniques are varied and some, e.g., hind-quarter amputation is often not only a test of anatomical knowledge and surgical skills but also a test of endurance on the part of the surgical team.

Metastatic bone tumours (Fig.7.14)

These are carcinomas that have arisen from primary tumours mainly of the thyroid, breast, lung, kidney, prostate and gastrointestinal tract. Of all these primary tumours, adenocarcinoma of the breast is the one most likely to metastasise to the skeleton. Two types of metastatic lesions are distinguished:

- *Lytic,* characterised by bone destruction. Metastases from breast, thyroid and kidney belong to this group.

- *Sclerotic,* characterised by reactive bone formation. Metastases from prostatic carcinoma are the classical example.

The distribution of lesions varies. Any bone may be affected but the spine and metaphysis of long bones of the extremities are more frequently involved than other bones. Carcinoma of the lung characteristically metastasises to the hand and foot.

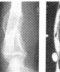

Fig.7.14. Metastatic tumour in the distal radius from a carcinoma of the kidney (hypernephroma) in a 60-year-old man

The patient is usually an adult past middle age and bone pain and/or pathological fracture are the commonest presenting features. X-rays may miss 20%-25% of skeletal metastases. Bone scan is the most accurate investigation, being over 90% sensitive. An MRI scan (Fig.7.15) provides helpful information, especially in spinal involvement. Fine needle biopsy is said to be 90% accurate in experienced hands.

The overall management of a patient with metastatic bone disease is best supervised by the Oncologist. Orthopaedic aspects include the management of pathological fractures. Fractures of the femoral neck are treated by hemiarthroplasty. Intertrochanteric fractures are treated by DHS-type fixation. Diaphyseal fractures are amenable to intramedullary nail fixation. Concomitant debulking of the tumour and radiotherapy is advised. Prophylactic reinforcement of bones afflicted with metastases and likely to fracture if left untreated should be considered in appropriate cases. Acrylic cement may be used to fill big defects, e.g., in the acetabulum. The treatment of spinal lesions can be complex. Metallic implants may be indicated.

Bone tumour centres

The diagnosis and treatment of bone tumours are a very specialised field of medical practice. Although the general practitioner and general orthopaedic surgeon are usually involved in the initial diagnosis, the specific investigation, diagnosis and treatment of these conditions are best left to specially trained and equipped teams of surgeons, physicians (oncologists), pathologists and supportive staff in specialised **bone tumour centres**. Such centres exist in a number of places and should be involved from the very beginning. Naturally, the best results of treatment are achieved by these centres. Even the relatively simple operation of bone tumour biopsy should ideally be carried out at such a centre. Patients should be advised to seek immediate medical advice and help if they or their charges suspect that they have a bone tumour, benign or malignant.

Further reading

Enneking WF, Spanier SS and Goodman MA. A system for the surgical staging of musculoskeletal sarcoma. *Clin Orthop 153:106, 1980.*

Lee FY, Mankin HJ, Fondren G et al. Chondrosarcoma of bone: An assessment of outcome. *J Bone Joint Surg 81A:326, 1999.*

Rougraff BT, Simon MA, Kneisl JS et al. Limb salvage compared with amputation for osteosarcoma of the distal end of the femur: A long-term oncological, functional and quality-of-life study. *J Bone Joint Surg 76A:649, 1994.*

Wong DA, Formnasier VI and MacNab I. Spinal metastases: the obvious, the occult and the impostors *Spine 15: 1, 1990.*

CHAPTER 8

BACK PAIN

Introduction

The back or spine is a complicated structure made up of vertebrae grouped into five regions - cervical (neck), thoracic (chest), lumbar (waist), sacral and coccygeal (tail). Altogether, there are 33-34 vertebrae – 7 cervical, 12 thoracic, 5 lumbar, 5 sacral and 4-5 coccygeal. The vertebrae of the neck, chest and waist have discs lying between them (intervertebral discs). Discs are shock absorbers made up of tough fibrous material and jelly. The vertebrae of the sacrum and coccyx are joined together, with no discs between them.

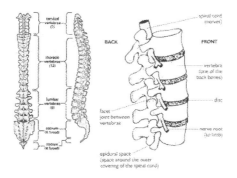

Fig.8.1. Two drawings of the spine showing the bones, discs and nerves

Back pain can be caused by injury, wear and tear of various components of the spine and various diseases affecting these components. It is important to know the cause of your patient's back pain as a prelude to successfully treating it.

ACUTE BACK PAIN

Sprains, Fractures, Dislocations and Slipped Discs. Most acute back pains are the result of trauma - Sprains, Fractures, Dislocations and Slipped Discs. Most injuries are mild and unrecognised. Sprains of the lumbar muscles through awkward or sudden unguarded movements, often associated with lifting heavy weights, are frequent causes of back pain, which usually radiates down to the knee level and not beyond.

Serious injuries to the spine may cause fractures, dislocations and "slipped discs". These are often dramatic in nature and cause severe and acute back pain, which force the patient to seek urgent medical attention. Most of those affected are young people in the 20-40 age bracket.

Diagnosis is based on the history, physical examination and results of investigations (X-rays, MRI and CT scans). Treatment depends on the injury and ranges from analgesics and non-steroidals to physiotherapy and surgery. The outcome may be poor, especially if there has been significant nerve damage caused by bone fragments, slipped discs or other soft tissues.

Whiplash is a special and important type of back pain. It is a sprain of ligaments and other soft tissues of the neck as a result of a sudden backward and then forward jerk of the head and neck. The commonest mechanism of whiplash is seen in vehicular collisions. The head of an occupant of a vehicle hit from the back by another vehicle is jerked first backward (hyperextension) and then forward (flexion). The degree of sprain of the soft tissues varies according to the magnitude of the collision and fractures of the vertebrae and nerve injury may occur in the more serious accidents.

Neck pain and stiffness are the usual symptoms of whiplash but an affected person usually does not feel these symptoms immediately after the accident; they come on gradually in the next 24-48 hours. Ligaments of the lower back may also be sprained at the time as the neck injury.

Treatment is with pain-killers, non-steroidal anti-inflammatory drugs and physiotherapy. Most whiplash injuries will resolve within three months but a minority of patients keep having symptoms for months or years after the accident.

PERSISTENT BACK PAIN

Persistent back pain, not attributable to a known trauma, constitutes a comparatively small percentage of cases but needs to be investigated to find the cause, which may be a life-threatening disease, such as a tumour. Let's summarise the possible causes of back pain:

Cervical Spondylosis (Fig.8.2)

Although, strictly speaking, cervical spondylosis is degeneration of the intervertebral disc and cervical osteoarthritis is degeneration of the facetal joints in the neck, cervical spondylosis is used to described the two conditions, which occur simultaneously. A better collective term may be "degenerative joint disease of the neck". So, we are talking of a diffuse wear-and-tear condition, which simultaneously involves the vertebral bodies, the discs between them and neighbouring joints and soft tissues. The resulting changes in the vertebrae (bony spurs) and discs (disc herniations) can cause pressure on the nerve roots behind the vertebral bodies, causing radicular pain, sometimes even nerve paralysis.

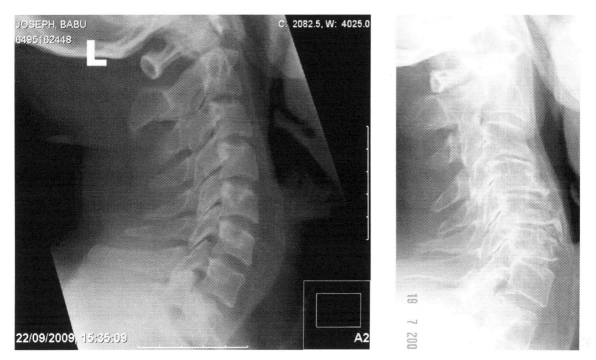

Fig.8.2. X-ray picture of a normal cervical spine and one afflicted with cervical spondylosis. An interesting point worth mentioning here is that not all patients with these X-ray signs of disease are symptomatic.

Diagnosis. The symptoms and signs are:

- The typical patient is an adult past middle age.
- The usual complaints are pain and stiffness in the neck.
- The stiffness is characteristically worse following periods of immobility of the neck and is relieved by motion.
- The pain is characteristically made worse by movements of the head and by certain sleeping positions.
- The pain may be localised in the neck or refer to the head, the shoulder(s) or front of the chest wall.

X-rays and MRI scans help to determine the extent of the disease and its special features in a given patient. Multilevel involvement is common. The lowermost two vertebral bodies and discs i.e. C5/C6 and C6/C7, are the most frequently affected.

Treatment. This is largely non-surgical. Physiotherapy in the form of massage, manipulation, moist heat, deep heat, support to the head and an exercise programme are useful. Anti-inflammatory tablets are also helpful. There may be a place for surgical treatment in the form of removing an identified cause of nerve root compression or fusing two or more neighbouring vertebrae for instability and this can be done from the front or back of the neck.

Lumbar Spondylosis (Fig.8.3)

What has been said about the pathology of cervical spondylosis applies to lumbar spondylosis. is the same as osteoarthritis of the lumbar spine or waist. As in the neck, it is a diffuse wear-and-tear condition, which simultaneously involves the vertebral bodies, the discs between them, neighbouring joints and soft tissues. It is an important cause of low back ache and pain. All of the five vertebral bodies in the waist region can be affected. Bony spurs and slipped discs are part of the wear and tear process and either of these can cause pressure on the nerves behind the vertebral bodies and cause severe pain in the legs (sciatica).

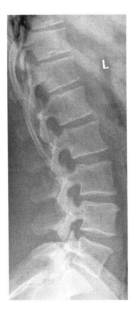 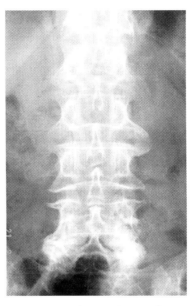

Fig.8.3 . X-ray picture of a normal lumbar spine and one afflicted with lumbar spondylosis

Diagnosis. It is probably true to say that most people over the age of 50 have osteoarthritis of the lower back. The main symptoms of this are:

- low back pain (or ache) and
- back stiffness.

Low back pain is sometimes referred to as *"lumbago"*. Stiffness is characteristically present first thing in the morning or following periods of prolonged sitting or other forms of inactivity. Gentle back movements tend to lessen low back symptoms but prolonged activity brings them back. Damp, cold weather worsens them. Quite often, lumbar pain refers to the buttocks and anterior upper thigh via connecting muscles and ligaments and also to the outer aspect of the knee. Osteophytes (bony spurs) are often formed as part of the wear-and-tear process and can impinge on nerves in the spine, causing the so-called *sciatica*, which is pain going down the leg or legs along the course of the sciatic nerve.

Investigation follows lines similar to those undertaken for cervical spondylosis. An MRI scan is mandatory if surgical treatment is planned. Again, multilevel involvement is common. The lowermost three vertebral bodies and discs are the most frequently affected.

Treatment

Non-surgical management

- Prescribe pain-killers and anti-inflammatory drugs. Advise on precautions and limitations of NSAIDs
- Advise patient to sleep on firm beds
- Advise patient to avoid bad posture as this is a recognised cause of back pain. Sitting, standing and lying in awkward positions should be avoided. Lift things "with your knee" rather than "with your back", that is, start the lifting from the kneeling position, rather than with the back bent.
- Advise rest and application of local heat.
- A physiotherapy programme aimed at pain-relief and maintenance of muscle tone and joint mobility should be instituted.
- Lumbar braces or corsets should be avoided as they tend to worsen stiffness.

Surgical management

The place of surgery is limited. The options include surgical removal of a herniated disc (please see below) and fusing two or more vertebrae to eliminate movement (and pain!). There may be a place for other forms of surgery.

Prolapsed intervertebral disc (PID) or "Slipped Disc" (Fig.8.4)

A slipped disc is a protrusion of disc material between any two vertebrae. Although this can happen anywhere in the spine, it is seen mainly in the neck and waist regions because they are the mobile segments of the spine. Slipped disc is seen mostly in young people and there is usually a history of significant trauma. In the elderly, it is usually secondary to wear and tear of the disc plus trivial trauma.

DIAGNOSIS

In the neck, disc herniations/protrusions are most common at the lowermost two levels -between C5/C6 and C6/C7 vertebral bodies. In the lumbar spine, it is most common also at the lowermost two levels - between L4/L5 and L5/S1 vertebral bodies.

The symptoms of a slipped disc in the neck are:

- local neck pain, which may go into the shoulder, arm, forearm and fingers and may also go to the front of the chest or shoulder blade area.

Similarly, in the lumbar spine, there is:

- low back pain, which refer to the buttock and back of the leg below the knee, sometimes going down as far as the toes. The term *sciatica* is used to describe this pain because it arises from irritation of the sciatic nerve.

In both locations, the pain is described as severe and sharp and is characteristically made worse by movements, coughing, sneezing and straining in the bathroom. There may also be some muscle weakness.

X-rays are useful but will only show narrowed disc spaces or bone changes, like osteophytes. The most fruitful investigation for a slipped disc is the MRI scan (Fig.8.4), which will show a disc protrusion and its relation to neighbouring nerve roots. A CT scan or myelogram can be used in place of an MRI scan.

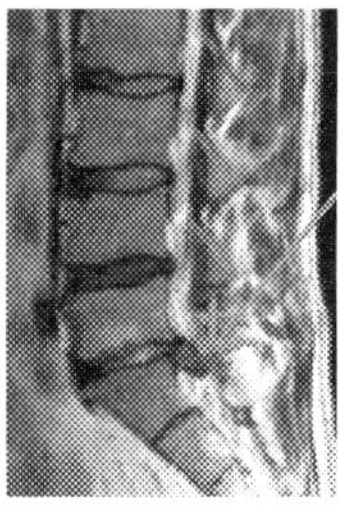

Fig.8.4. An MRI scan of the lumbar spine showing a prolapsed disc at L5/S1 intervertebral disc space.

TREATMENT

Non-surgical management

- If acute pain is present, a temporary collar may be useful for neck pain, whilst a lumbar corset may be useful in low back pain.
- Strong analgesics, NSAIDs and muscle relaxants are usually required to control the pain.
- Moist heat applied locally is also useful.
- Leg traction may be indicated to ease pressure on a nerve root. This probably works by enforcing bedrest.
- Progress or lack of must be monitored.
- Manipulation of the spine for acute PID is dangerous and should not be attempted.

Surgical management

Surgical treatment may be indicated in some patients to free compressed nerve roots but only after non-surgical treatment has been given a fair trial and has failed to relieve the patient's symptoms. Surgical options include

- *open disc excision* (open discectomy) and *microdiscectomy* through a small incision or endoscopically.

- *Chemonucleolysis* with chemopapain injection into the disc is said to be effective in 70% of patients with acute disc prolapsed. There are also newer methods of removing the disc by suction.

OTHER CAUSES OF BACK PAIN

- **Inflammatory arthritis**
  Neck pain is common in rheumatoid arthritis, discussed further in Chapter 3. Ankylosing spondylitis, also discussed earlier in Chapter 3, is also a well-known cause of back pain.

- **Osteoporosis**
  Osteoporosis, discussed in more detail in chapter 4, causes hunchback, which may cause back pain.

- **Infections of the spine**
  Bacterial and TB infections of the spine cause back pain. The affected individual is likely to feel unwell and may have fever. Infections are dealt with in greater detail in Chapter 5.

- **Back pain from tumours** of the spine: this could be benign or malignant. Most of the malignant tumours are cancers of various organs of the body which have spread to the spine.

- **Back pain from blood diseases** e.g. lymphomas are common examples.

- **Diseases a person was born with.** Congenital diseases e.g. wry neck and Sprengel shoulder are associated with back pain but these conditions are usually recognisable in infancy or in the first two years of life.

It is apparent from this list that the causes of back pain are varied and that all age groups are affected. When presented with a patient suffering from back pain, the doctor should seek to make a diagnosis on the basis of which they will manage the condition. It is reassuring that most diseases that cause back pain can be successfully treated.

PART III
FRACTURES

CHAPTER 9

INTRODUCTION TO FRACTURES

It is important that doctors who manage fractures speak "a common language", otherwise confusion will result which may compromise the comparison of results of various treatment options, clinical audit and the learning process.

DEFINITION OF A FRACTURE (Fig.9.1)

A fracture is a break in the continuity of bone, caused by trauma. It is important that the element of trauma is included in the definition because it then excludes those breaks in the continuity of the bone, which are obviously not fractures, for example, a congenital pseudoarthrosis of the clavicle. The term "spontaneous fracture" is sometimes used, especially in relation to pathological fractures. This is erroneous and should be avoided. In pathological fractures, the trauma is usually mild but is there nevertheless.

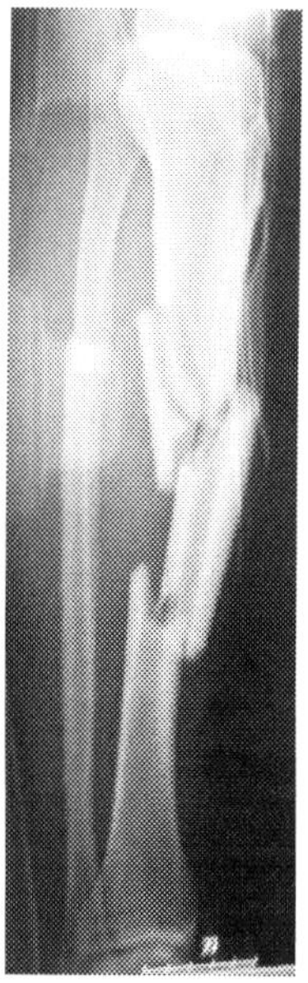

MECHANISMS OF FRACTURES (Fig.9.2)

Fig.9.1 A fracture is a break in the continuity of bone caused by trauma

The key factor in the origin of fractures is trauma, by which is meant physical violence. Fractures do not come about spontaneously. Even fractures through bone weakened by disease or previous injury (pathological fractures) still require some physical violence. Such violence can arise from activities of daily living, sports and various types of accidents. In spite of this diversity in origin and nature, their action on the affected bone can be classified into direct and indirect.

Direct trauma. The injuring force acts directly on the bone and the site of fracture corresponds to the site of application of the injuring force. Sources of such a force include direct kicks on the shin during football and blows with sticks or other hard objects.

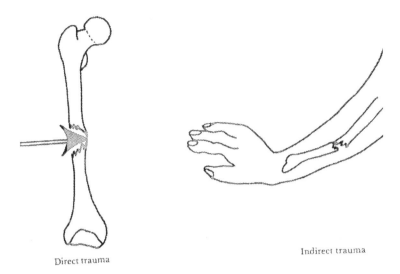

Fig.9.2. Mechanisms of fractures (a) direct injury (b) indirect injury

Indirect trauma, in which there is a distance between the point of application of violence and the site of the fracture. Such a force may be predominantly angulatory, rotator/torsional, compressional, traction (tension,) in nature or may be a combination of two or more of the above, producing fractures that are correspondingly described:

DESCRIPTION OF FRACTURES (Fig.9.3)

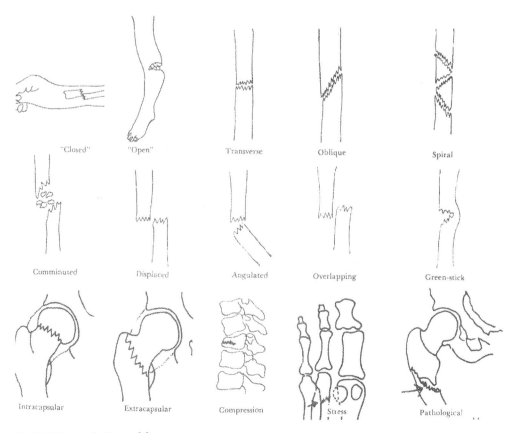

Fig.9.3. Description of fractures

Fractures are described in many ways using established terms, which are summarised below.

- **Closed or Open /Simple or Compound? (Fig.9.4)**
  i.   **Closed fracture** is one that is not in communication with the outside environment via an associated wound.
  ii. **Open fracture.** This is also called "Compound" fracture. It is one in which the fracture site is in communication with the outside via a wound. In most cases of open fractures, this communication is potential rather than direct because muscles usually interpose between the fracture fragments and the outside.

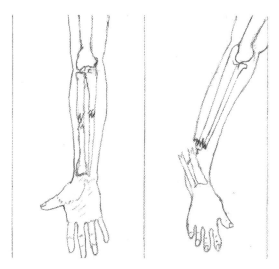

Fig.9.4. Closed and open fracture

- **Based on the presence or absence of displacement (Fig.9.5)**
  i.   Undisplaced
  ii. Displaced (these can be angulated, rotated, overlapping or overriding)

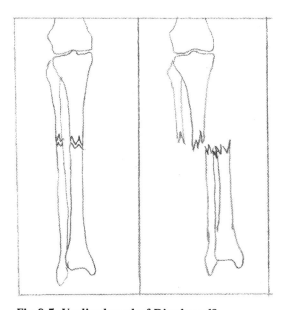

Fig.9.5. Undisplaced of Displaced?

- **Based on the site of fracture (long bones mainly)**
  i. Fracture in the proximal one-third of the shaft (of a long bone).
  ii. Fracture in the middle one-third of the shaft.
  iii. Fracture in the distal one-third of the shaft.
  iv. Fracture involving the metaphyseal or epiphyseal regions.

- **Based on the direction of the fracture line**
  i. Transverse
  ii. Oblique (short or long)
  iii. Spiral

The injuring force can be guessed from the direction of the fracture line(s). A direct tapping force or a bending force usually causes a transverse fracture. Bending plus axial loading produce oblique fractures. Rotational forces produce spiral fractures whilst axial loading produce compression or impacted ones.

- **Based on the number of fracture fragments**
  i. *Two-/3-/4-fragment fracture.* Sometimes this is associated with a tiny third fragment called a *butterfly* fragment. The term *"segmented fracture"* is also used to describe a three or more fragment fracture.
  ii. *Comminuted.* Here, there are more than two fragments. A variety of this type is the so-called *segmented fracture* in which a long bone is broken in two or more places, giving rise to three or more sizeable fragments.

- **Based on the alignment of the main fragments**
  A fracture is said to be in alignment if the longitudinal axes of its major fragments are more or less parallel. If not, it is said to be out of alignment.

- **Fractures near or involving joints**
  Intracapsular
- Involving articular cartilage e.g. T- and Y-shaped condylar fractures of the distal femur and humerus; Bennett's fractures of the thumb
- Not involving articular cartilage e.g. transverse femoral neck fractures.
  Extracapsular e.g. trochanteric fractures of the femur; Colles fracture.

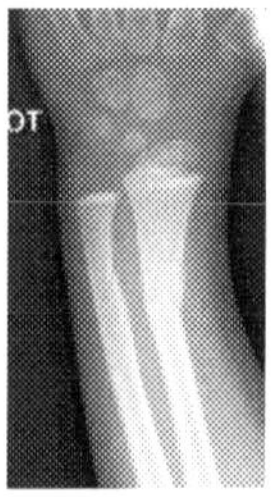

OTHER DESCRIPTIVE TERMS

Complete or Incomplete? (Fig.9.6). A complete fracture is one in which the break is through and through. An incomplete one is one in which, on an X-ray, a part of the cortex is intact. A green-stick fracture seen in children is an example of an incomplete fracture.

Fig.9.6. Greenstick fractures of the radius and ulna in a child are examples of incomplete fractures

Stress Fracture. This is described as a fracture of bone trabeculae (micro-fracture). There is usually no history of obvious trauma; it is thought to result from fatigue from repetitive stress. Relatively common in the metatarsals, it is common among young army recruits, hence the term *"march fracture"*. This fracture is diagnosed definitively only with the help of an X-ray taken some 2 or more weeks later on which it shows as a thin-lined crack surrounded by a cloud of callus. A bone scan will also show this fracture.

Crush or compression or impacted fracture. These occur characteristically in cancellous bones and are common in vertebrae, the neck of femur, proximal tibia and distal radius. The injuring force may be a fall from a height or the hammer action of one bone on its neighbour e.g. the lateral humeral condyle on the radial head and the amount of compression/impaction depends on the magnitude of the injuring force.

Pathological Fracture. This is a fracture through a bone already weakened by disease or previous injury. Common examples are fractures through metastatic deposits or through screw tracks.

The 'named' Fractures - Many fractures have become named after the doctors who first described them. Although many orthopaedic surgeons have been fighting this idea, most still prefer to retain them, perhaps as evidence of some special knowledge of the fractures concerned. Common examples include Bennett's, Colles', Galleazzi, Monteggia and Pott's fractures.

CLASSIFICATIONS OF FRACTURES

Quite apart from description, various fractures have been individually classified by various authors. Many of these classifications bear their names e.g. Salter-Harris classification of fractures involving the growth plates in children or Garden's classification of femoral neck fractures. Classifications of fractures are complicated and are not emphasised in this book as they may turn off the beginner. The AO classification, which is all-embracing, classifying nearly all fractures in a systematic way, is summarised below (Fig.9.7):

The AO Classification of fractures

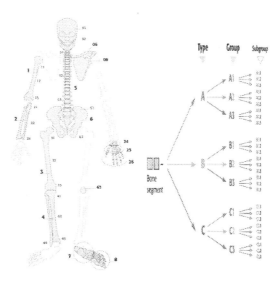

Fig.9.7. The AO Classification of fractures

143

The AO classification of fractures is based on the following principles:

Each long bone or group of bones (forearm and lower leg), as well as the spine and pelvis, is allocated a number as follows:

Humerus	1	Spine	5
Radius/ulna	2	Pelvis	5
Femur	3	Hand	7
Tibia/fibula	4	Foot	8

- Each long bone is divided into 3 zones as follows:
  1. Proximal metaphyseal/epiphyseal zone
  2. Shaft or Diaphysis
  3. Distal metaphyseal/epiphyseal zone

An exception is made for the ankle joint mortise where a 4th zone is allocated. Accordingly, a malleolar fracture complex is designated as 44: 4 for the tibia/fibula and 4 for the malleolar zone.

- For each zone of each bone, the fractures are divided into 3 groups –A, B and C - in ascending order of severity and difficulty in management.
- Furthermore, within each A, B or C group, there are 3 additional subgroups, 1, 2 and 3. For example, a severe distal humeral fracture would be 13-C3.
- There are further subdivisions for more precise coding of fractures.

EXAMPLES

- An injury coded "11" represents a fracture of the humerus in the epiphyseal or metaphyseal region.
- An injury coded "32" represents a fracture of the femoral shaft.
- An injury coded 33C.3 represents a complex fracture of the femur in the distal epiphyseal/metaphyseal region.

HEALING OF FRACTURES (FIG.9.8)

Fracture healing is usually divided into three phases: *inflammatory, reparative and remodelling*, but it must be emphasised that these phases usually overlap.

INFLAMMATORY PHASE (0 – 5 days)

This can be divided into two sub-phases:

- ***Formation of Haematoma* (the first two days following fracture).**
  A so-called *fracture haematoma* is formed as soon as a bone breaks. Its sources are ruptured blood vessels of the periosteum, bone cortex and marrow and of the surrounding soft tissues. Platelets in the clot release growth factors such as transforming growth factor-beta (TGF- beta) and platelet-derived growth factor (PDGF), which regulate cell proliferation

and differentiation. The ends of the ruptured vessels soon clot and there is little bleeding into the fracture site at 24 hours. The ends of the fractured bone, which have been stripped of their periosteum are avascular.

- **Organisation of fracture haematoma and invasion of it by inflammatory cells (Day 2 – 5 after fracture).** The haematoma begins to organise within a few hours of its formation. At the same time, it is invaded by inflammatory cells, notably multinuclear phagocytes and monocytes, which start to phagocytose necrotic tissue and other debris. This process of phagocytosis continues for days or weeks, depending on the amount of tissue to be removed.

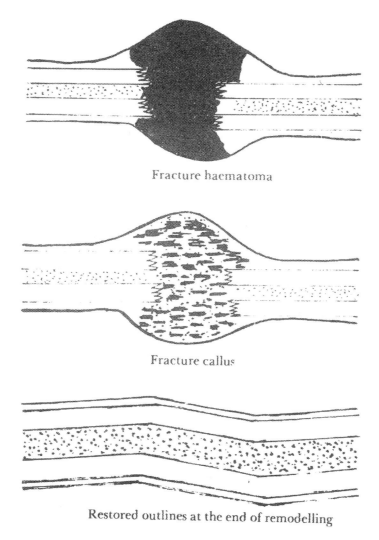

Fracture haematoma

Fracture callus

Restored outlines at the end of remodelling

Fig.9.8. Stages of fracture healing

REPARATIVE PHASE (DAY 5 – 40).

During this phase, a *fracture callus* forms and transforms into mature bone. *Callus is an immature bony structure* of "impure" composition - woven bone, cartilage and fibrous tissue. *The source of callus is pluripotential mesenchymal cells,* which arise from the periosteum, perivascular and vascular endothelial cells, muscle, fascia and the bone marrow. *They transform into osteoblasts, chondroblasts and fibroblasts, which form osteoid, cartilage and collagen respectively.* Growth factors such as bone morphogenetic protein (BMP) and cytokines such as interleukin (IL) -1 and -6 are active throughout this phase.

The early stages of callus formation are sometimes called the *sticky phase of fracture healing.* It is attained at about 3 weeks from the time of the fracture and represents the clinical stage in which the fracture can still be moved but cannot be widely displaced by a moderate deforming force. This is the phase in which a functional brace can be safely applied.

REMODELLING PHASE (from day 40)

This phase is the longest ans slowest. It may last as long as nine years after the fracture. The osteoclasts are the major performers, resorbing unneeded trabecular bone from the fracture callus. Osteoblasts lay down new and better orientated trabeculae in more functionally appropriate sites. The Haversian system is restored in the cortical bone; the medullary canal is restored, with better quality trabeculae replacing the coarse ones of the fracture callus.

From the clinical view-point, angular deformities may correct to a greater or lesser extent during the remodelling phase, depending on the age of the patient. In general, children do better than adults. Rotational deformities, however, correct little, even in children, hence the teaching that in the reduction of fractures rotational deformities must be corrected completely or reduced to their barest minimum.

CLINICAL FACTORS INFLUENCING FRACTURE HEALING

Age of the patient. As a general rule, fractures heal faster in children than in adults. This is because of the greater healing potential in the former. Healing and remodelling is also faster and more complete in childhood fractures.

Degree of displacement and associated soft-tissue damage. Fractures associated with considerable displacement and soft-tissue injury heal slower than those without.

Type of bone involved. Fractures through cancellous bones tend to be stable and heal faster than those through cortical bone.

Bone Loss. This retards fracture healing because more new bone will be required to fill the gap created. Obviously, the bigger the lost piece, the bigger the problem. In losses of segments more the 2-3 cm long, the need may arise to bone-graft the defect.

Presence of infection. This retards fracture healing due to depression of osteogenesis by toxic products and also to actual dissolution of formed new bone by them. Furthermore the presence of infection usually excludes certain treatment methods e.g. internal fixation of the fracture.

Pathological fractures. Those occurring through primary or secondary malignant lesions usually heal poorly. Fractures through bones affected with non-malignant conditions may or may not heal normally e.g. fractures through simple bone cysts heal normally but those in Paget's disease heal slowly.

Intra-articular fractures. These heal relatively slowly. This is at least partly due to the fibrinolytic effect of synovial fluid on the initial fracture haematoma.

Intact "fellow bone". In the forearm and leg where there are two long bones, when one is fractured and the other is intact, the healing of the fractured bone may be retarded by the strutting up action of the intact one e.g. an intact fibula frequently struts up a fractured tibia.

Smoking and fracture healing. Fracture healing relies on blood supply to the broken bone. Nicotine causes constriction of the small blood vessels around the fracture site. Carbon monoxide in smoke decreases the amount of oxygen delivered to the fracture site. Together the lack of oxygen and decreased blood flow retards the healing process. A recent study looked at the effects of smoking on healing of ankle fractures. It was found that ankle fractures of smokers were 16 times more likely not to heal than in non-smokers. Another study showed a 40% risk of failure of fusion for low back pain in smokers compaired to non-smokers.

Other Factors. Many other factors facilitating or retarding fracture healing have been identified. They cannot all be mentioned here. Suffice it to state that the effect of the vast majority of them, including those outlined above, has been demonstrated mainly in experimental studies involving animal models and cell cultures. In clinical practice, their effects, especially separately, have not been demonstrated. The practising orthopaedic surgeon relies more on the clinical circumstances of a given fracture to predict the likely outcome of healing, and takes steps to prevent likely complications.

Complications of Fracture Healing. The specific complications of fracture healing are mal-union, delayed union and non-union. These are discussed in some detail in relevant chapters.

CHAPTER 10

DIAGNOSIS AND TREATMENT OF FRACTURES

DIAGNOSIS OF FRACTURES

In the diagnosis of fractures, a systematic approach is imperative as it is the surest way to avoid embarrassing and sometimes dangerous mistakes. This systematic approach begins with first aid (when indicated), goes through good history-taking, physical examination, radiographic and laboratory investigations and ends with a definitive diagnosis on which treatment can be based. It can be summarised with the common phrase "do first things first".

FIRST AID

Team approach to first aid gives the best results. Therefore, it is important that you seek immediate help from your colleagues. Don't play the hero!

Life-threatening injuries must be contained before engaging in accurate diagnosis of fractures. Doctors who are required to manage patients with severe injuries are required to attend courses on and imbibe the principles of the Advanced Trauma Life Support (ATLS). The basic teachings of ATLS can be summarised with the abbreviation ABCDE, where A=Airway, B=Breathing, C=Circulation, D=Disability, E=Exposure.

In other words, to have a life patient, such a patient must be breathing and must have an intact circulation. "Disabilty" alludes to examining to exclude neurological injury and "Exposure" alludes to carrying out a full examination of the patient from head to toe, the so-called *secondary survey*. Additional measures include securing a venous access for blood and fluid transfusion, taking blood for baseline tests, grouping and cross-matching blood, splinting of fractures (Fig.10.1) and generally making the patient comfortable with adequate analgesia.

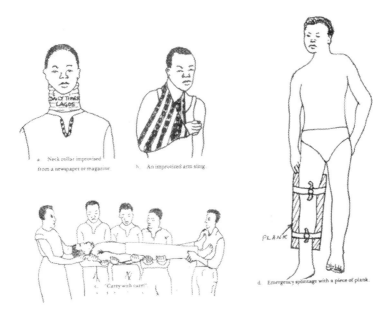

Fig.10.1. Some methods of first aid splintage of fractures
a. Neck collar improvised from a newspaper or magazine
b. An arm sling improvised from a scarf
c. "Carry with care!"
d. Temporary immobilisation of a lower limb fracture with a plank

HISTORY

Every event has a story behind it, so also do fractures. Good history-taking is so important that it can be over-emphasised. Invest in good history-taking and you and your team will laugh all the way to the bank of accurate diagnosis and effective treatment! (Fig.10.2).

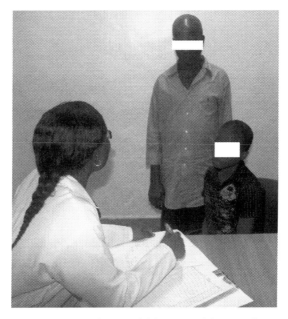

Fig.10.2. Invest in good history-taking and you and your team will laugh all the way to the bank of accurate diagnosis and effective treatment!

One of the effective ways of obtaining a good history is to begin with the patient's COMPLAINTS. An acute fracture patient will complain of or have one or more of the following symptoms:

Complaints/Symptoms of Fractures

- **Pain.** This is usually severe and made worse by any movements of the affected limb or part which is transmitted to the fracture site. Pain is not manifest in the unconscious patient.

- **Loss of function.** In most cases, the patient is unable to use the broken bone normally - because of structural discontinuity and because of pain. In a few cases, for example, in impacted fractures (usually of the neck of femur or humerus) the patient may still be able to move the broken bone. Pain is still present, however.

- **Swelling.** This is mainly due to a local haematoma and associated soft-tissue injury, and usually increases in size with the passage of time. Swelling is usually not obvious in fractures of deep-seated bones like the spine and pelvis.

- **Deformity.** Continuity in the line of long axis of the affected bone is broken at the fracture site and together with the accompanying swelling constitute a deformity which could be angulatory, rotatory or both. Deformity could also result from over-riding (or overlapping) fracture fragments.

HISTORY OF SYMPTOMS

Patients' symptoms/complaints usually arise from trauma. Such trauma could be serious, moderate, mild or even unnoticed by the patient. Details of such an injury must be sought by the doctor because knowledge of them usually aids management. The details sought must include the time of the accident and any treatment received by the patient before arriving in the hospital.

PAST MEDICAL/SURGICAL HISTORY (PMH)

The patient's past medical history must also be sought. They may have a medical condition like hypertension or diabetes, which could influence the management of his fracture. History of previous injuries or operations should be sought as it is commonly omitted by patients because of anxiety.

SOCIAL HISTORY (SH)

Their social history is also important. He/she may be a hard drinker, a fact that may be important when anaesthetising them for reduction or fixation of their fracture. Their cultural attitudes may influence their attitude to hospitalisation. The social status, occupation, earning capacity, number of children and financial commitments to relatives are all factors that could influence management, as are the requirements of their religion. These aspects are particularly important in countries like Nigeria where healthcare is not free and patients or their relatives bear the burden of hospital charges. The physician must patiently seek out and document these details. Current medications and history of allergy to drugs, food or other substances must also be noted.

PHYSICAL EXAMINATION

This part of fracture management is very important and the temptation to cut ends must be resisted, no matter how obvious or simple a case may appear. Physical examination must be systematic. First, a quick routine general examination of the body, system by system, is carried out. This is then followed by a more thorough examination of the affected part.

General Examination

It is essential to carry out a general examination of every fracture patient. The aim is to elicit any abnormal condition in the patient as a whole that might affect the management of their injury. Not infrequently, such a condition was in existence before the injury, for example, anaemia of various origins, and cardiac, respiratory or other insufficiencies. Should the patient come to surgical operation, the anaesthetist will be very interested in knowing their fitness for anaesthesia. Any significant finding must be noted and recorded.

In summary, a general examination could reveal signs of shock or haemorrhage, of injury to the central nervous system e.g. paraplegia or a possible pre-disposing cause of a fracture e.g. malignancy, as well as signs of chronic cardiac, pulmonary or hormonal disease, all of which will affect the management of their fracture.

Local Examination

This elicits the local status (status localis). In injuries involving a limb, comparison of the affected limb with the unaffected one is vital. Again, local examination must be systematic:

- **Look!** A careful look will reveal a deformity, swelling, bruises and wounds, if present. The nature of a wound is important. If it is at the fracture site, the fracture is likely to be an open (compound) one, in which case its size is important. A puncture wound "from within" has been caused by a bone spike and is less likely to be heavily contaminated whereas a wide and irregular wound is likely to have originated "from without" and likely to be contaminated with dirt. Scars or any other abnormality in the affected part should also be sought; they may be pointers to a pathological fracture.

- **Palpation.** This is the procedure of examination with the hand. It includes touching, feeling and sometimes, exerting firm pressure with the fingers, thumb or clenched fist. It will define the bounds of a swelling, determine its texture or consistency and define points or areas of tenderness.

- **Movement.** Testing for the presence or absence of movement in an injured part is fundamental to the physical examination of an injured patient. Testing for active movement is more important than for passive movement. The patient is asked to move the injured part. Usually, if a fracture is present (except an impacted fracture), he will not be able to do so, but in limb fractures it is important to ask the patient to move the joints distal to the site of the fracture, especially the fingers or toes. Absence of movement in these parts may denote significant nerve or tendon injuries.

Passive movement usually causes severe pain but a gentle effort to determine the presence or absence of movement (pathological mobility) at a site of suspected fracture is acceptable. No determined effort to elicit a crepitus is allowed; the contribution of such an effort to diagnosis is too little to justify the usually severe pain associated with it.

INVESTIGATIONS

Investigations are needed for the confirmation of clinical diagnosis.

RADIOGRAPHIC IMAGING

Conventional X-rays

An X-ray picture of the suspected fracture site is imperative. Usually, two views, an anteroposterior (AP) and a lateral view, are sufficient but oblique views may sometimes be necessary. In limb fractures, it is usually necessary to insist on the inclusion on the X-ray of *one joint above* and *one joint below* the fracture. Special views, which home in on particular areas or structures, may be necessary, although most have now been rendered obsolete by CT, MRI and ultrasound scans. However, not every hospital have these scan, so I will summarise some of these views here:

Special X-ray views

- *axial* and *"Y" views* (for the humeral head and glenohumeral joint)
- *tunnel views* (of the wrist for hamate fractures and of the knee joint for condylar fractures and loose bodies)
- *stress views* (for the diagnosis of ligament injuries in the knee, ankle and digits)
- 15 degree oblique views of the tibial plateau
- 60 degree pelvic inlet and outlet views for pelvic fractures
- 45 degree Judet views for acetabular fractures.

A chest X-ray may be indicated in the elderly, mainly for anaesthetic purposes. Special care is needed in the interpretation of X-rays of suspected fractures in children. The beginner must avoid interpreting every translucent line as a fracture as most represent growth plates.

Tomography

This is a conventional X-ray imaging in which the beams are concentrated on a small area of interest – "cone view". This method has been largely overtaken by computed tomography.

Computerised Tomographic (CT) scan (Fig.10.3)

This provides a cross-sectional image of a given bone and can be very useful in the diagnosis of fractures in deep parts of the body, especially the skull, spine, pelvis and intra-articular fractures. A 3-dimensional recontruction is particularly useful in intra-articular fractures.

Magnetic Resonance Imaging (Fig.10.3)

This is particularly useful in elucidating *soft-tissue injuries* involvement by fractures. It is very useful in the finer diagnosis of spinal and intra-articular fractures.

Ultrasonography

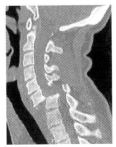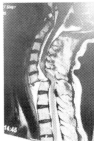

Fig.10.3. CT and MRI studies of the cervical spine showing a C6-C7 dislocation-dislocation. The CT clearly demonstrates the fracture-dislocation whilst the MRI clearly demonstrates the relationship between the fraction-dislocation and the surrounding soft tissues, especially the spinal cord.

This investigation is particularly helpful in the diagnosis of muscle, tendon and rotator-cuff injuries.

Isotopic Bone Scan

A radiolabelled *phosphorus-based compound* e.g. Technetium 99, Gallium 67 or Indium 111 gets taken up by bone and can therefore be used as a physiological marker to detect abnormalities of bone metabolism. The uptake is determined by blood flow, so any condition characterised by increased blood flow e.g. injury, inflammation, infection, tumours, will cause increased uptake, which can be depicted on a film

Arthrography

With the advent of MRI scanning, this investigation now has limited indications e.g. in the investigation of ligamentous injuries in the ankle.

Venography/Arteriography

A venogram is useful in the diagnosis of deep vein thrombosis which may complicate fracture management. An arteriogram may be required when an arterial injury is suspected.

Laboratory Tests

In patients with open fractures and associated external bleeding and in those whose fractures require open reduction, the haemoglobin (Hb) level must be determined. In appropriate cases, it is wise to at least group and save serum in case of subsequent need to transfuse the patient.

There may be specific indications for other laboratory tests e.g. blood gases, serum urea, electrolytes and proteins, etc.

Electrocardiography

An ECG may be indicated in the elderly or in patients with a history of heart disease.

TREATMENT OF FRACTURES

The definitive treatment of most fractures does not constitute a surgical emergency. The patient's general condition must therefore be satisfactory before the treatment of their fracture is undertaken. It is worthwhile repeating here that in major bone fractures and in injuries involving the head and neck, the ATLS principles (ABCDE) must be applied.

The aims of treatment of a fracture are to restore the anatomy and function of the broken bone to a perfect or as near-perfect as possible state. These aims are achieved through three procedures: reduction, maintenance of reduction (immobilisation) and rehabilitation. This implies and means that **only displaced fractures need reduction.**

REDUCTION OF FRACTURES

By reduction is meant bringing together the fracture ends (or pieces in case of a comminuted fracture) in such a way as to restore the anatomy of the bone at the fracture site.

To achieve *a perfect reduction* is the dream of every orthopaedic surgeon but in practice he often is forced by circumstances to accept less-than-perfect reductions. It is common to hear the terms "satisfactory" or "acceptable" being used to describe reductions.

A satisfactory or acceptable reduction must at least:

(a) achieve a total or near-total correction of all deformities (angulatory or rotatory) present at the fracture site and
(b) achieve the apposition and contact of at least 75% of the cross-sectional
(c) area of the fracture ends or pieces.

Methods of achieving reduction

A fracture can be reduced by "closed" or "open" methods.

1. CLOSED REDUCTION AND IMMOBILISATION
    The classical methods of closed reduction are illustrated on Fig.10.4:

    (a) manual traction plus manipulation
    (b) continuous gravity-assisted traction
    (c) continuous traction using weights attached to the end of a rope attached to a bandage applied to skin or a pin inserted into bone.

An external fixator can also be used to achieve the same purpose (Fig.10.5). Closed fracture reduction can be difficult and requires a degree of mastery.

A simple balanced traction using a traction frame (The IWOT frame) invented by the author is illustrated on Figs.10.6.

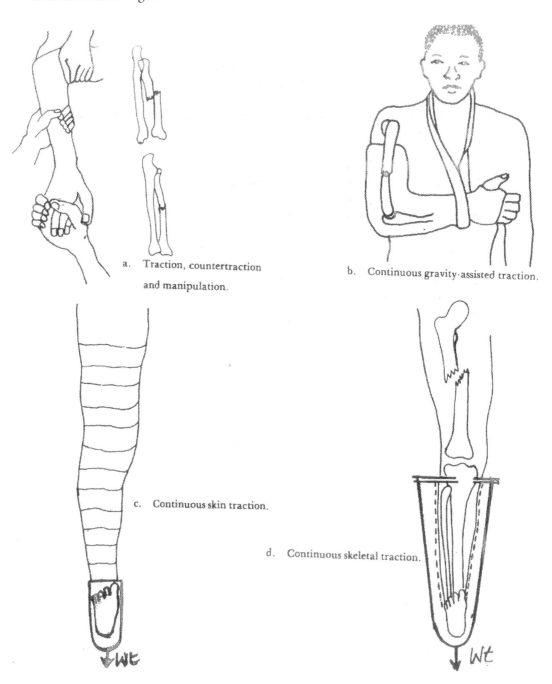

a. Traction, countertraction and manipulation.

b. Continuous gravity-assisted traction.

c. Continuous skin traction.

d. Continuous skeletal traction.

Fig.10.4. Methods of closed reduction of fractures: (a) by manual traction plus manipulation (b) continuous gravity-assisted traction (c) continuous traction using weights attached to a bandage (Skin traction) or to a pin inserted into bone (Skeletal traction)

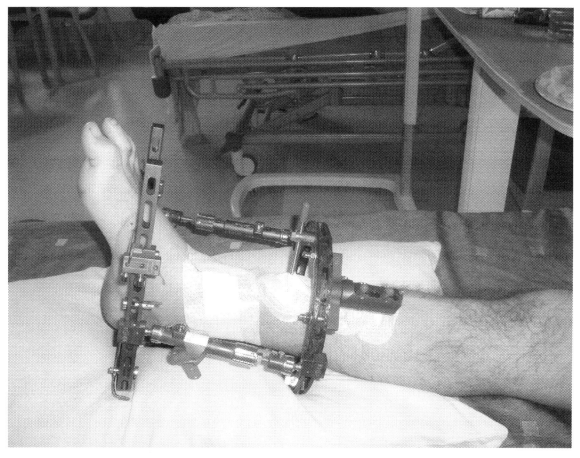

Fig.10.5. Closed reduction can also be achieved using an external fixator.

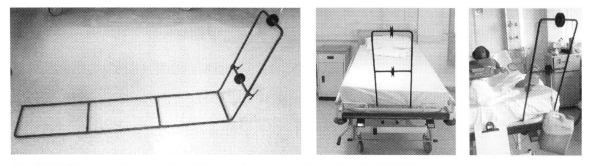

Fig.10.6. Closed reduction by skin traction using the author's IWOT frame

2. OPEN REDUCTION AND INTERNAL FIXATION (Fig.10.7)
   Technique of ORIF

Briefly, the fracture site is exposed and the fracture fragments identified. The fracture is reduced by the surgeon under direct vision by manipulation and by using various instruments. This is then followed by fixation (immobilisation), using appropriate fixation devices and methods. Open fracture reduction can be difficult and requires a degree of mastery.

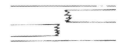

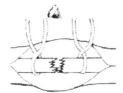

Fig.10.7. Open reduction of fractures: the fracture site is opened up and reduction is carried out under direct vision using various instruments, followed by fixation (immobilisation) using various fixation devices and methods.

The indications for ORIF are:

(a) failure of the closed methods just described
(b) intra-articular fractures in which accurate reduction is desirable for good joint function
(c) lower limb fractures in the elderly in whole early mobilisation is desirable from a general health point of view
(d) in multiple fractures to facilitate the management of the patient overall
(e) pathological fractures to prevent further fractures
(f) associated arterial injury to protect and facilitate arterial repair.

Contra-indications to Internal Fixation of Fractures

Contaminated or infected open fracture. In principle this is an absolute contra-indication. Implants are foreign bodies and as such are bound to facilitate and perpetuate infection. However, other factors such as the need to have some measure of stability may justify fracture fixation in this situation.

Severely comminuted fractures. These are technically difficult to fix. Such fixation, if attempted, is usually unsound.

Fractures in children. Most diaphyseal fractures in children can be adequately managed by closed methods. Intra-articular fractures are exceptions.

Timing of Internal Fixation

Immediate or early (within 24 hours) fixation is ideal for all fractures in which ORIF is indicated. It is particularly indicated in intra-articular fractures. When delayed beyond this time, inflammatory reaction around the fracture (soft-tissue swelling; softening of bone fragments) may make the achievement of successful internal fixation and skin closure difficult.

Delayed internal fixation (within 2 weeks) has been advocated by some in diaphyseal fractures. Smith of the Birmingham Accident Hospital, England, showed that the incidence of delayed and non-union is much lower in patients so treated than in those in whom immediate or early fixation was carried out. However, nowadays, delayed internal fixation is often forced upon the surgeon by circumstances beyond their control, ranging from medical co-morbidities to reservations about high risk of infection from poor skin at the proposed operation site.

Advantages of ORIF

- early mobilisation of the fractured bone (and the patient) and
- early discharge of the patient from hospital.

METHODS OF MAINTAINING REDUCTION (IMMOBILISATION)

Reduction must be maintained, otherwise, the fracture will displace or re-displace. This is the case in the vast majority of fractures. A common exception is the fractured clavicle, which heals despite lack of reduction. Methods of maintaining reduction are illustrated in Figs 10.8 to 10.12.

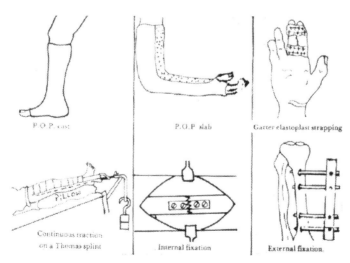

Fig.10.8. Methods of maintaining reduction – with a plaster of Paris (P.O.P) cast; POP backslab; garter elastoplast strapping; continuous traction; internal fixation using a plate and screws; with an external fixator.

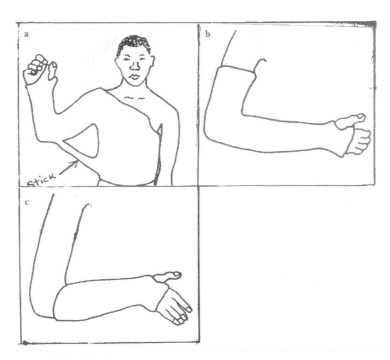

Fig.10.9. Methods of maintaining reduction: Cast immobilisation of fractures of the upper limb fractures
a. Shoulder spica: suitable for fractures of the shoulder girdle or proximal humerus
b. An above-elbow cast (axilla to knuckles): suitable for fracture of the radius or ulna or both
c. A below-elbow cast is suitable for fractures of the radius or ulna close to the wrist joint

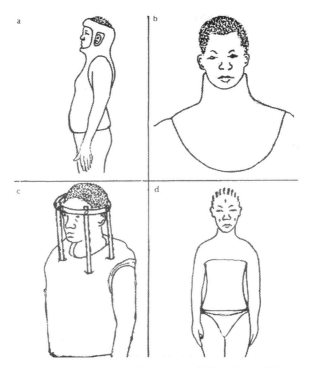

Fig.10.10. Methods of maintaining reduction: Cast immobilisation of fractures of the spine
a. A Minerva jacket is used to immobilise fractures of the cervical spine
b. A POP neck collar may also be used to immobilise a cervical fracture
c. A halo-body jacket is also suitable for cervical fractures
d. A POP jacket is suitable for fractures in the thoraco-lumbar and lumbar regions of the spine

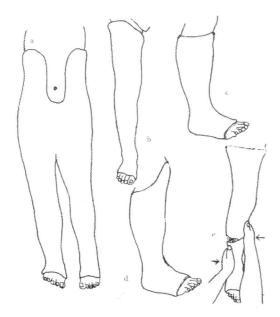

Fig.10.11. Methods of maintaining reduction: Cast immobilisation of fractures of the lower limb
a. A hip spica is used in pelvic or proximal femoral fractures
b. A groin to toes (long-leg) cast is used for fractures of the tibia
c. A tibial tubercle to toes (short-leg) cast is used for fractures around the ankle joint
d. A patella-bearing cast (Sarmiento) cast is a special cast used for some proximal tibial fractures
e. "Wedging" is a very useful method of correcting residual angular deformities

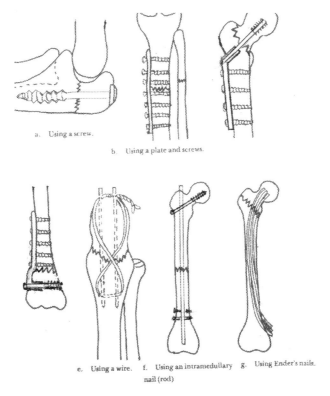

Fig.10.12. Methods of maintaining reduction: Internal fixation of various fractures using various metallic devices.

FUNCTIONAL BRACING OF FRACTURES

In general, a brace is an external splint and the term "functional" is used to denote that it is made and applied in such a way as to allow movement in the neighbouring joints, unlike the conventional plaster casts. For example, if a POP-casting is chosen for the treatment of a fracture at the upper end of the tibia, it is a applied from the toes to the groin, which eliminates movement in the ankle and knee joints. Cast-brace treatment of the same fracture allows movement in the knee joint by using hinges to join the two casts below and above the knee (Fig.10.13).

The main advantage of functional bracing, therefore, is that the involved joint retains its freedom of movement, which accelerates fracture healing and the regaining of function. A cast-brace can be made from P.O.P. or other material. The essential prerequisite for cast-bracing is that the fracture should be in the "sticky" phase of healing. This phase is attained around 3 weeks after the fracture.

Advantages of cast-bracing over conventional P.O.P. casting include:

- Fracture healing is faster.
- Regaining of movement in neighbouring joints takes place faster.
- Because of both the above advantages patients requiring admission leave hospital earlier.

Advantages of cast-bracing over operative methods of Treatment include:

- there is no risk of post-operative infection and
- freedom from possible anaesthetic problems and
- freedom from post-operative complications

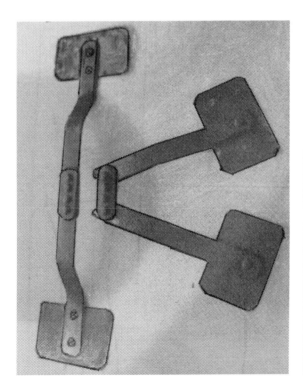 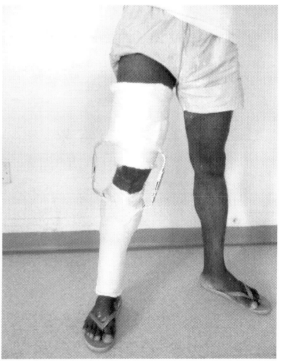

Fig.10.13. The Zaria Metal hinges suitable for functional bracing of lower limb fractures were designed by the author in the 70s. Here, a fracture of the upper end of the tibia was "braced" three weeks down the line using the hinges.

TRACTION METHOD OF MAINTAINING FRACTURE REDUCTION (FIG.10.14)

As mentioned under the section on reduction of fractures, continuous traction can also be used to maintain a reduction. It can be used for shaft fractures - femoral, tibial, humeral and also for peri and intra-articular fractures. All forms of traction require counter-traction. In the lower limb, this is achieved by raising the bottom of the bed so a part of the body weight provides the counter traction weight.

Advantages of traction include

- It maintains the reduced position.
- The patient is more comfortable and is able to exercise the muscles

The main disadvantage of traction as a definitive method of fracture treatment is that the patient has to be in bed and in hospital, risking bedsores, pin-track infection (skeletal traction) and incurring more hospital charges

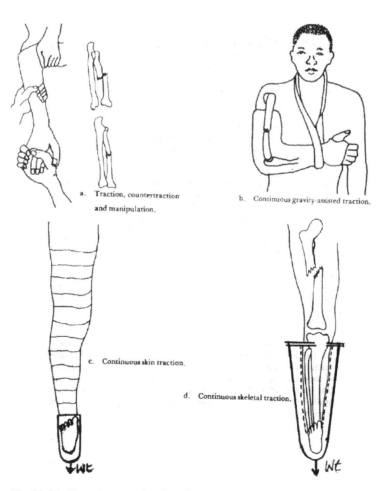

a. Traction, countertraction and manipulation.

b. Continuous gravity-assisted traction.

c. Continuous skin traction.

d. Continuous skeletal traction.

Fig.10.14. Traction methods of maintaining reduction – gravity traction (U-slab; hanging cast), skin traction, skeletal traction

"FIXED" AND "BALANCED" TRACTION (FIG.10.15)

Fixed traction is more important historically than in terms of present-day use. Classically, it was used in the treatment of femoral shaft fractures. A Thomas-type splint is essential. The traction itself can be on skin or bone. The traction cord is tied under tension to the distal end of the splint while the ring of the splint rests on the base of the limb. Thus, the traction weight is the tension on the cord while counter-traction is provided by the tension in the thigh muscles. The tendency of the ring to produce sores in the perineal and ischial tuberosity areas was countered by anchoring the lower end of the Thomas' splint by tying it to the bed or by applying traction to it.

Balanced Traction

In fixed traction an attempt is made to prevent the pressure sores mentioned above by applying traction to the lower end of the splint. However, this often fails to solve the problem satisfactorily. The traction weight may pull the patient down towards the foot of the bed. If unchecked, this will continue until the splint comes to rest on the end of the bed or traction pulley. To counter this, the foot of the bed is raised thereby allowing a part (an upward component) of the body weight to balance the traction weight; hence the term 'balanced' traction. There are many interesting and complicated methods of achieving this balance using several cords passed through rollers placed at several points on a Balkan beam but the basic principle in all is the same.

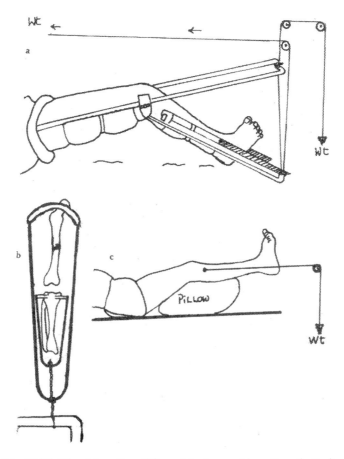

Fig.10.15. Fixed traction (b) and balanced traction (a & c)

OPEN REDUCTION AND INTERNAL FIXATION (ORIF) OF FRACTURES

The Indications for Open Reduction and Internal Fixation of fractures

The indications for open reduction of fractures were enumerated above. Following an open reduction of a fracture, the reduction is held by internal fixation using of an orthopaedic implant, usually a metal but sometimes a plastic, to hold a reduced fracture.

PRINCIPLES OF DIAGNOSIS AND TREATMENT OF OPEN FRACTURES

Classification

The most popular classification is the modified Gustilo and Anderson classification:

Type I: puncture wound less than 1 cm long with minimal soft- tissue damage.

Type II: wound more than 1 cm long with moderate soft-tissue damage.

Type IIIA: large wound typically > 10cm, extensive muscle damage but adequate skin cover (Fig.10.16).

  IIIB: additional extensive periosteal stripping and skin defect requiring reconstruction.

  IIIC: additional vascular injury requiring repair.

It has long been realised that it is not the size of the visible wound that is important but the mechanism of injury and degree of soft-tissue damage and wound contamination.

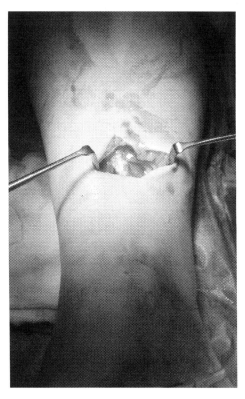

Fig.10.16. An open fracture of the tibia in the distal one-third. The wound is larger than 10cm, there is significant muscle damage but adequate skin cover is available

Diagnosis

Diagnosis is easy because of the presence of an open wound. Investigation follows established lines. Possible vascular injury may necessitate additional imaging, mainly angiography.

Treatment

Orthopaedic surgeons have learnt by bitter experience to accord the highest respect, if not fear, to open fractures. The populace has also come to realise the difference between closed and open fractures. Even in the rural areas of the developing countries, the so-called traditional bone setters are beginning to direct patients with open fractures to the orthodox doctors, having had to face the ghastly consequences of treating open fractures with dirty concoctions and in dirty environments.

The most important problem posed by open fractures is the *increased risk of infection.* Infective organisms gain access to the fracture site at the time of the injury or later through the wound and can multiply very rapidly in a suitable medium. Devitalised tissue, a frequent accompaniment of open fractures, especially comminuted ones, provides such a medium. Therefore, after the administration of *first-aid treatment,* which must include covering the wound with an antiseptic-drenched swabs, definitive treatment is begun with measures directed at preventing bacteria from entering the wound and at dealing with those that have already gained access.

"EMERGENCY" MEASURES IN THE MANAGEMENT OF OPEN FRACTURES

Prophylactic antibiotics

This is imperative. A broad-spectrum antibiotics plus another effective against bacteroides are usually chosen. Intravenous Cefuroxime or Flucloxacillin and Metronidazole is a popular combination. Erythromycin is given in place of Flucloxacillin, if there is allergy to penicillin. Anti-tetanus toxoid is also given, if indicated.

Treatment of soft tissues

A ***primary wound toilet and excision – debridement*** is an absolute necessity. The main aim of this procedure is to get rid of all dead tissues and foreign bodies in the wound. It is carried out under general anaesthesia. If a limb is involved, the use of a tourniquet should be avoided as it may make it difficult to recognise devitalised tissue.

Under sterile conditions, with assistants helping when necessary, the wound is given a copious washout with a bland antiseptic such as Cetavlon or Savlon. In cases with gross contamination, a sterile brush may be used to scrub the wound edges. The table may need to be re-draped after this. Next, after haemostasis has been procured, the wound is re-examined and re-assessed. All obviously dead tissue at the edges of the wound is removed. All foreign bodies e.g. pieces of clothes, are also removed. The wound may need to be extended to provide a more adequate exposure. If the wound is very contaminated and tendons or nerves have been cut, they should be left un-sutured but marked with black silk for easy identification later. Bone ends should be thoroughly inspected to make sure that no dirt is left behind in them. Only totally detached (from soft-tissues) and small bone fragments should be removed as significant bone loss is difficult to make good and predisposes to delayed and non-union.

If a joint is involved, it is copiously washed and sparingly debrided. The synovial membrane and capsule are sutured. It is safest to leave the wound unsutured, dressing it with greased gauze (Vaseline, Jelonet, Sufra-tulle, Paraffin gauze). It is wise to put in a drain. The help of vascular and plastic surgeons may be necessary.

Fracture stabilisation

Classically, immediate internal fixation (screw fixation, intramedullary nailing, plating) is permissible only if fracture contamination has been minimal. However, many surgeons, backed by studies suggesting that one may be able to get away with internal fixation in even Type III injuries, are resorting to this option more and more. ***External fixation is a popular middle-ground procedure.*** If, for any reason, none of the above options can be used, a P.O.P. cast, appropriately "windowed" over the wound to permit daily dressings, can be used.

Post-operative care

Elevation is vital in all limb fractures but is particularly so in open fractures in which soft-tissue injury could be particularly extensive. Antibiotic therapy based on culture and sensitivity studies is continued. Wound inspection is carried out at 48 hours and later as necessary. If it is clean, delayed primary suture can be carried out, if feasible; otherwise split-skin grafts are applied. Where available, plastic surgical help should be sought early.

Definitive Treatment of the fracture

Once the danger of infection has been overcome, the fracture, to all intents and purposes, has become a closed one and can then be treated as such along lines previously outlined.

Complications of open fractures

The incidence of **infection** is quoted as 1.5-2.5% for Type II fractures and as high as 19-28% for Type IIIB fractures. There is also a high incidence of **delayed** and **non-union.**

PRINCIPLES OF DIAGNOSIS AND TREATMENT OF FRACTURES IN CHILDREN

INTRODUCTION

Increased activity level and decreased understanding of risk

Fractures and injuries to soft tissues of the musculoskeletal system are common in children, not only because they are so active but also because they have a diminished understanding of risk. The leading cause of death in children aged 1 to 14 years is accidental trauma.

Apart from birth injuries, the crawling baby and toddler, oblivious of the danger posed by the stairs, the younger child jumping up and down beds, steps, the trampoline and fences and the older child enthralled by the excitement of ball games, cycling and other physical activities, are all exposed to an increased risk of musculoskeletal injuries.

The overall ratio of boys to girls who sustain a single fracture is 2.7:1. The peak incidence of fractures for boys is at the age of 16 for boys and 12 for girls. The management of these injuries pose special problems for the doctor, care staff and parents/carers.

Diagnosis can be difficult. Getting an accurate history of the injury is difficult in the first 7-8 years of life. Examining a young child (younger than 5) is difficult. Ordinary x-rays are not useful in certain situations e.g. in a baby with suspected ankle injury, since most of the bones in this region are in cartilage at this age and do not show up on x-rays. Ultrasound scanning can be used to identify epiphyseal separation in an infant.

The presence of growth plates and secondary centres of bone formation similarly pose diagnostic difficulties for the trainee surgeon. X-raying the unaffected limb for comparison is helpful here.

Why fractures in children are different from adult fractures

1. Children's bones are more **porous and elastic** and have a **thicker periosteum** than those of adults. This produces patterns of injuries/fractures that are different from those seen in adults (Please see below).

2. Children's bones possess **growth plates**, otherwise called growth discs or physes. The growth plate is a unique type of cartilage where growth in length takes place. Its thickness varies, depending on the given bone and the age of the child. The physis is weaker than bone and so injury tends to occur through it rather than through bone when subjected to bending and rotational injuring forces. Injuries involving growth plates may retard the growth of the involved bones or produce deformities.

3. Ligaments in children are functionally stronger than bones. Therefore, their bones give in/ break before ligament injury occurs, unlike in adults.

PATTERNS OF INJURIES/FRACTURES IN CHILDREN

Fractures of children's bones have characteristic patterns as follows:

*   The green-stick fracture
*   Torus fracture
*   Plastic bowing
*   Growth plate injury/fracture
*   Adult-like fractures in adolescent and older children

THE GREEN-STICK FRACTURE

A green-stick fracture is a uni-cortical fracture in a young child; the opposite cortex and periosteum remain intact. It looks like a kink in the bone. Green-stick fractures are caused by bending forces. Typical examples are seen in the distal radius and ulna (Fig.10.17).

Diagnosis is not difficult. There is usually a history of trauma, witnessed and unwitnessed. The child is upset and must be handled with care. Swelling may be apparent and there is no need to palpate for fear of causing pain. X-rays will show the kink, which may be subtle or obvious.

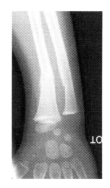

Fig.10.17. A green-stick fracture is an incomplete fracture in which only one cortex is broken on the X-ray

Treatment: Most fractures will not require manipulative reduction as most surgeons will accept an angulatory deformity of up to 20 degrees in a young child on the grounds that they will remodel in the ample growth period left. Angulation greater than 20 degrees should by corrected by MUA. In either case, POP immobilisation will be required. The kind of cast depends on the bone involved.

THE TORUS FRACTURE

A torus fracture is a fracture caused by compression forces and is most commonly seen at the junction of the metaphysis and diaphysis. There is no fracture line or gap, only a sideways protrusion or "blob" of bone at the site and the injury is stable.

PLASTIC BOWING

Plastic bowing: the affected bone bends from a compressive load. If the elastic limit of the bone is exceeded, the deformity does not correct with the cessation of the load.

GROWTH PLATES INJURIES

Growth plate injuries have long been recognised and classified. The Salter-Harris classification is the best known and has been enhanced by other authors.

Contentious cases of possible growth plate injuries can be resolved by X-raying the unaffected limb for comparison.

SALTER-HARRIS CLASSIFICATION OF EPIPHYSEAL INJURIES (Fig.10.18)

This classification recognises five types of injury as follows:

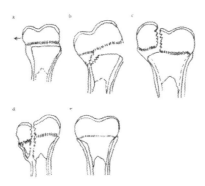

**Fig.10.18. Salter-Harris classifi-
cation of epiphyseal injuries**

Type I: **Separation of the epiphysis**
Type II: **Separation plus fracture involving the metaphysis**
Type III: **Fracture and separation of part of the epiphysis**
Type IV: **Fracture going through both the metaphysic and epiphysis**
Type V: **Crushing of the growth plate**

Extended follow up is needed to exclude and deal with any significant deformity arising from growth plate injuries

ADULT-LIKE FRACTURES IN ADOLESCENT AND OLDER CHILDREN

Adult fracture patterns are seen in children when the injuring forces are of great magnitude, especially if rotational forces are also included (Fig.10.19)

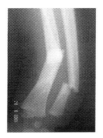 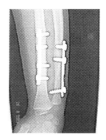

**Fig.10.19a&b. Adult pattern frac-
tures of the radius and ulna in a
child treated by plating.**

REHABILITATION FOLLOWING MUSCULO-SKELETAL INJURIES

Rehabilitation can be defined as the sum total of all therapeutic measures carried out on the injured part and on the patient as a whole with the aim of restoring the function of the injured part to its pre-injury status or as close to it as possible. It has to do with the reactivation of a movement temporarily paralysed by injury, surgery for it or reaction to both and must therefore start as soon as safely possible after the patient's admission. The main drivers of rehabilitation are the patient, the physiotherapists, occupational therapists and the Social Services (where they exist!).

Successful rehabilitation will result in:

- Restoration and maintenance of the range of movements in affected joints.
- Prevention of muscle atrophy in the affected part and maintenance of muscle power.
- Enhancing the rate of fracture healing by the beneficial effects of motion.
- The return of the patient to his job as early as possible.

Further reading

Iwegbu, C.G. Cast-Bracing of Femoral Fractures: Further Experience With The Zaria Metal Hinge Joint. E Afr Med J 63(4): 228, 1986.

CHAPTER 11

COMPLICATIONS OF FRACTURES AND OF FRACTURE TREATMENT

SUMMARY

Fractures are attended by many complications. Some, like shock, cardiac arrest and pulmonary embolism, can be life-threatening. A way to remember fracture complications is to group them into general and local. Under general complications come *shock, cardiac arrest, deep vein thrombosis and pulmonary embolism, fat embolism, tetanus and delirium tremens.* Under local complications come *skin injury, muscle injury, vascular injury, nerve injury, crush syndrome, infection, compartment syndrome, Volkmann's contracture, the complications of fracture healing, namely, mal-union, delayed union and non-union; avascular necrosis of bone, Sudeck's atrophy(reflex sympathetic dystrophy), post fracture osteoarthritis, joint laxity, joint stiffness. Then come* the complications of treatment: *tight casts and cast sores, operative technical complications, wound infection, bone infections and implant breakage. These and a few others more are discussed in greater detail below.*

GENERAL COMPLICATIONS

The most important are shock, cardiac arrest, deep vein thrombosis (DVT) and pulmonary embolism (PE), fat embolism and tetanus. The crush syndrome is also important and minor complications include delirium tremens and the so-called fracture fever.

SHOCK

Shock can be defined as a state of deranged cardiovascular function characterised by significantly reduced circulating blood volume with resultant hypotension and reduced capillary blood flow in vital tissues. There are four main types of shock - neurogenic, cardiogenic, hypovolaemic, septic, cardiogenic and anaphylactic. Hypovolaemic, cardiogenic shocks are the most likely to be encountered in fractures.

Hypovolaemic Shock

This is also called *oligaemic, haemorrhagic, traumatic, wound or surgical shock*. In this type of shock, the reduction in the circulating blood volume is due to actual escape (loss) of whole blood or plasma from the vascular space. Such blood loss occurs to a greater or lesser extent in every fracture, being the source of the fracture haematoma.

Shock results from a rapid loss of 20% or more of the circulating blood volume (5 litres in an adult). Such a significant blood loss can occur in major fractures, especially of the pelvis, femur and tibia.

Diagnosis. The classical signs of hypovolaemic shock are hypotension, tachycardia, pallor and prostration. The degree of shock and the corresponding symptoms and signs are given on Table 11.1.

Table 11.1. Degree of shock with symptoms and signs

Degree of shock	Amount of blood loss	Symptoms and signs
I	<750ml (15%)	Minimal
II	750-1,500ml (15-30%)	Tachycardia>100, decreased pulse pressure, tachypnoea, pale, sweaty, cold peripheries
III	1,500-2,000ml (30-40%)	Tachycardia>120, hypotension, tachypnoea, pale, cold peripheries, decreased LOC, oliguria
IV	>2,000ml (40%)	Real danger of cardiac arrest and death: Tachycardia>140, hypotension, tachypnoea, pale, cold peripheries, 50% unconscious, oliguria

Treatment. Prevention is better than cure. A high index of suspicion is necessary to identify a patient in danger of going into shock.

In fracture patients, arrest of bleeding and replacement of lost blood, splintage of the fracture, relief of pain and apprehension and avoidance of rough handling of the affected part may prevent shock.

When hypovolaemic shock has become established, the most important treatment measure is early and adequate blood transfusion to restore the volume of circulating blood. Group O Rh-negative blood may be used in an emergency until cross-matched blood is available. Plasma and plasma substitutes could be used as a stop gap before blood becomes available but blood for grouping and cross-matching must be taken before such infusion is commenced.

Resistant shock. Shock is described as resistant if apparently adequate blood replacement fails to bring about significant improvement in the patient's condition or if there is remission after an initial improvement.

Resistant shock could be due to a number of factors, including continuing blood loss, brain injury, intrathoracic injury interfering with ventilation or circulation, a ruptured viscus, prolonged tissue hypoxia due to inadequate blood supply and coincident disease e.g. cardiac or pulmonary disease. *Resistant shock* can only be effectively treated by treating its cause e.g. dealing with a chest or abdominal injury.

Neurogenic shock

Neurogenic shock, otherwise called *primary shock, fainting or syncope*, is due to a rapid pooling of blood in the splanchnic bed and skeletal muscles as a result of dilatation of their arterioles in response to sudden outflow of autonomic impulses. It is encountered in fracture situations and spinal cord injuries (transection).

Neurogenic shock is self-limiting. The recumbent position, which the patient assumes as of necessity, constitutes an essential part of treatment. The patient should be encouraged to rest in this position or in a head-down position for a few minutes. Elevation of the legs in a recumbent patient speeds up recovery. In the presence of trauma involving significant blood loss to the circulation, neurogenic shock usually becomes replaced or complicated by hypovolaemic shock.

Cardiogenic Shock

This is due to an acute decrease in the cardiac output secondary to an intrinsic cardiac disease or state e.g. myocardial infarction, cardiac tamponade, tension pneumothorax or massive pulmonary embolism. It may be precipitated by trauma. *It is important to recognise cardiogenic shock because intensive fluid replacement, which forms the basis of treatment of the other types of shock, is contra-indicated in cardiogenic shock.* Treatment consists of relief of pain, administration of oxygen and treatment of the underlying cardiac condition.

Septic Shock

This is also called *vasogenic, toxic* or *endotoxic shock*. It is more commonly associated with other causes (diabetes, diseases of the genitourinary, hepatobiliary and intestinal tracts, haematological malignancies and immunosuppressive states, etc.) than with fractures but it remains a real threat to the patient with multiple injuries and fractures. The hallmark of septic shock is the presence of sepsis and hypotension despite adequate fluid replacement.

Septic shock is usually caused by gram-negative organisms (Escherichia coli; Klebsiella, Proteus, Pseudomonas and Bacteroides) but gram-positive organisms can be responsible in up to one-third of cases.

Septic shock is commonest in the very young and the very old and should always be suspected when a febrile patient has chills associated with a falling (low) BP. Laboratory and X-ray investigations are hardly helpful but serial blood cultures must be done. A clinical diagnosis should be made early and treatment must be started forthwith.

Treatment. Treatment is best provided in an Intensive Care Unit, if available and consists of combination antibiotic therapy and adequate fluid replacement plus ventilation support, if needed. Gentamycin, Carbenicillin and long-acting, broad-spectrum cephalosporins e.g. Rocephin are commonly used. The Microbilologist should be invoved. The source of the sepsis must be drained.

CARDIAC ARREST

Cardiac arrest is a sudden cessation of the heartbeat secondary to acute myocardial hypoxia, toxicity or conduction disturbance. Blood supply to vital organs stops immediately after. Since only about 5 minutes of cerebral ischaemia is all that is needed for the patient to acquire a permanent brain damage (if he survives at all), it is obvious that something must be done before the arrival of a cardio-pulmonary resuscitation team.

It is the duty of every doctor to acquaint themselves with the nature and management of cardiac arrest but this need assumes an imperative nature in the circumstances of medical practice in most hospitals in Africa and the rest of the Third World where cardio-pulmonary resuscitation teams hardly exist. Doctors and other trained medical personnel working in these regions must therefore be able to at least promptly recognise the condition and initiate treatment.

In the context of musculo-skeletal trauma, cardiac arrest can occur secondary to any of the types of shock discussed earlier, especially neurogenic and hypovolaemic shock. Furthermore, it can occur during the induction of anaesthesia for fracture treatment or in the course of an operation.

Diagnosis. The premonitory signs of cardiac arrest are irregular heartbeats, slowing down of the heart rate and a rapid fall of the blood pressure. The pathognomonic signs are absent pulse and absent heart sounds.

Treatment. Treatment will be meaningful only if instituted immediately and adequately and this means that the doctor must be familiar with the Advanced Trauma Life Support (ATLS) principles. Briefly:

- Ensure a clear airway and establish ventilation by mouth-to-mouth breathing until oxygen under pressure can be given by mask. Get an anaesthetist.

- Start closed cardiac massage: Place the heel of the palm of one hand over the lower half of the sternum. Then place the palm of the second hand over that of the first. Then exert compression on the chest wall sufficient to force the sternum down about 4-5cm (less in children) - at the rate of one compression per second. Four simultaneous compressions are alternated with one mouth-to-mouth breathing. The above procedures must be continued until spontaneous respiration and circulation are restored.

It is not possible to discuss the details of heart-lung resuscitation in this text. Suffice to say that resuscitation can hardly be successful from the effort of one doctor or person alone. Assistance is needed from other trained hospital personnel. An E.C.G machine is necessary (to diagnose the presence of ventricular fibrillation), a defibrillator, preferably the D.C. type, is necessary to treat ventricular fibrillation and cardiopulmonary resuscitative drugs (adrenaline, sodium bicarbonate, calcium chloride or gluconate) are also necessary. Open cardiac massage by a competent qualified doctor via a thoracotomy could be considered (in operating theatre only) if closed massage and other adequately administered measures fail to restore cardiac function. All said, only an efficient team has a good chance of achieving a successful resuscitation.

Successful resuscitation will result in the restoration of cardiac, pulmonary and central nervous system function. Many patients have survived but with compromised CNS. Central nervous system function in some of them is so poor that they are referred to as "vegetables".

DEEP VEIN THROMBOSIS (DVT) AND PULMONARY EMBOLISM (PE)

Pathogenesis

Deep vein thrombosis is a well-recognised complication of fractures and bone surgery, especially in the pelvis and lower limbs. Many aspects of the pathogenesis are still not fully understood but Virchov's triad: hypercoagulability of blood, intimal damage and stasis still lie at the root of the pathology. Hypercoagulability occurs as a result of the activation of factor X by thromboplastins released from damaged tissues.

The true incidence of this condition is not known. Most are silent; only 25% are symptomatic. It is certainly more common in patients of the European stock than in Africans or Asians. Even though reliable statistics are not available, it can be stated that it is rare in Nigeria. In the author's 10 year clinical experience in Zaria, for example, there was only one established case of DVT and PE - in an obese post-patellectomy male patient. The incidence of pulmonary embolism in patients with deep vein thrombosis is uncertain. Figures of up to 10% are quoted but fatality from the condition is under 1%.

Diagnosis

The typical patient is a multiple injury patient, obese, middle-aged or older and female, especially one on the contraceptive pill and with a history of cardiovascular or pulmonary disease.

An affected limb may be swollen, warm to touch and tender along the affected veins and there may be constitutional signs such as slight pyrexia and tachycardia. Clinical features are more reliable in thigh vein thrombosis where swelling, pain and tenderness may be severe. In the calf, pain may be present on dorsiflexion of the foot (positive Homan's sign) but this is by and large unreliable and its absence does not exclude the condition. The current diagnostic test of choice is duplex ultrasonography, which demonstrates obstruction to venous outflow by a thrombus. Other tests include contrast venography and MRI scan but venography is invasive and requires the use of potentially harmful contrast agents. On the other hand, MRI is expensive and does not give results superior to those of venography. D-Dymer testing is used in some centres but a positive D-dimer does not confirm the diagnosis of DVT and false-positive levels are seen in patients with malignancy, trauma, recent surgery, infection, pregnancy and active bleeding. 125 I-labelled fibrinogen uptake test (FUT) is no longer popular.

Small emboli to the lungs cause few symptoms and signs (pleuritic pain, often with a transient friction rub, a dry cough, haemoptysis, local rales, X-ray evidence of a small amount of pleural fluid and of pleural consolidation). Massive pulmonary embolisms which almost always originate from pelvic or thigh veins present dramatically with shock, dyspnoea and cyanosis or with a choking chest pain. There may be a transient premonition of death and involuntary defaecation; death could set in within a few minutes. Useful tests in the diagnosis of PE include lung perfusion scanning, ventilation scanning and selective pulmonary angiography.

Treatment

The best treatment of DVT and PE is their prevention. This approach is particularly important in situations where the luxury of modern diagnostic tests is not available, drugs needed for full treatment of the established case are unavailable or unaffordable and the possibility of treatment by pulmonary embolectomy absent. Doctors practising in environments where the condition is rare will do well to realise that rarity does not mean total absence. In fact, it should invite more vigilance on the part of the doctor and this can only be possible if he knows as much about the condition as possible.

PROPHYLACTIC TREATMENT OF DVT

This should be instituted in high-risk patients. These include those who have sustained pelvic or femoral fractures and in addition are obese, females on the pill as well as patients with malignant disease or a previous history of thromboembolism. General prophylactic measures include adequate hydration, avoiding local calf pressure and early postoperative mobilisation.

Pharmacological prophylaxis of hypercoagulability and increased platelet aggregation can be achieved with low molecular weight heparin and Dextran whilst stasis can be tackled with mechanical devices (calf compression devices used during surgery or compression stockings used pre-, intra- and post-operatively.

TREATMENT OF ESTABLISHED THROMBOEMBOLISM

The treatment of established thromboembolism is by intravenous heparin: 10,000 i.u. 6 hourly, for 48 hours. At the time of the first dose (which procures almost immediate anticoagulation), a loading dose (30-40mg) of Warfarin, a prothrombin depressant, is given by mouth. This becomes effective at 48 hours when the heparin is discontinued. The monitoring of anticoagulation with heparin is done by determining the clotting time, which should not exceed 18 minutes. The monitoring of anticoagulation with Warfarin is done by serial prothrombin time determinations. The prothrombin time is kept to about 1.5 - 2 times the normal with daily administration of Warfarin. Treatment is continued for 3-6 months.

TREATMENT OF PULMONARY EMBOLISM

Acute pulmonary embolism is initially treated by closed cardiac massage, immediate anticoagulation with Heparin, positive pressure ventilation and administration of vasopressor drugs. Pulmonary embolectomy may be indicated if the patient survives. Even in places with adequate manpower and facilities, the prognosis is not good and only the occasional patient survives pulmonary embolectomy.

FAT EMBOLISM AND THE ADULT RESPIRATORY DISTRESS SYNDROME

This entity is perhaps best conceptualised as a syndrome characterised by respiratory insufficiency and mental confusion as a result of the lodgement of fat globules in the lungs and brain. Fat globules released from the bone marrow from major bone fractures are the obvious cause but it is now thought that abnormal fat metabolism as a result of trauma is the more likely mechanism. Formed fat globules are carried in the blood vessels and get lodged in various organs on their way, clogging their vessels and causing a reduction in their blood flow, with resultant symptoms.

DIAGNOSIS

The incidence of fat embolism following long bone fractures is quoted as 0.5 – 2% and up to 10% following polytrauma. The classical patient is a young male with multiple lower limb (tibial or femoral) fractures or an old (past middle age) patient with pelvic or hip fractures, but single fractures, intrathoracic, intra-abdominal, intracranial, soft-tissue or major arterial injuries are also frequent causes of fat embolism. Therefore, a patient with a combination of fractures and considerable soft-tissue injuries stands a good chance of having this complication. The symptoms of breathlessness, restlessness and mental confusion may appear within a few hours of the injury. A mild pyrexia and an increase in the pulse rate are early warning signs. Long tract signs may be present and urinary incontinence may occur. Petechiae appear in the conjunctivae and can also be seen across the front and back of the chest in light-skinned patients. These may disappear after a few hours.

The measurement of blood gases is the most important single investigation in fat embolism. In fact, other laboratory tests (platelet estimation, estimation of the amount of fat in the urine; serial chest X-rays; E.C.G.) and biopsies (lung, kidney, skin) are said to be of doubtful value. PaO2 values below 60mm Hg (8kPa) indicate significant pulmonary hypoxaemia and serial determinations of the PaO2 should be used to monitor the response to treatment.

Differential diagnosis

It is necessary to distinguish the pulmonary insufficiency due to fat embolism from that due to other pulmonary conditions, especially the adult respiratory distress syndrome (ARDS or shock lung), pulmonary contusion or pulmonary oedema from overhydration. These conditions are characterised by acute respiratory failure, with tachypnoea, hypoxia, decreased lung compliance and diffuse pulmonary infiltrates on chest X-ray and there are known causative factors which will help to distinguish them from FE (Table 11.2.).

Table 11. 2. Causes of ARDS

Pathology	Details
Infection	Septicaemia
Inhalation	Smoke, water, vomit, chlorine ammonia, O2
Embolism	Fat, air, fluid e.g. amniotic
Brain injury	Head injury, intracranial haemorrhage
Drugs	Barbiturates, opiates
Others	Major trauma with shock, blood transfusion, DIC

NB: DIC = disseminated intravascular coagulation

The clinical features of fat embolism (dyspnoea, tachycardia, mental confusion, petechial rash), the low PaO2 and demonstration of fat globules in a cryostat frozen section of clotted blood will help in this differential diagnosis.

TREATMENT

This can be discussed under general and specific measures.

General measures. These include the maintenance of the airway, control of bleeding when present, splinting of fractures and avoidance of unnecessary movements of the patient, restoration of the blood volume and maintenance of fluid and electrolyte balance.

Specific treatment. The most effective treatment is the giving of oxygen. This can be given by a face mask (in mild cases) or by ventilatory assistance (in severe cases). Treatment with oxygen must be started as soon as the diagnosis has been made. The aim is to achieve a PaO2 of 70mm Hg or above. Serial blood gases determinations are necessary for good treatment. Renal support may be necessary.

Other treatment measures that have been used include:

Cortiscosteroids. These have been used in massive doses over a short period for their anti-inflammatory properties. They depress inflammation in the alveoli thereby improving gaseous exchange in them. For example, 500-1000mg of Methylprednisolone can be given 6 hourly for 24 hours.

Heparin. This can be given subcutaneously in doses of 5,000 i.u. 8 hourly for one week - for its lipolytic and anticoagulant properties.

Low-molecular-weight Dextran can also be used to improve the microcirculation.

Intravenous alcohol has also been used in treatment but its effectiveness has not been apparent.

PROGNOSIS

This depends on the severity of the condition. Mild to moderate cases are hardly symptomatic and moderate cases have a very good chance of survival with treatment. Patients with severe pulmonary and cerebral symptoms have a poor prognosis but may also survive if effective treatment is begun early. Mortality figures of 10 to 50% are quoted.

TETANUS

This dreadful disease can complicate open fractures but it is important to emphasise that the size of the skin wound is irrelevant: small cuts or abrasions associated or unassociated with a fracture can also be complicated by tetanus. Because most people in most African countries are not immunised against the disease, doctors working in such environments will do well to bear this in mind each time they are treating patients with even the smallest skin wound.

The causative organism is Clostridium tetani, an anaerobic gram-positive bacillus present in environments contaminated by faecal matter of domestic animals or humans. Its spores, which are quite resistant to heat and other adverse conditions, are frequently found on human skin, hence the ease with which they contaminate wounds.

Clostridium tetani is a non-invasive organism, tending to remain localised in wounds. Dead tissue provides the best environment for its rapid multiplication. Its adverse effects are due to the toxins it produces which have affinity for nervous tissue, access to which they gain via the bloodstream and lymphatics. In particular, the toxins have affinity for the anterior horn cells of the spinal cord to which they fix themselves.

DIAGNOSIS

Local pain and tingling at the site of the wound may be the first symptoms of the disease. This local form usually has a good prognosis. The symptoms of the more common generalised form are tonic contractions (which later become clonic) of skeletal muscles, especially those of the jaw (hence the alternative name, lock-jaw) and later, those of the neck and trunk (giving the classical picture of opisthotonus). The ultimate involvement of the diaphragm and the intercostal muscles can lead to death by asphyxia.

TREATMENT

The chances of successful treatment are slim. It is better to prevent the disease by immunisation. However, in the author's experience, quite a few patients do survive the established disease. Anti-tetanus serum is given intravenously in a single dose of 30,000 units and supportive therapy in the form of heavy sedation and administration of muscle relaxants is instituted. Endotracheal intubation and controlled respiration may become necessary.

PROPHYLAXIS

Active immunisation of at least all children under the age of 16, if not the whole population, should be undertaken. An immunised patient should be given a booster dose of tetanus toxoid (0.5ml intramuscularly) on presentation to hospital with an abrasion or a cut. An unimmunised patient is given the same dose on presentation, repeated 6 weeks and 6 months later - in addition to wound toilet. If the wound is considered to merit antibiotic therapy, injectable penicillin should be included for the first 2 days.

DELIRIUM TREMENS

This is characterised by an acute psychotic behaviour in a post-fracture chronic alcoholic patient. Such a patient could be violent and harmful to both himself and other patients. With heavy sedation (usually with chlorpromazine) he usually settles down after a few days.

FRACTURE FEVER

This should not really be considered a complication in itself. Many consider it to be part of the complex of symptoms of the fat embolism syndrome. Pyrexia persisting for more than 48 hours after a major fracture should be presumed to be due to infection and treated with antibiotics.

THE CRUSH SYNDROME

Crush fractures could be accompanied by the crushing of a large mass of muscles and if a crushed limb remains trapped for more than 6 hours by the crushing agent, the crush syndrome should be assumed. The pathology of the syndrome is that the crushing agent e.g. wreckage of a vehicular crash; a fallen wall or tree from a tornado or an earthquake, or a tight tourniquet, causes a breakdown of muscle tissue. One of the breakdown products, acid myohaematin, formed from myoglobin and the haeme moiety of haemoglobin, on reaching the kidneys (via the circulation) blocks the tubules, leading to their necrosis and resultant low-output uraemia. Renal hypoperfusion and acidaemia secondary to initial inadequate fluid resuscitation would also result in prerenal failure.

DIAGNOSIS

The diagnosis is obvious from the history. The released limb is pulseless, swollen and covered in blisters. There may also be loss of sensation and power in the limb. Oliguria with dark brownish red urine is present. Electrolyte abnormalities include hyperkalaemia due to muscle cell damage and potassium release from the intracellular space and hypocalcaemia due to deposition of circulating calcium in damaged areas. The presence of myoglobinuria (pigmenturia) points to a good chance of the patient developing acute renal failure. In surviving patients, renal function recovers within one week. However, many patients become increasingly uraemic and die within 14 days.

TREATMENT

In a diagnosed case, aggressive fluid resuscitation is the mainstay of treatment. A balanced crystalloid solution should be administered to maintain a urine output of at least 100ml/hour. If indicated, amputation, carried out proximal to the site of compression before the compression is released, is the effective treatment. Supportive treatment includes the establishment of a diet regime. Carbohydrate intake is encouraged while giving an anabolic steroid and neomycin reduces protein catabolism. Renal dialysis is essential in severe cases.

SOFT-TISSUE COMPLICATIONS OF FRACTURES

Skin wound is a complication of open fractures, especially of the limb bones. Its management has been discussed earlier.

Muscle and tendon injuries often accompany fractures, depending on their sites. Furthermore, disuse atrophy of muscles occurs with most limb fractures, its degree being directly proportional to the period of immobilisation and the amount of active exercise given to the part. Late tendon ruptures are also know to occur, the classical example being the late rupture (at about 6 weeks) of the extensor pollicis longus tendon following an undisplaced Colles-type fracture. Aseptic inflammation of tendons (tendinitis) also occurs after fractures of adjacent bones.

Nerve injuries are common. Classical examples include injury to elements of the brachial plexus in clavicular fractures, to the radial nerve in proximal humeral shaft fractures and to the sciatic nerve in fracture-dislocations of the hip joint. The degree of damage varies. It could be a neurapraxia (nerve bruising with only temporary loss of function), an axonotmesis(cut of axons but with intact axon sheaths so that nerve regeneration is possible) or a neurotmesis (cut of whole nerve; functional return will only occur with nerve repair or graft).

Arterial complications. Arteries supplying a limb may be cut, compressed or contused at a fracture site with compromise of the blood supply. Untreated severe arterial ischaemia leads to either gangrene or compartment syndrome (Volkmann's ischaemia) depending on its speed of development.

Gangrene. This is the necrosis of a part, usually a limb, as a result of total and sustained cut-off of its blood supply. Usually the most distal part of the limb i.e. the toes or the fingers, are first affected, proximal progression being determined by the level of the arterial injury and the state of collateral circulation in the region.

The distal limb is cold, pulseless and discoloured. It may be dry (dry gangrene) if exposed to dry atmospheric conditions or wet (wet gangrene) if not, as can happen if it is wrapped in wet cloth or bandage.

Wet gangrene is prone to infection. Therefore, antibiotic therapy must be instituted when it is present. With time a demarcation line (which is really a product of inflammatory reaction between dead and living tissues) appears. This line must be established to have stopped advancing before the level of amputation, the only effective treatment, is undertaken.

COMPARTMENT SYNDROME (VOLKMANN'S ISCHAEMIA).

PATHOGENESIS

This is a syndrome characterised by an increase in the pressure in an osteofascial compartment of a limb caused by an injury or tight casts and bandages, with resulting ischaemia of the tissues, especially muscles and nerves. The key elements in the pathogenesis are trauma, muscle ischaemia, oedema formation and increased intramuscular pressure as described by Eaton and Green in 1972 (Fig.11.1).

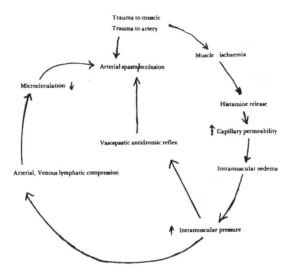

Fig. 11.1. The trauma-oedema cycle (Eaton and Green, 1972)

The syndrome was first described by Volkmann in 1872 in connection with tight bandages and P.O.P. casts applied on the forearm as treatment for supracondylar fractures of the humerus. The compartment syndrome has since been known to occur in the lower limb as well and to be caused by injuries to a compartment other than fractures. The most commonly affected compartments are those of leg (anterior, lateral, deep posterior and superficial posterior compartments and the forearm (anterior and posterior aspects) (Fig.11.2).

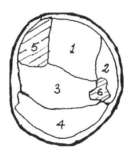

Fig.11.2. Osteofacial compartments of the leg
1. **Anterior compartment**
2. **Lateral (peroneal) compartment**
3. **Deep posterior compartment**
4. **Superficial posterior compartment**
5. **Tibia**
6. **Fibula**

DIAGNOSIS

In practical terms, the diagnosis of compartment syndrome in an awake patient is a clinical one and its treatment is an emergency. There is no need to wait for compartment pressure measurements and monitoring, the facilities for which are lacking in many places, certainly in the Third World.

The patient is usually a child but adults are also commonly affected. There is a definite history of trauma which, although usually a fracture, could also take the form of soft-tissue contusion, burns, bullet wounds, arterial catheterisation and even drug overdose. The hallmark symptom is **pain**, which is excruciating, unrelenting, poorly localised and increases with any passive movement of the limb that involves excursion of the tendons of the affected muscles e.g. extension of the fingers or of the toes. **Peripheral nerve deficit** (motor and sensory and loss of two-point discrimination) is also an early sign. **Pulselessness** is another sign but the presence of the pulse does not exclude the syndrome. **Cyanosis** is an early sign but is of significance only in light skinned patients. **Pallor** is also present but should be sought in black people in the conjunctivae.

Compartment pressure measurement

In the normal situation, the difference between the mean arterial blood pressure and the pressure in a given compartment is around 40 mm Hg. If this difference is less than 40mm Hg, it means the compartment pressure is high and compartment syndrome is likely to be present.

Compartment pressure measurements are confirmatory of the diagnosis and particularly useful in the unconscious or anaesthesised patient. They can be carried out with a wick catheter. The figure obtained is subtracted from the mean arterial blood pressure to obtain the deltaP, which should not be less than 40mm of Hg. For example, compartment syndrome is presumed if delta P is 30mm.

TREATMENT

This must be instituted within six hours of the commencement of symptoms if muscle necrosis and contracture are to be prevented. All constrictive bandages, dressings, P.O.P casts must be removed immediately and surgical decompression (fasciotomy and epiphysiotomy) of the affected compartment must be carried out without undue procrastination.

Successful decompression is usually followed by the return of the relevant pulse. If this does not happen, the artery must be explored – by a vascular surgical colleague. Arterial surgery should be preceded by internal fixation of the fracture (which caused the arterial injury in the first place!). Ischaemic muscles must be excised peacemeal until they bleed. The wound is left open and a delayed primary suture performed about five days later. Prolonged post-operation physiotherapy is usually required to minimise the muscle contracture that is bound to follow muscle ischaemia.

VOLKMANN'S CONTRACTURE (FIG.11.3)

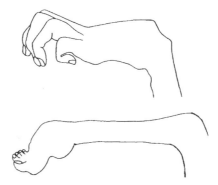

Fig.11.3. Volkmann's ischaemic contracture of the hand, foot and the lower leg.

Volkmann's contracture is a contracture of ischaemic muscles and a common complication of the compartment syndrome. Now very rare in the developed countries, the examples shown on Fig.11.3 are still seen in the developing countries. Initially the affected muscles undergo fibrosis and then gradually contract. Whole muscles or only part of them may be involved. Related nerves whose blood supply has also been compromised are also involved in the fibrotic process. Contracted muscles cause deformities of joints distal to them.

The flexor compartment of the forearm is a classical site of Volkmann's contracture. Here, the forearm becomes thin due to muscle contracture and shrinkage and the fingers are flexed at the proximal and distal interphalangeal joints (claw hand). The fingers can be extended only if the wrist is flexed. Similar deformities are present in the leg and foot in ischaemic contracture of the calf muscles (Fig.11.3). Nerve involvement manifests in diminished or absent sensation.

Treatment is based on the pathology, which is a massive infarction of muscles (and nerves). All fibrotic muscles and nerves should be excised and whatever is left reconstructed to minimise expected functional deficits. Tendon transfers and nerve grafts may be necessary. A long period of physiotherapy is usually required after operative treatment.

BONE COMPLICATIONS OF FRACTURES

Local bone complications include:

- **Avascular necrosis.** Any bone completely deprived of its blood supply undergoes avascular necrosis but common sites are neck of humerus and femur, the scaphoid and the talus.

- **Complications of bone healing**

    1. **Mal-Union.** This is union in deformity. The most important cause of mal-union is non-reduction or inaccurate reduction. In general, mal-union is more tolerable in the upper limb, which is non-weightbearing, than in the weightbearing bones of the lower limb

where malalignment is bound to cause abnormal stresses on joints, with resultant pain, stiffness and secondary osteoarthritis. *Cross-union* is a form of mal-union occasionally seen between the radius and the ulna and between the tibia and fibula.

Treatment may be non-operative in mild cases e.g. a shoe raise to lessen the effect of lower limb shortening or operative treatment. Arthrodesis may be necessary for mal-union at the ankle.

2. **Delayed Union.** The time various fractures take to heal enough to be able to withstand normal stresses varies. Delayed union is when a fracture has not healed in one and half times the normal healing time. ***Important possible risk factors for delayed union include*** *the age of the patient, degree of fracture displacement and associated soft-tissue damage, type of bone, bone loss, inadequate immobilisation, excessive traction (distraction), soft-tissue interposition, presence of infection, pathological fracture, intra-articular fracture and fracture of a bone strutted by an intact fellow bone (forearm and leg).* Treatment is directed at rectifying the cause.

3. **Non-Union (Fig.11.4).** Non union is said to have occurred if painless movement can be elicited at the fracture site, signifying the presence/formation of a false joint (*a pseudarthrosis*). On X-ray, the fracture line is still visible and the bone ends are sclerotic, sealing off the medullary canal. Non-union may be (a) ***hypertrophic:*** The bone ends are bulbous, indicating that osteogenic activity is still present or (b) ***atrophic*** when there are no signs of new bone formation. Briefly, hypertrophic non-union should be treated by surgical fixation alone as healing potential exists whilst the treatment of atrophic non-union is by surgical fixation plus bone grafting.

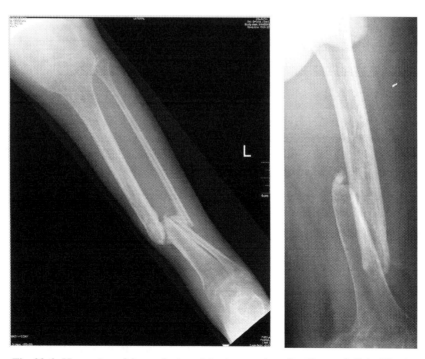

Fig.11.4. Hypertrophic and atrophic non-union (ipsilateral tibia/fibula and femur in the same patient)

Joint stiffness is common and could be due to direct injury, immobilisation, myositis ossificans, mal-union, infected compound fracture and post-traumatic osteoarthritis. Treatment is directed at the cause plus physiotherapy.

Joint Laxity. This may result from injury to the ligaments e.g. at the knee, from muscle weakness secondary to prolonged immobilisation for a fracture or from bone loss in or adjacent to a joint. Treatment depends on the nature of a given case.

OTHER LOCAL COMPLICATIONS OF FRACTURES

- **Post-traumatic reflex dystrophy (Sudeck's atrophy)**
  This condition of unclear pathogenesis is characterised by the appearance of pain, hyperaesthesia, swelling and decreased range of movements in the wrist or hand or in the ankle or foot a few weeks after a forearm or leg injury. This injury could be due to a fracture or soft-tissue injury and is usually minor. The pain has characteristic features: it is burning or aching in nature, increases with motion and such external stimuli as noise, laughter, vibration and emotional upsets and is usually out of proportion to the severity of the causative injury.

  The physical findings are also characteristic. The affected hand or foot is glossy in appearance, cold to touch and the joint movements are limited. X-rays show osteoporosis, which is at first diffuse but later becomes patchy in nature. Symptoms are progressive and could be present for several months.

  Treatment is mainly by physiotherapy, consisting of elevation, heat and graduated exercises. The observed emotional overlay in many of the patients also needs treatment. Sympathetic ears, reassurance and small doses of tranquillisers are helpful in this regard. Many patients with mild forms of the condition will recover with this treatment but others may need sympathetic blocks. Local anaesthetic injections, corticosteroids, hormones, etc, have also been tried.

- **Infection**
  Open fractures are always in danger of becoming infected. Infection is best prevented than treated. Prevention is by prompt wound toilet, debridement, immobilisation and prophylactic antibiotic therapy. Established infection is treated according to its characteristics. Prolonged wound dressing and operative intervention are usually necessary.

- **Bone growth disturbances**
  Fractures involving the growth plates in children, the so-called Salter-Harris injuries, can cause growth disturbances. A crush injury of the whole plate will in all likelihood retard growth and cause shortening. Injury to only a part of the plate could cause deformity later through unequal growth. Early and accurate reduction gives the best chance of preventing this. Children with injuries involving the growth plates should be followed up for as long as is necessary to exclude growth disturbance. This usually takes several years.

COMPLICATIONS OF FRACTURE TREATMENT

All fracture treatment options are associated with complications. It is the duty of all hospital personnel involved in the treatment of fractures to strive to prevent all possible complications.

Briefly, these are the complications

- **Injury to vital structures** during fracture reduction – muscles, nerves or blood vessels

- **Bandages and casts.**
  Tight bandages and casts used in the treatment of certain fractures classically cause *Volkmann's ischaemia and contracture*. Prolonged immobilisation of a patient could cause joint stiffness, chest infection, generalised osteoporosis, renal calculi, and depression. These can be prevented or controlled by appropriate measures. The patient must be mobilised as early as possible.

  The cast syndrome is seen in patients being treated with P.O.P. jackets, hip spicas or on P.O.P beds. Characterised by vomiting, shock and prostration, it is said to be due to duodenal compression by the superior mesenteric artery. Treatment is by removal of the cast, gastric suction and fluid replacement.

- **Operative complications.**

  1. *Technical Complications.* These include intra-operative fractures and soft-tissue damage that could pre-dispose to delayed and non-union.
  2. *Infection.* Open reduction can be complicated by infection. *Pin track infection* is a common complication of skeletal traction. Rarely, it may lead to full-blow osteomyelitis. Daily pin-track care usually suffices in preventing it. Good operative technique, incorporating aseptic and gentle handling of tissues, correct use of instruments and implants will all help to minimise the possibility of infection. Prophylactic antibiotics must also be given.
  3. *Implant failure.* Internal fixation devised such as plates, screws, rods, nails and wires sometimes break. Implant corrosion is sometimes a problem too.

THE SO-CALLED "TRADITIONAL BONE SETTERS"

In most African countries, India and other similar environments, there is an undeclared war between the orthodox doctors and the so-called traditional or native doctors on the subject of fracture treatment. The foregoing chapters show that neither the orthodox nor the native doctor heals fractures. Fractures heal themselves by virtue of an intrinsic endowment from Nature. The role of the doctor is therefore restricted to reducing and holding the fracture in the reduced position and in encouraging all measures which will facilitate the early return of normal function to the injured part (rehabilitation). The issue, therefore, is: which of the two groups of practitioners is better trained and equipped to bring about these desired results?

Ischaemic complications, especially associated with supracondylar humeral fractures in children, mal-united fractures of both the upper and lower limbs in children and adults, unreduced dislocations of the hip, shoulder and elbow are common complications of traditional bone setting. A lot of valuable time and of the meagre resources of hospitals in the developing countries is spent on correcting the mistakes of "traditional bone-setters". Governmental intervention is needed to tackle this problem. This intervention can take many forms, including:

- Sponsorship of serious research into the problem
- Provision of adequate manpower and facilities for the treatment of fractures in orthodox hospitals
- Enlightenment of the population on the dangers of treatment of fractures by unqualified personnel

CHAPTER 12

PRINCIPLES AND MANAGEMENT OF SOFT-TISSUE AND NERVE INJURIES

SPRAINS AND RUPTURES OF LIGAMENTS

Definitions and classifications

A sprain is a partial tear of a ligament. Three degrees of severity of ligament tear are recognised as follows:

- *Mild:* Mild stretch of the fibres of a ligament with snapping of a few fibres. Affected joint remains completely stable.

- *Moderate:* More severe stretch of the fibres of a ligament causing more fibres to snap. A mild degree of joint instability can result.

- *Severe:* Even more severe stretch of the fibres of a ligament causing most of them to snap fibres to snap. This degree of sprain can cause significant joint instability

Tears allow joints to dislocate partially – "subluxation" or completely – "dislocation".

A rupture is a complete tear of a ligament (Fig.12.1). In contrast to a sprain, a rupture is always associated with instability of the affected joint. The type of instability (subluxation or dislocation) that results will depend on the anatomy of the joint and the severity of the ligamentous damage.

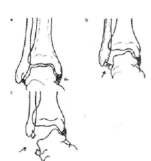

Fig.12.1. Definition of sprain and rupture of a ligament
a. normal joint ligaments
b. a sprain is a partial tear of a ligament
c. a rupture is a complete tear. It may occur at any site in the ligament

191

Mechanisms of injury

Forces stretching the ligaments to breaking point usually cause sprains and ruptures. They can come from any direction. Sports and road traffic accidents are the most frequent causes. A ligament may tear at its point of origin, point of insertion or between these two points. If either of the first two applies, there may be an associated avulsion fracture. The ankle joint is probably the most frequently sprained or ruptured joint, followed by the knee, wrist, fingers and other joints. In terms of causative injuries,

Clinical features

There is usually a helpful history of the causative injury. *Pain* is always present but its severity may not correspond to the severity of the injury. For example, partial tears i.e. sprains, are known to be sometimes more painful than complete tears (ruptures). This is particularly true of the knee joint. During physical examination, it is important to determine to point of maximum tenderness, as this will indicate the point of tear.

Swelling is an important symptom and can be verified objectively. As it may be due to haemorrhage (haemarthrosis), increased amount of joint fluid or soft-tissue injury.

Skin discolouration (bruise) due to bleeding into subcutaneous soft tissues may be visible in light-skinned patients.

Instability is the most important single symptom and sign of ligamentous injury. It manifests as either subluxation of varying magnitude or as frank dislocation. Stressing the affected ligament (stress test) can elicit joint instability but, as this is usually very painful, it is best done after an injection of a local anaesthetic into the tender areas. It is important that the uninjured joint is tested at the same time as the injured for comparison so that a previously lax ligament is not diagnosed as pathological. The stress test is reliable only within one or two hours after the injury.

Investigations

Routine X-ray views are rarely helpful; *stress views* in which the affected ligament is stressed maximally and then X-rayed are more helpful, especially in the ankle joint. In other joints, special positioning of the patient, the X-ray tube and the film may be necessary. Examples include the so-called *axillary view* used in the diagnosis of a posterior subluxation or dislocation of the shoulder joint and the tangential view of the sternoclavicular joint which is useful in the diagnosis of instability in this joint.

An X-ray of a joint into which a dye has been injected, *arthrography*, and inspection of the joint with a fibre optic instrument, *arthroscopy*, may be useful, especially in differentiating ligamentous injuries from associated intra-articular injuries.

Treatment

The key factor in treatment is the state of stability of the injured joint. If the ligamentous injury has not resulted in instability of the joint, i.e. if it is a mild sprain, no specific treatment is prescribed.

Local applications such as cold compress applied within the first 2 hours following the injury or one of the ant-inflammatory/anti-oedema gels or creams may be useful.

On the other hand, moderate to severe sprains, which have caused instability as well as all grades of, ruptures which always cause instability usually need specific treatment, which can be surgical (open repair) or non-surgical (splintage).

Complications

The most significant complication of ligamentous injuries is chronic instability manifesting as recurrent subluxation or dislocation. This occurs frequently in the shoulder joint. Painful secondary osteoarthritis may also eventually result.

SUBLUXATIONS AND DISLOCATIONS OF JOINTS

Definitions and Classifications

A dislocation is a total loss of contact (really, loss of apposition) between two or more articulating surfaces. A subluxation is a partial or incomplete dislocation (Fig.12.2). Although a dislocation or subluxation may result from other causes, e.g. congenital joint laxity, septic arthritis or paralytic disease, most of them result from injury to tissues maintaining the integrity of joints (traumatic subluxation or dislocation).

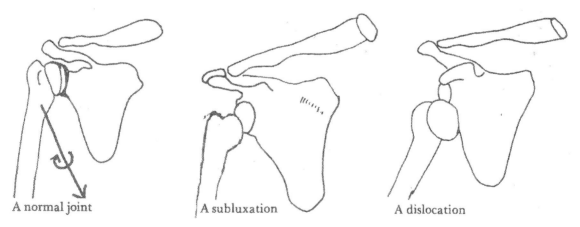

A normal joint   A subluxation   A dislocation

Fig.12.2. Subluxation and dislocation of a joint

Mechanisms of injury

The relative ease or difficulty with which a dislocation (or subluxation) occurs in a given joint depends on the inherent stability of the joint. The shoulder joint dislocates more easily than the hip joint. Both indirect and direct forces may be responsible. For example, an anterior dislocation of the shoulder joint can result from both a fall on the abducted and externally rotated arm (indirect force) and a direct fall on the point of the shoulder.

Diagnosis and Treatment

History

As with more other injuries, the history of the causative injury is important. The mechanism of injury may suggest the diagnosis. The possibility of an injury being a recurrent one should always be borne in mind when one is confronted with a case of suspected dislocation; leading questions in this direction should be asked. This is particularly true of the shoulder joint and the patella.

Clinical features

Pain: Pain is a constant feature of acute dislocations and usually persists until reduction is effected.

Attitude: In some cases, the appearance of the affected part of the body may be diagnostic. For example, in posterior dislocation of the hip joint, the limb is held flexed, adducted and internally rotated; in anterior dislocation it is held abducted and externally rotated. Similarly, in anterior dislocation of the shoulder joint, the affected arm is usually held in slight flexion, abduction and external rotation.

Loss of normal contour: The normal shape of the affected joint is changed. Usually there is flattening in the area of the joint normally occupied by the dislocated articular surface and fullness in the area in which it comes to lie.

Loss of movement: Movement in a dislocated joint is either totally impossible due to an anatomical block or grossly limited by it or by pain.

Investigations

An X-ray examination is necessary even if a dislocation has been correctly diagnosed by physical examination. This is in order to exclude or confirm associated fractures, many of which cannot be diagnosed clinically. This is particularly important in dislocations of the hip and shoulder joints, which are often complicated by fractures of neighbouring bones.

Treatment

The principles of treatment of dislocation (and subluxations) are exactly the same as those of treatment of displaced fractures, namely, reduction, immobilisation and exercises (Fig.12.3). The methods of reduction, immobilisation and exercises are also similar and will not be repeated here.

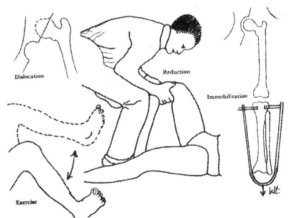

Fig.12.3. Principles of management of dislocations: reduce, immobolize, exercise.

Complications of Subluxations and Dislocations

These include:

1. Associated fractures.
2. Nerve injury
3. Vascular injury
4. Recurrent dislocation
5. Myositis ossificans
6. Avascular necrosis
7. Joint stiffness
8. secondary osteoarthritis

PERIPHERAL NERVE INJURIES

TYPES OF INJURY TO PERIPHERAL NERVES

Three types of peripheral nerve injury are classically distinguished: *neurapraxia, axonotmesis* and *neurotmesis.* To this may be added root avulsion in case of nerve plexus injury.

Neurapraxia. Usually, the nerve has been subjected to a stretch injury. There may be a minor injury to the myelin sheath but the axons are intact. Motor loss may at first be total due to predominant affection of the larger motor fibres; sensory loss is rare but spontaneous recovery of all deficit usually occurs.

Axonotmesis. The axons are damaged but their endoneurial sheaths remain intact. Accordingly, the potential for regeneration is retained. Initially clinically indistinguishable from a complete division (neurotmesis), reinnervation of muscles distal to the injury occurs in most cases as the proximal stumps of the divided axons grow into the intact distal endoneurial sheaths.

Neurotmesis. This is a complete cut of the nerve; no nerve function is retained and spontaneous regeneration cannot be expected. The same effect is obtained if there is mangling of the nerve at a point but no actual cut. A neuroma formed by sprouting axons is a common complication of this injury.

Root avulsion is a special injury involving nerve plexuses. It is discussed further later in this section.

REGENERATION OF A DIVIDED NERVE

The complex structure of a peripheral nerve helps us to understand why nerve regeneration and therefore functional recovery is hardly complete after a division. Following a division, the axons and their sheaths distal to the division degenerate completely (Wallerian degeneration), losing their power of conduction within 2 - 4 weeks. Proximally, a similar degeneration occurs but only for a short distance to the next node of Ranvier. The endoneurial tubes then grow from the proximal stump, followed by their axons until the end-organ is reached.

DIAGNOSIS OF PERIPHERAL NERVE INJURY

The diagnosis of peripheral nerve injuries follows the established route of history-taking, physical examination and investigations. Knowledge of the nerves likely to be injured, the likely sites of injury and clinical features of individual nerve injury is also essential. These issues are addressed in the discussion of individual nerve injury. To summarise here, injury sites and the nerves commonly injured are shown in Table 12.1. Nerve injuries cause motor and sensory deficits, the grading of which is summarised in Table 12.2 and 12.3 respectively.

Table 12.1. Common sites of peripheral nerve injuries

Site	Injury	Nerve(s) likely to be injured
Shoulder	Birth and traction injury	Brachial plexus
Shoulder	Anterior dislocation	Axillary nerve
Upper arm	Proximal humeral fractures	Radial nerve
Elbow	Dislocations; supracondylar fractures; cuts	Median and ulnar nerves
Wrist	Knife/glass cuts	Median and ulnar nerves
Palm	Knife/glass cuts	Digital nerves
Hip	Posterior dislocation of the hip; surgery	Sciatic nerve
Knee	Traction or pressure injuries; sugrery	Common peroneal nerve

Table 12.2. Grades of sensory loss

Grade 0	Total anaesthesia
Grade 1	Pain perception only
Grade 2	Pain and some touch perception
Grade 3	Pain and normal touch but no two-point discrimination
Grade 3+	Same as grade 3 plus some two-point discrimination
Grade 4	Normal sensation

Table 12.3. Grades of motor loss

Grade 0	Total paralysis
Grade 1	Muscle contraction insufficient to bring about movement in relevant joint
Grade 2	Contraction sufficient to bring about movement with gravity eliminated
Grade 3	Contraction sufficient to bring about movement against gravity.
Grade 4	Contraction able to move a joint against some external resistance.
Grade 5	Contraction able to move a joint against considerable external resistance (Normal power).

Investigation of nerve injury

Magnetic resonance Imaging (MRI). Abnormal changes can be seen as early as four days post-injury, which is significantly earlier than changes detected on electromyography.

Electromyography. When muscle fibres contract, they generate electric current, which can be displayed on a cathode-ray oscilloscope, heard via a loud speaker or recorded on paper. This current takes the form of action potentials, which differ, for normal, denervated and reinnervating muscle, hence the diagnostic and prognostic importance of this investigation. It is unfortunately limited by the fact that the action potentials of denervated muscle, called fibrillation potentials, do not appear until 2-4 weeks after a nerve injury.

Nerve conduction studies. The conduction velocity of an injured sensory or motor nerve can be measured and compared with that of the normal nerve. The velocity is obviously impaired by injury. The practical value of the test is however limited by the fact that it is unreliable in the first 10 days following injury.

Surgical Exploration. Most of the investigations listed above are of limited value in early (i.e. within a few days) diagnosis of a nerve injury. Where facilities for MRI and electrophysiological investigations are not available, as in many hospitals in the Third World, surgical exploration is an invaluable diagnostic tool.

Treatment of nerve injuries

Neurapraxia. A wait and see policy is appropriate in a neurapraxia.

Axonotmesis. In axonotmesis, the waiting period can be estimated by measuring in millimetres the distance between the site of the nerve injury and the nearest muscle innervated by the nerve and assuming a rate of regeneration of 1mm a day. During the waiting period, splintage, exercises and electrical stimulation of paralysed muscles should be instituted.

Neurotmesis. A divided nerve must be repaired if useful regeneration is to be expected. Nerve division associated with an open wound should be sutured at the same time as the wound is being toileted and debrided. This is called *primary nerve suture.* If primary suture cannot be carried out for one reason or the other, secondary suture can be done at a later date. *Nerve grafting* becomes indicated when, after the removal of a damaged nerve segment, mobilising the ends cannot bridge the resulting gap.

In practice, the axons grow at a speed of about 1mm a day. The practical implication of this is that if a peripheral nerve innervating a group of hand muscles is cut at the axilla, 30cm away from the hand, the axons will reach their end-organ in 300 days. Accordingly, if the end-organ is not kept viable by constant and meticulous exercises in the meantime it will surely atrophy and be of no use by the time its innervation is re-established.

Monitoring of Nerve Regeneration

The most handy method is the Tinel test: gentle tapping with the tip of a finger is carried out along the course of the nerve. At a certain point, the patient feels 'pins and needles' in the distribution of the nerve. This point represents the ends of growing axons; it gradually moves distally as recovery proceeds.

BRACHIAL PLEXUS INJURIES

MECHANISMS OF INJURY

Most injuries occur through the indirect mechanisms of traction and compression. Falls off motor cycles are frequent causes. Direct injury by stabbing or missiles e.g. bullets are relatively rare.

DIAGNOSIS

A working knowledge of the anatomy of the brachial plexus (Fig.12.4) is obviously helpful in understanding injuries to it but this is rather complicated and can be acquired later in your career. Briefly, the plexus is located in the lower part of the posterior triangle of the neck and the upper part of the axilla and is formed by the anterior rami or roots of the 5th, 6th, 7th and 8th cervical and 1st thoracic nerve. The roots then give rise to the trunks, divisions, cords and main nerve branches in this order.

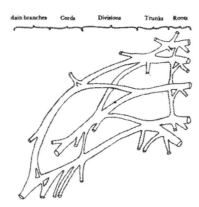

Fig.12.4. The brachial plexus

From the clinical view-point, the most fruitful approach is to use the classification of all brachial plexus injuries into *preganglionic and post-ganglionic*. The explanation is as follows: the peripheral nerves are mixed nerves formed by the dorsal (or posterior) sensory roots and the ventral (or anterior) motor roots. The *posterior sensory roots* have their cell bodies in the *dorsal root ganglia* (the singular is *ganglion*). In an injury situation, the segment that has the cell body retains its functional capacity. Please note this. Fig.12.5 illustrates an injury (tear) of the roots before they reach the dorsal root ganglion(=*pre-ganglionic lesion*) and another injury occurring after the dorsal root ganglion(= *post-ganglionic lesion*). This is the basis of the *axon reflex:*

The axon reflex. A stimulus such as a drop of histamine or a cold object applied to an area of the skin reflexly causes vasodilation of the skin. This manifests as redness in light-skinned people. This reflex is mediated at the level of the posterior root ganglion. Accordingly, the axon reflex test is positive in a pre-ganglionic (root avulsion) lesion in which the dorsal root ganglion remains in continuity with the axon, but negative in a post-ganglionic lesion in which this connection has been severed.

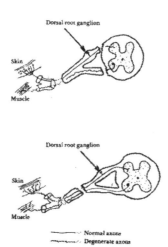

Fig.12.5. The axon reflex. This reflex is mediated at the level of the dorsal root ganglion. Accordingly, it is positive in a pre-ganglionic lesion (root avulsion) in which the ganglion remains in continuity with the axon and negative in a post-ganglionic lesion in which the ganglion is disconnected from the lesion.

A positive axon reflex denotes root avulsion and a bad prognosis. *As this test is applicable only in light-skinned people, it is therefore of limited value in many African or Asian environments. Measuring the sensory nerve action potentials (SNAPs) works on the same principle and can be used for dark-skinned people.*

HORNER'S SYNDROME

The cervical sympathetic nerve chain can be injured in brachial plexus injuries. Fibres to the 1st thoracic sympathetic ganglion arise from T1 root and carry the sympathetic supply to the ipsilateral half of the face. *Avulsion of T1 root* will therefore interrupt this sympathetic supply, producing the so-called *Horner's syndrome*. This is characterised by *unilateral ptosis, enophthalmos, miosis and absence of sweating in the face, neck and upper chest.* The presence of Horner's syndrome signifies a T1 root avulsion and a bad prognosis.

INVESTIGATIONS

Conventional X-rays are needed to diagnosis or exclude associated fractures. *MRI scanning, Radiculography, Electromyography, Nerve conduction tests, measurement of SNAPs* are all good diagnostic tools with their specific indications.

Electrical stimulation of muscles. The paraspinal muscles receive innervation from the posterior roots, which have a common origin with the anterior roots, which form the brachial plexus. Therefore, in root avulsion, corresponding paraspinal muscles will be robbed of their innervation. This can be detected by their failure to respond to electrical stimulation. Furthermore, the plexus can be stimulated directly and the response (or absence of it) noted.

Surgical exploration is an important diagnostic tool too. It is indicated in post-ganglionic lesions and affords an opportunity to distinguish between lesions in continuity and cuts or ruptures.

TREATMENT

Early exploration is indicated in postganglionic lesions. If the plexus is found to be visually intact at surgery, neurapraxia or axonotmesis is assumed and the wound is closed. This causes no significant harm. If elements of the plexus are found to be ruptured, an end-to-end nerve suture may be practicable. Nerve grafting may be required.

In a complete plexus lesion with a flail and anaesthetic arm, amputation is indicated but this does not cure a pre-existing pain in the arm.

Physiotherapy is compulsory instituted following surgical or conservative treatment. This may include direct Faradic and galvanic stimulation of the muscles is given to maintain their tone.

PROGNOSIS

As stated earlier, the prognosis for avulsion lesions is generally hopeless. In a neurapraxia, recovery may occur within a few weeks but an axonotmesis regenerates more slowly, roughly at the rate of 1mm a day. The rate of regeneration following nerve suture is similar. Accordingly, evidence of reinnvervation will appear first in the proximal muscles of the shoulder and upper arm and last in those of the wrist and hand. It is therefore imperative that dedicated physiotherapy is instituted and maintained in order to keep affected muscles and joints supple while reinnervation is awaited; re-innervation is useless to an atrophied and fibrosed muscle and a stiff joint! In general, the prognosis for recovery of function of distal muscles, especially the intrinsic muscles of the hand, is poor because of the long distance between them and the site of the lesion.

NAMED BRACHIAL PLEXUS SYNDROMES

Erb's (or upper arm) palsy

This is also known as obstetrical palsy because of its frequent association with birth trauma (head presentation). It is a traction injury to C5 and C6 roots; sometimes C7 is also affected. There is paralysis of shoulder abduction and external rotation, of elbow flexion and forearm supination. The whole arm is therefore held internally rotated beside the trunk with the elbow extended and the forearm pronated, hence the allusion to *waiter's tip position*. The elbow may develop flexion contracture in longstanding cases but the forearm remains pronated (Fig.12.6).

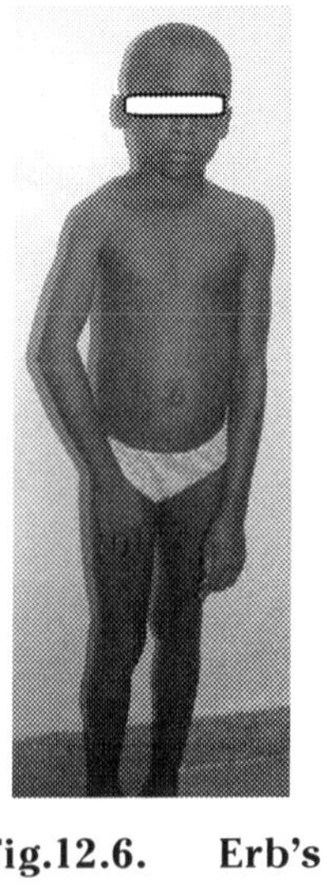

Fig.12.6. Erb's palsy of the right upper limb in an 8-year-old boy.

Up to three-quarters of cases recover spontaneously but as it is not known which given case will recover and which will not, all cases should be treated.

Treatment consists of applying a shoulder spica, which holds the arm in abduction and external rotation and the forearm in supination, for six weeks. Muscle massages and range of motion exercises are carried out prior to and after POP immobilisation. The current trend in management is early exploration and microsurgical nerve repair, if there are no signs of recovery in the first three months or so. Good results are claimed.

Klumpke's palsy

This is also an obstetrical palsy but this time acquired during a breech delivery. It is much rarer that Erb's palsy. The lower roots, C8 and T1 are injured, hence the alternative name "lower arm palsy". Clinically, the intrinsic muscles of the hand and the flexors of the fingers are paralysed, with severe clawing of the affected hand. Sometimes there is associated sensory loss in the ulnar part of the forearm and hand or a Horner's syndrome. The fingers should be kept supple by physiotherapy in hope of reinnervation. The prognosis is however poor largely because of the long distance between the sites of nerve injury and the muscles innervated.

Complete brachial plexus palsy

This is otherwise called the whole-arm type of paralysis. The muscles of the arm, forearm, hand and some of the scapula are paralysed. The limb is almost completely anaesthetic.

In management, early exploration is indicated in all cases except if root avulsion has been established. Prolonged and enlightened physiotherapy is indicated in all patients. For a flail and anaesthetic arm, an above-elbow amputation is probably the best treatment.

INDIVIDUAL PERIPHERAL NERVE INJURIES

Axillary nerve

This nerve supplies the deltoid and teres minor muscles, the shoulder joint and a patch of skin in the so-called regimental badge area of the arm. The most common cause of injury is traction on the nerve during an anterior shoulder dislocation or during surgery in the shoulder joint region.

The main clinical features are loss of shoulder abduction and anaesthesia in the regimental badge area. Most traction injuries tend to recover over a period up to 6 months. While recovery is awaited the deltoid should be held in a relaxed state with an abduction frame and stimulated electrically. Daily active shoulder exercises should also be encouraged. If the nerve has been divided, suture should be carried out but this is technically difficult except if it is the main nerve that is involved. The result of such suture is unpredictable.

Radial nerve

The major muscle supplied by the radial nerve in the arm is the triceps. Further down, it supplies the anconius, brachioradialis, extensor carpi radialis longus and brevis, extensor carpi ulnaris, supinator, adbuctor policis longus and brevis, extensor policis longus and extensor indicis. In terms of sensory function, the nerve innervates the posterior and posterolateral areas of the arm, the posterior third of the forearm and at the first web space. The motor and sensory deficit resulting from a given injury depends on its level.

Most injuries are caused by the jagged edge of a fracture fragment in the spiral groove of the humerus, the lateral intermuscular septum also playing a compressive role in this situation. Delayed palsy may result from enclosement of the nerve in the callus of a healing fracture. Gunshot and stab wounds are rarer causes of radial nerve injury.

In a classical case, the patient suffers a *wrist drop*. S/he holds the limb at the side of the body with the elbow slightly flexed, the forearm pronated, the hand dropped at the wrist, the fingers dropped at the metacarpophalangeal joints and the thumb dropped unto the palm. The patient is unable to make a fist because of the dropped wrist and thumb. In case of an incomplete division, causalgia is experienced in the distribution of the nerve. Electrodiagnostic tests are adjunctive to clinical findings.

In an acute injury with immediate and complete paralysis, exploration is indicated. Nothing is lost if the nerve is found intact. On the other hand, if a division is found early primary suture gives the best results. A causalgic lesion should be explored. The neuroma should be excised and an end-to-end suture carried out. Physiotherapy is indicated in both operative, and conservative treatment. A so-called 'lively' splint based on the Brian Thomas' splint holds the metacarpophalangeal joints straight and the thumb straight and abducted and can be made locally from elastic strips of rubber (catapult splint).

Median nerve

The median nerve does not have any branches in the arm. In the elbow region, it supplies the pronator teres. In the forearm, it supplies the flexor digitorum profundus (slips to the index and middle fingers only), flexor digitorum superficialis and pronator quadratus. In the hand, it supplies the thenar muscles (opponens pollicis, abductor pollicis brevis). From its five palmar digital nerves arise motor branches to the lumbricals of the index and middle fingers and sensory branches which supply the thumb, index and middle fingers and the radial half of the ring.

The functional deficit or deficits arising from a given injury will therefore depend on the level of such injury. Division above the elbow will result in loss of flexion of the thumb, index and middle fingers. In trying to make a fist, the hand is held with the index finger standing straight (*the pointing index sign*) and the middle, ring and little fingers flexed. This is due to the fact that the ulnar nerve supplies the ring and little finger flexors; the middle finger is able to flex because its deep flexor, though paralysed, is joined anatomically to the unparalysed half of flexor digitorum profundus.

Wrist flexion is weak and the hand is deviated towards the ulna from unopposed action of flexor carpi ulnaris (supplied by the ulnar nerve). Forearm pronation is lost from paralysis of the pronators and the thenar muscles atrophy from paralysis such that the hand acquires a flat appearance resembling the hand of the monkey (*simian hand*).

Division at the level of the wrist paralyses the flexor pollicis brevis (the thumb cannot be brought far forward opposite the index finger), the opponens pollicis, the superficial part of abductor pollicis brevis and the lumbricals to the index and middle fingers. Loss of sensation occurs in the thumb, index, middle and radial half of the ring finger. Trophic changes are seen mainly in the index finger, which becomes thin with a cone-shaped tip.

Treatment. Suture is indicated in complete divisions. It is usually possible to mobilise the nerve enough to bridge small gaps. The result of early nerve suture is generally good. Nerve graft e.g. with the sural nerve, is required in large gaps. Partial divisions or irritative lesions should be explored. Usually neuromas are found in such lesions; they can be excised and direct nerve suture can be effected.

Ulnar nerve

The ulnar nerve does not supply any muscle in the arm. In the forearm, it supplies the flexor carpi ulnaris and the medial half of flexor digitorum profundus. At the wrist and hand levels it supplies palmaris brevis, the 3 hypothenar muscles (abductor, flexor brevis and opponens digiti minimi), the lumbricals to the ring and little fingers, the 7 interossei and the abductor pollicis. The sensory supply is to the ulnar portion of the palm, the little finger and the ulnar half of the ring.

Injuries to the nerve can occur at any level. Trying to work out the functional deficits resulting from injury to the nerve at various levels is an interesting and complex example of the relation between anatomy and physiology. Try this out; you don't have to cram it all:

- At and above the elbow, the nerve is particularly vulnerable at the elbow where it lies right on the posterior aspect of the medial epicondyle and is prone to injury in fractures involving this area.

- A non-united fracture of the lateral condyle leads to cubitus valgus and this can cause delayed ulnar palsy. At the wrist glass cuts may involve the nerve.

- In injuries above the elbow or at the elbow level (*high lesions*), loss of flexor carpi ulnaris function results in radial deviation of the hand on attempting to flex the wrist.

- Paralysis of flexor digitorum supply to the ring and little fingers results in loss of flexion at their distal interphalangeal joints. *This can be demonstrated by asking the patient to place the fingers flat on the table and scratch the surface with the fingernails; they are unable to do this with the ring and little fingers.* Atrophy of both muscles leads to thinning of the ulnar aspect of the forearm.

- Further down, the ring and little fingers are extended at the metacarpophalangeal joints and flexed at the proximal interphalangeal joints, due to loss of lumbrical action.

- The hypothenar eminence is thinned due to paralysis of its muscles and the interdigital spaces are hollowed due to paralysis of the intrinsics supplied by the nerve. Abduction and adduction of the fingers are weak or lost completely and the patient is unable to grip a piece of paper between them. The index and middle fingers may still abduct because the median nerve supplies their lumbrical muscles.

- Paralysis of adductor pollicis permits over-action of flexor pollicis longus which results in loss of the ability to stabilise the thumb at the carpometacarpal joint and consequently in loss of power of pinch. This can be demonstrated in a unilateral lesion by the **Froment test:** *a sheet of paper is placed on the two palms held flat and the patient is asked to hold it with the thumbs and to resist its being pulled away by the examiner. When the paper is gradually pulled away, the patient is able to hold the paper with the normal hand but not with the one with ulnar nerve injury in which the thumb is seen to go into flexion at the interphalangeal joint - paralysis of pinch action.*

- Sensory deficit expresses itself in loss of sensation in the ulnar areas and also in tropic changes in the ring and little fingers.

- *In low lesions* occurring after the flexor carpi ulnaris and the ulnar half of the flexor digitorum profundus have been innervated, ulnar forearm atrophy does not occur and the ring and little fingers are flexed (not extended) at the distal interphalangeal joints. There is, therefore, *true clawing* of these fingers. All the other changes in the hand described in respect of high lesions are present in low lesions.

Treatment follows lines described for the radial and median nerves. Mobilisation for suture can be enhanced by flexion of the elbow and wrist joints. At the elbow, anterior transposition of the nerve can also be carried out to aid suture.

Recovery of function may take over a year. While this is awaited the innervated muscles must be splinted in a relaxed position. In the hand, this means holding the metacarpophalangeal joints in flexion and the interphalangeal joints in extension. In permanent paralysis, tendon transfers can be done. Various surgical procedures are also available for the correction of clawing and their functional effects.

LUMBOSACRAL PLEXUS

The lumbar plexus is formed by the ventral rami of L1 - L3 and part of L4 spinal nerves, with a small branch from the subcostal nerves in half the cases. The so-called lumbosacral plexus is formed by the contribution from L4 and the ventral rami of S1-S4 spinal nerves. Elements of the two plexuses supply the whole lower limb and the distal part of the trunk.

Because of their location, these plexuses are rarely injured per se. Only a few of their elements are frequently injured. These are discussed here.

SCIATIC NERVE

Division of the main nerve is rare. Traction injury may occur during operation on the hip joint, posterior dislocation of the hip or due to pelvic fractures.

Clinically, a sciatic nerve division manifests in paralysis of all muscles below the knee with *thinning of the calf and the leg* and a *foot drop*. Knee flexion is weak because of paralysis of the hamstrings. Sensation is absent below the knee with the exception of the medial side of the leg and trophic ulcers may develop on the sole of the foot.

Suture should be carried out if possible. Functional recovery usually takes a long time. While this is awaited, splintage should be effected with below-knee irons or a toe-raising spring.

In the more frequently seen traction injuries, most are neurapraxias and recover in several weeks with non-operative treatment.

LATERAL POPLITEAL NERVE

This is otherwise called the common peroneal nerve. Because of its close anatomical relationship to the neck of the fibula it is frequently injured in upper tibial fractures, upper tibial osteotomies (usually for genu valgum) and from compression by tight P.O.P casts.

Most lesions are high and manifest as foot drop and inability to invert the foot due to paralysis of tibialis anterior, extensor hallucis longus and extensor digitorum longus. These muscles are innervated by the deep (profoundus) branch of the nerve which also supplies the extensor digitorum brevis and the peroneus tertius.

A low lesion may paralyse only the peroneals so that when the foot is dorsiflexed it goes into varus.

Sensory deficit may result from paralysis of the other two branches of the nerve - the lateral sural cutaneous and the superficial peroneal nerves. In the former, there is anaesthesia in the posterior and lateral surfaces of the leg; in the latter, in the medial side of the big toe, the adjacent sides of the 2nd and 3rd, 3rd and 4th, and 4th and 5th toes.

Where possible a divided nerve should be sutured. While recovery is awaited, the foot must be splinted and exercised as in sciatic nerve palsy. If recovery does not occur, tendon transfer can ameliorate the effects of foot drop e.g. tibialis posterior can be detached at its insertion into the navicula, mobilised and threaded through the interosseous membrane and reattached to the dorsum of the foot. Alternatively, ankle fusion can be carried out.

MEDIAL POPLITEAL NERVE

This is otherwise called the tibial nerve. It supplies both gastrecnemii, the soleus, popliteus, plantaris, tibialis posterior, flexor digitorum longus and flexor hallucis longus. It enters the sole of the foot behind the medial malleolus and then divides into the medial and lateral plantar nerves which supply the small muscles of the toes and most of the skin of the sole (except the extreme medial and lateral borders).

A cutaneous branch, the sural nerve, is given off at the level of the popliteal fossa. It descends superficially in the calf, occupying a roughly middle position down the leg and supplying the middle of the back of the leg and the lateral part of the ankle.

In contrast to the lateral popliteal nerve, the medial popliteal is rarely injured. A complete division results in paralysis of plantar flexion of the ankle and clawing of the toes due to paralysis of the intrinsics.

Further reading

Flores AJ, Lavernia CJ and Owens PW. Anatomy and physiology of peripheral nerve injury and repair. *Am J Orthop 29(3): 167-173, 2000.*

Goddard NJ and Fixsen JA. Rotation Osteotomy Of The Humerus For Birth Injuries Of The Brachial Plexus. *J Bone Joint Surg 66B: 257, 1984.*

Hems TEJ and Glasby MA. Prospects For The Treatment of Spinal Cord and Peripheral Nerve Injury. *J Bone Joint Surg 78B: 176-177, 1996.*

Robinson LR. Traumatic injury to peripheral nerves. *Muscle nerve 23(6): 863-873, 2000.*

Sedel L. The Results of Surgical Repair of Brachial Plexus Injuries. *J Bone Joint Surg. 64B: 54, 1982.*

CHAPTER 13

INJURIES OF THE SHOULDER AND HUMERUS

INJURIES OF THE SHOULDER GIRDLE AND SHOULDER JOINT

THE SHOULDER GIRDLE

The shoulder girdle consists of the scapula and the clavicle, which are joined to each other by the acromioclavicular joint and the coracoclavicular ligaments (Fig.13.1). The clavicle occupies a horizontal position, articulating with the sternum at the stenoclavicular joint and functioning as a bony strut between the sternum and the shoulder. The scapula is attached to the posterior chest wall and spine by muscles - the serratus anterior, the rhomboids, the levator scapulae and the trapezius.

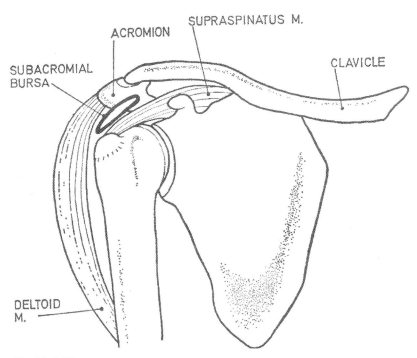

Fig.13.1. The shoulder girdle and proximal humerus

FRACTURES OF THE CLAVICLE

INTRODUCTION

Fractures of the clavicle are quite common, accounting for about 5% of all fractures. They are seen in all age groups: they are common birth injuries and remain common in childhood and adulthood. The average age of patients with fractures of the clavicle is about 40 years. A simple, practical classification is based on dividing the clavicle into three parts – medial one-third, middle one-third and lateral one-third – and grouping the fractures according to their sites in these three segments. 70-80% of the fractures occur in the middle one-third.

MECHANISM OF INJURY

- **Indirect injury**
  - (a) Most clavicular fractures (87%) result from falls on the point of the shoulder during normal walking or running, contact sports and other activities.
  - (b) Lesser numbers (about 6%) result from falls on the out-stretched hand
  - (c) Road traffic accidents are also important causes.

- **Direct injury**
  Direct blows to the point of the shoulder or other points along the bone cause about 7% of the fractures.

Most injuries are low-energy injuries. High energy injuries such as are encountered in falls from heights, construction site injuries and road traffic accidents probably produce less than 25% of fractures. Associated injuries may involve the scapula, the ribs, lungs and neighbouring neurovascular bundles.

DIAGNOSIS

The history is helpful in imagining the mechanism. There is swelling and deformity at the fracture site; the proximal fragment is usually more prominent than the distal. The shoulder droops and is shorter in width than the unaffected side. The fracture site is tender to palpation. Conventional X-rays usually provide sufficient details of the fracture (Fig.13.2). A CT scan may be needed to provide more details in medial third and distal-third intra-articular fractures.

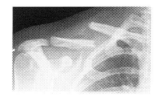

Fig.13.2. A severely displaced fracture of the clavicle in the middle one-third

TREATMENT

Anatomical peculiarities of the clavicle make the reduction of its fractures difficult and their immobilisation almost impossible. Fortunately, accurate reduction of these fractures, though desirable for cosmesis, is not essential for good functional results. Most fractures are treated non-operatively. Treatment methods are shown on Fig.13.3.

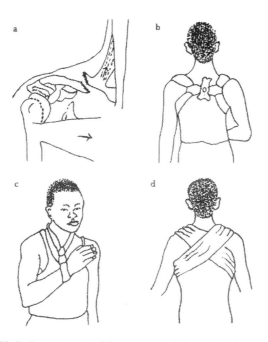

Fig.13.3. Treatment of fractures of the clavicle
a.   **Fracture of the clavicle in the middle one-third**
b.   **Treatment with axillary loops joined posteriorly**
c.   **Treatment with a collar and cuff sling**
d.   **Treatment with a figure-of-8 bandage**

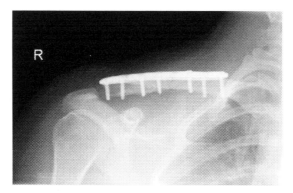

Fig.13.4. Treatment of clavicular fractures: ORIF of a severely displaced fracture of the clavicle in the middle one-third.

Exercises are important in the treatment of clavicular fractures. Right from the start, the elbow, wrist and fingers must be exercised to avoid stiffness, which easily occurs if exercises are not instituted. Active shoulder joint movements should also be encouraged so that full movements can be quickly regained after immobilisation is discontinued.

COMPLICATIONS

- *Nerve injury* to elements of the brachial plexus can occur in open fractures.
- *Vascular injury* to the subclavian or axillary arteries) may occur in open fractures.
- *Mal-union* is a common complication.

- *Non-union* is rare.
- *Shoulder stiffness* is common but can be prevented or cured by exercise.
- *Post-traumatic osteoarthritis* may occur in the acromioclavicular (more commonly) and sternoclavicular (rare) joints following intra-articular fractures.

FRACTURES OF THE OUTER END OF THE CLAVICLE

These occur distal to the coracoclavicular ligament and may involve the acromioclavicular joint, so, the distal fragment remains attached to the acromion. They can be displaced or undisplaced. Undisplaced fractures not spreading into the AC joint can be treated by immobilisation in a collar and cuff for about two weeks, with gradual exercises commenced thereafter. ORIF may be indicated for intra-articular fractures. Non-union may result.

INJURIES OF THE ACROMIOCLAVICULAR JOINT

The acromioclavicular joint is a synovial joint between the clavicle and the acromion, with a fibrocartilaginous disc in-between, similar to the knee meniscus. A whole spectrum of injuries to the joint, ranging from a simple sprain to frank dislocation and fracture-dislocation, is possible.

A history of a fall on the point of the shoulder may be suggestive of an acromioclavicular joint injury. In all injuries except a simple sprain, there is a deformity at the site consisting of a step between the outer end of the clavicle (which is prominent) and the acromion. There is localised tenderness in all fresh injuries. X-rays show the injury type and special views may be necessary.

Treatment naturally depends on the type of injury. With minor injuries (sprain and subluxation), initial ice and immobilisation in a broad arm sling is sufficient to make the patient comfortable.

For more severe injuries, reduction may be indicated. Non-operative reduction may be possible but its maintenance by non-operative means is virtually impossible. Operative treatment involves open reduction and internal fixation. Muscle transfer can also be used.

COMPLICATIONS

The main complication is post-traumatic osteoarthritis of the joint with resultant pain. This can be treated by excision of the outer 2cm of the clavicle.

DISLOCATIONS OF THE STERNOCLAVICULAR JOINT

INTRODUCTION

The sternoclavicular joint is a "limited" ball-and-socket synovial joint, which also has an intervening disc dividing it into two separate joint spaces. Its stability depends mainly on the surrounding ligaments.

A point of interest in sternoclavicular joint injuries is the fact that the epiphysis of the medial end of the clavicle does not begin to ossify until the age of 18 years or so and fuses with the rest of the bone only at about the age of 25 years. Accordingly, many of the sternoclavicular dislocations occurring before the age of 25 years could be epiphyseal injuries.

Dislocations of the sternoclavicular joint are rare, accounting for only 3% of all shoulder girdle dislocations.

CLASSIFICATION

Two types of dislocations are distinguished –

- **anterior**, accounting for about 95% of all dislocations and
- **posterior**, which accounts for the remaining 5%.
- **atraumatic dislocations**) are also recognised. These could be congenital, voluntary/habitual or senile.

MECHANISMS OF INJURY

Road traffic accidents are responsible for most injuries but an indirect force transmitted to the joint during a fall on the shoulder or a fall on all abducted and outstretched arm can also cause anterior and posterior dislocations. Some posterior dislocations may result from a direct hit, kick or pressure to the joint in an anteroposterior direction.

DIAGNOSIS

The clinical features depend on the given injury. In a sprain, the patient complains of pain, which increases, with movement of the arm. The joint may be swollen and tender to palpation. There is no evidence of instability. With subluxation, the pain and swelling are more marked.

In anterior dislocation, the "step" in the sagittal plane between the medial end of the clavicle and the manubrium sterni is more prominent.

In posterior dislocation, there is more pain, the "step" is absent and pressure of the clavicle on the great vessels at the root of the neck may cause venous congestion in the neck, respiratory difficulties and difficulty in swallowing. Anterior or posterior subluxation can be seen by comparing the injured with uninjured joint.

X-ray examination and its interpretation are not easy. X-rays may show an associated fracture of the medial end of the clavicle in a patient aged between 18 and 25 years in whom the medial clavicular epiphysis may have ossified.

CT and MRI are useful in defining the position of the medial end of the clavicle in relation to the sternum; the CT scan is probably the best imaging option.

TREATMENT

Sprain. In the first 12 hours a cold compress may be useful. Analgesics are also useful. A broad arm sling may also be helpful.

Anterior dislocation. Reduction can be achieved by closed or open method but immobilisation afterwards is difficult. As the deformity is usually slight, the patient may be persuaded to accept it rather risk injury to the great vessels and pericardium attendant on ORIF.

Posterior Dislocation. It is important to exclude the possible serious complications of this injury e.g. injury to the lung or great vessels, before embarking on specific treatment. Reduction can usually be achieved closed under a general anaesthetic. Closed reduction can sometimes be achieved by getting the patient to lie supine with a sandbag between the shoulder blades and then pulling on the abducted and extended arm. Immobilisation can be achieved with a figure-of-eight bandage.

Recurrent and old unreduced dislocations. These are usually anterior dislocations and are best treated by operation.

COMPLICATIONS

Complications occurring at the time of the dislocation are related mainly to the posterior variety and involve compression or injury to the vital structures lying behind the medial end of the clavicle. Recurrent dislocation (from instability) is the most important late complication.

FRACTURES OF THE SCAPULA

INTRODUCTION

Fractures of the scapula are uncommon. This may be due to its rather obscure (and protected) location and its muscular cover. The scapula may be fractured in any of its different parts. The frequency of fractures differs in the different parts of the bone. More frequently fractured are the body and the parts related to the humeral head and the clavicle - the neck, glenoid cavity, the acromion and the coracoid process. Although some of these fractures may look frightening on X-rays, the outcome in most scapular fractures is generally good.

DIAGNOSIS

Most patients have been involved in polytrauma. If mobile, some patients walk into the Accident and Emergency unit holding the affected limb (arm) adducted. Pain, swelling, bruises and tenderness are usually present. The patient will not allow the shoulder joint to be moved; abduction is particularly resented. If associated chest injuries are present, corresponding additional symptoms and signs are present.

The physical signs of scapular injury may be masked in a patient with severe multiple injuries. Possible associated fractures of neighbouring bones should be sought as they may modify treatment.

Conventional X-rays will show most fractures and their characteristics; a CT scan may be helpful in delineating complex fractures.

TREATMENT

The standard treatment of most scapular fractures is immobilisation in a broad arm sling and control of pain with analgesics, followed by gradual mobilisation as soon as acute symptoms subside, usually within 2 weeks of the injury. The regime can be modified accordingly for patients who have to lie in bed because of associated injuries. Open reduction and internal fixation has been advocated for some displaced fractures but, in the long term, the results of surgical treatment have not been shown to be superior to those obtained with simple immobilisation of the arm in a broad arm sling followed by physiotherapy.

DISLOCATIONS OF THE SHOULDER JOINT

INTRODUCTION

Dislocations of the shoulder joint are common because the joint is essentially an unstable one, formed by the shallow and relatively small glenoid cupwhich covers only one-third of the large spherical articular surface of the humerus. Therefore, unlike the hip joint, there is little bony basis for stability in the shoulder joint. Stability derives mainly from the surrounding muscles and ligaments.

Dislocations of the shoulder joint is a very popular topic in orthopaedic trauma because they are quite common; in fact it is the most commonly dislocated joint in the human body. This popularity dates back into ancient times. Ancient history dating back to over 1000 years BC contains evidence of knowledge of shoulder dislocation and its treatment.

The shoulder joint is capable of 90 degrees of active abduction. After the first 30 to 60 degrees of it, the scapula begins to rotate anticlockwise, covering one degree for every two degrees of shoulder joint abduction so that at full elevation (of 180 degrees) the scapula has rotated through 60 degrees to the shoulder joint's 120 degrees. Simultaneously, movements occur at the acromioclavicular joint (20 degrees) and the sternoclavicular joint (40 degrees) - at full elevation.

CLASSIFICATION

The most enduring classification is based on the position of humeral head in the antero-posterior plane relative to the glenoid cup and other neighbouring anatomical landmarks. It groups them into *anterior* and *posterior dislocations*. There is a further group termed *atraumatic dislocations,* which are pathological in the sense that they occur without significant trauma.

ANTERIOR DISLOCATION OF THE SHOULDER JOINT

MECHANISMS OF INJURY

Indirect forces generated during falls on the outstretched abducted and externally rotated arm is the commonest mechanism. Direct injury such as heavy blow or kick on the posterolateral aspect of the shoulder in the postero-anterior direction can sprain supporting ligaments and cause a subluxation or tear them sufficiently to cause a frank dislocation.

DIAGNOSIS

Anterior dislocation of the shoulder is the commonest form of shoulder joint dislocation, accounting for about 95% of all dislocations of this joint. The commonest type of anterior dislocation is the subcoracoid variety (Fig.13.5), followed by the subglenoid type.

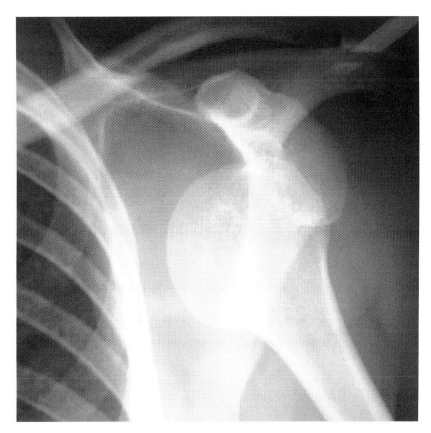

Fig.13.5. Subcoracoid anterior dislocation of the shoulder

The history of the injury should be obtained. Physical examination should be done with the patient appropriately undressed so that the two shoulders can be compared. Inspection reveals slight abduction and external rotation deformity at the shoulder. Viewed from the front, the acromial process is unusually prominent, while the deltoid prominence is reduced; there is an unusual fullness in the anterior aspect of the shoulder so that the coracoid process is no longer easily seen or palpated. The shoulder span is shorter than on the opposite (normal) side.

Palpation confirms most of these visual features, especially in children and thin adults. Movement of the shoulder is painful and should be avoided. Because the circumflex branch of the axillary nerve (sensory) is commonly injured in anterior dislocations, its function should be tested routinely if anterior dislocation is suspected. The test consists of testing for sensation to pin-prick in the regimental badge area of the shoulder and for voluntary abduction of the shoulder after the dislocation has been reduced. If this test is not carried out, injury to the nerve from the original injury may be blamed later on the treating surgeon.

An X-ray examination of the shoulder is needed to confirm the clinical diagnosis and exclude or confirm associated fractures, some of which may be important enough to warrant modification of the treatment of the dislocation. Positioning the arm for X-rays can be difficult because of pain but an axial view will show the dislocation.

TREATMENT

The dislocation must be reduced and as early as possible. The method of reduction may be modified if there are associated fractures. Reduction under intravenous or intramuscular sedation usually suffices. Various authors have invented many methods of reduction; some of them gained popularity but most did not. The most popular ones to date happen to be among the most ancient or their modifications. The author's preference is for the Kocher's method (Fig.13.6) which he has consistently used over the years and which has neither failed him nor has been, in his experience, associated with significant complications.

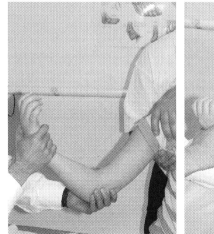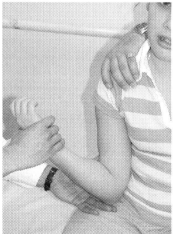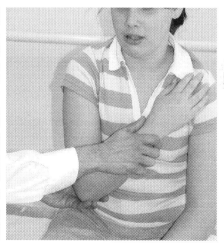

Fig.13.6a-c. Kocher's manoeuvre for reduction of an anterior dislocation of the shoulder: abduct and pull the arm against counter-traction, then adduct, then internally rotate it.

Other methods of reduction of anterior shoulder dislocation include the Hippocrates' Method (c500 BC) and the Stimson method (1900) (Figs.13.7 and 13.8). Both methods have the advantage that they can be carried out without sedation.

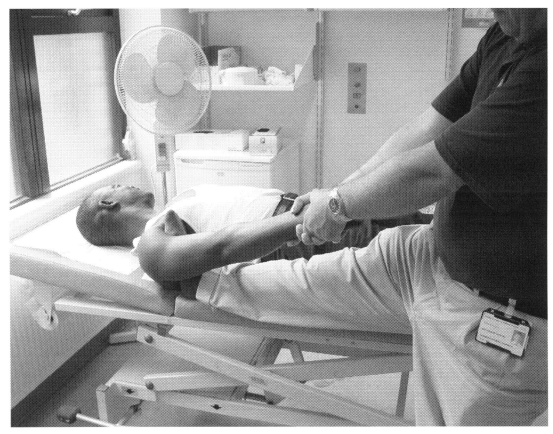

Figs13.7. The Hippocrates method: put the foot across the axilla, then pull on the arm, then lever the humeral head into the glenoid with the foot

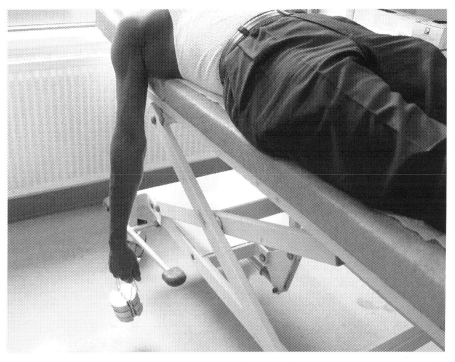

Fig.13.8. The Stimson method: a weight of about 5 lbs on the wrist gradually effects reduction in 10-20 minutes.

Post-Reduction Management

This consists of immobilisation in a body bandage (Fig.13.9) for three weeks and physiotherapy.

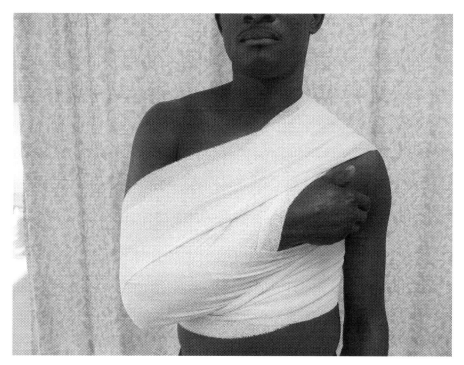

Fig.13.9. Immobilisation of the arm in a body bandage after reduction of anterior shoulder dislocation.

Indications for Open Reduction of Anterior Dislocation

Irreducibility is the commonest reason for open reduction. Irreducibility is usually due to soft-tissue (a part of the rotator cuff, the capsule or triceps tendon) interposition. Other indications for ORIF include associated fractures: (a) displaced greater tuberosity fracture (b) fracture of the surgical or anatomical neck of the humerus, (c) glenoid rim fractures bigger than 5 cm in size.

Luxatio Erecta

This rare type of anterior dislocation occurs with the arm in the elevated (hyperabducted) position. The humeral head impinges against the acromial process, which levers it inferiorly out of the glenoid cup. If the arm drops, the humeral head will assume its usual upright orientation and the dislocation usually becomes a subcoracoid one.

A diagnosis is made on the basis of the characteristic position of the arm and the X-ray findings. Reduction is usually achieved by pulling on the arm in its abducted position and swinging it into adduction. Immobilisation is as for other types of anterior dislocation.

COMPLICATIONS OF ANTERIOR SHOULDER DISLOCATION

Early complications include

- **Associated fractures:**
  (a) Banchart's lesion (fracture of the anterior rim of the glenoid
  (b) Hill-Sach's lesion(a dent in the posterolateral aspect of the humeral head)
  (c) greater tuberosity fracture and rotator cuff tears (in elderly patients mainly).

- **Injury to neighbouring nerves** is common. Elements of the brachial plexus may be injured and the **axillary nerve** being the most frequently injured. Other nerves that may be injured are the radial and **musculocutaneous nerves**; injury to the **median or ulnar nerves** or to the entire plexus may also occur but is rare. Axillary vessels may also be injured.

Other complications include **recurrent dislocation,** ossification of soft tissues around the joint (myositis ossificans), shoulder joint stiffness and arthritis.

RECURRENT ANTERIOR DISLOCATION

This is easily the most serious of all the complications, early or late. It can be defined as dislocation occurring 2 or more times after the initial dislocation. The first recurrence may occur within a few months of the initial dislocation, most will occur within the first 2 years but some may occur as late as 5 years later. The dislocation is mainly anterior, very occasionally posterior. The main causes of anterior dislocation are (a) glenoid rim fractures (Bankart and Hill-Sachs' lesions)(Fig.13.10) (b) inadequate immobilisation after the first dislocation. It has a high incidence - quoted as being up to 90% in some papers.

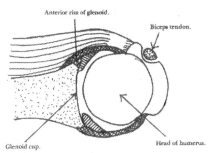

a. Cross-section of a normal shoulder joint

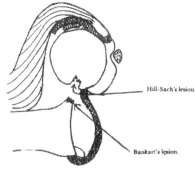

b. A dislocated joint showing a Bankart's and a Hill-Sach's lesion

Fig.13.10. Recurrent dislocation of the shoulder joint: cross-section of normal and dislocated shoulder showing Bankart and Hill-Sach lesions

DIAGNOSIS

The diagnosis of recurrent dislocation is not difficult. There is a history of previous dislocations. In most patients, the dislocation would have reduced itself by the time they are seen by the doctor. Physical findings include a positive apprehension test: on passively putting the shoulder into abduction, extension and external rotation, the patient tenses themselves up to avoid the shoulder coming out. Appropriate X-ray views, CT and MRI scans can show Bankart and Hill-Sach lesions.

TREATMENT

Several treatment procedures have been invented. They include:

- Procedures which tighten the muscles and joint capsule e.g. the Putti-Platt operation,
- Procedures that repair the Bankart lesion e.g. the Bankart operation and
- Procedures that use bone to block further dislocation e.g. the Helfet operation

POSTERIOR DISLOCATION OF THE SHOULDER JOINT

Posterior dislocation is much rarer than anterior, accounting for less than 5% of all shoulder dislocations. The dislocation is almost always partial (i.e. a subluxation) but the term "dislocation" is traditionally used.

MECHANISMS OF INJURY

The injury is usually caused by an indirect force - forced internal rotation of a flexed and adducted arm as can occur in a fall on the out-stretched hand. Another common indirect force is violent muscle contraction such as occurs in accidental or therapeutic electric shocks, convulsions or tetanus; this latter cause is important in the tropics. A direct blow or hit to the anterior shoulder can also cause a posterior dislocation.

DIAGNOSIS

Possibly because of its rarity but probably because of a reduced index of suspicion and disregard for routine history-taking and physical examination on the part of the doctor, this injury is often missed. This is hardly justifiable because the features of the injury are quite characteristic. The history is often suggestive of the diagnosis – an epileptic fit, a hit on the shoulder in the anterior to posterior direction. There is complaint of severe pain and of inability to abduct or externally rotate the arm.

On examination, the arm is held in adduction and internal rotation, the anterior aspect of the shoulder is flat and the coracoid process more prominent compared with the opposite side. The posterior aspect of the shoulder is "full". These visual signs are best elicited with the patient seated and the surgeon standing and looking from the side and then from the back. Abduction is severely limited and external rotation completely blocked.

On AP X-ray, the humeral head may appear in its socket but a more careful look may reveal absence of a normal joint space (Fig.13.11). The so-called axillary view (Fig.13.12) is the most helpful view for diagnosis but as positioning the arm for it usually causes a lot of pain, one can make do with a transthoracic (lateral) view which does show the outline of the humeral head to lie posterior to the glenoid cup. The vast majority of posterior dislocations are subacromial in position; the odd case may be subglenoid or subspinous (spine of the scapula).

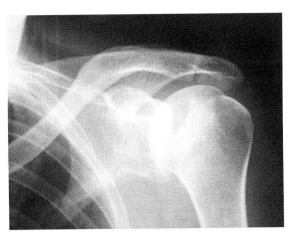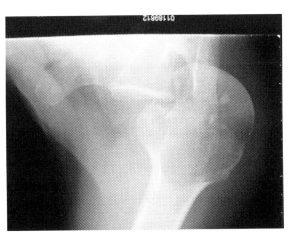

Fig.13.11a&b. Posterior shoulder dislocation: On an AP X-ray, the humeral head may appear in its socket but a more careful look may reveal absence of a normal joint space
Fig.13.12. Posterior shoulder dislocation: the axillary view shows a posterior position of the humeral head

TREATMENT

Reduction is imperative. This can be done under intravenous diazepam as in anterior dislocation but general anaesthesia is best. The arm is pulled, rotated externally as the humeral head is pushed forward. If the reduction is stable, the arm is immobilised in a body bandage and sling for 3 weeks as with anterior dislocation. If it feels unstable, a shoulder spica is applied for the same period with the arm is moderate abduction, extension and external rotation. Exercises are then begun.

COMPLICATIONS

A posterior dislocation may be complicated by associated fractures of the posterior glenoid rim, lesser tuberosity and of the proximal humerus. These may warrant modification of treatment. Recurrent dislocation also occurs and may require surgical treatment with a reversed Putti-Platt or a reversed Bankart operation. Joint stiffness, myositis ossificans and secondary osteoarthritis may also occur.

ATRAUMATIC DISLOCATIONS OF THE SHOULDER JOINT

It is important to remember that this class of shoulder dislocations exists, if only for differential diagnostic purposes. These dislocations are:

Voluntary (Habitual) dislocation. This may be anterior or posterior. There is no history of trauma.

The patient is able to sublux or dislocate the shoulder at will. Some of the patients can also dislocate other joints and use this to entertain others for money or fun.

For treatment purposes two groups of patients are distinguished: those psychiatrically normal and those psychiatrically abnormal. Treatment, which is mainly operative, may succeed in the former group; in the latter, it is not worthwhile as the patients are bound to wreck the repair sooner or later. Most have been known to do so sooner rather than later - just after recovery from anaesthesia.

Congenital dislocation. This could be anterior or posterior. It is rare and due to various anatomical defects involving both the bones, especially the glenoid cup, and the soft-tissue elements, including the rotator-cuff muscles and the ligaments. Reconstructive procedures are usually needed, the type depending on the causative defect.

FRACTURES OF THE PROXIMAL HUMERUS

Constituting 5–7% of all adult fractures, proximal humeral fractures are relatively common in elderly patients, especially females, in whom osteoporosis is an important factor.

Anatomy

The proximal part of the humerus can be divided into four segments (Fig.13.12).

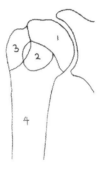

Fig.13.12.The four segments of the proximal humerus
1. The humeral head
2. The lesser tuberosity
3. The greater tuberosity
4. The proximal part of the humeral shaft

COMMON FRACTURE TYPES

AVULSION FRACTURE OF THE GREATER TUBEROSITY (Fig.13.13)

The usual mechanism is a fall on the shoulder. The fragment may be pulled off (avulsed) by the supraspinatus tendon. Clinically, there is swelling and fairly localised tenderness. Minimally displaced fractures are treated with immobilisation of the arm in a collar-and-cuff sling for about 2 weeks,

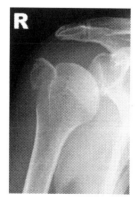

Fig.13.13. Fracture of the greater tuberosity of the humerus

followed by physiotherapy. Some displaced fractures can be reduced by closed manipulation followed by percutaneous fixation with a screw. Others may require ORIF.

FRACTURES OF THE SURGICAL NECK

These are seen in adults following falls on the outstretched arm. Direct forces such as direct blows or hits are rare and tend to cause comminuted fractures.

DIAGNOSIS

The history of the causative injury can be helpful. The main complaint is of pain and limited ability to abduct the arm. Physical examination may reveal swelling, ecchymosis and tenderness; abduction is painful, limited or absent. Examination should include a search for possible neurological injury (seen in 36% of patients) and vascular injury (seen in 5% of patients.). X-ray evaluation should include AP, scapular and axillary views. Various fracture patterns are seen.

TREATMENT

This depends on the fracture type

(a) Minimally displaced or impacted fractures of the surgical neck are treated with immobilisation of the arm in a collar-and-cuff sling for about 2 weeks, followed by physiotherapy.
(b) Comminuted fractures that can be reduced are treated by plate fixation.
(c) Comminuted fractures with head fragments that are unlikely to survive are best treated by hemiarthroplasty.

- *Physiotherapy*
  Irrespective of the method of treatment employed, an active exercise programme must be instituted immediately under the supervision of the physiotherapist. Particular attention must be paid to exercises in the elderly patient because they are in particular danger of developing shoulder joint stiffness.

COMPLICATIONS

- Associated dislocation of the shoulder
- Nerve and vascular injury
- Shoulder stiffness

FRACTURES OF THE SHAFT OF THE HUMERUS (FIG.13.14)

Introduction

The humeral shaft starts at the proximal metaphysis and ends at the distal metaphysis. It is worth noting here that humeral shaft fractures can injure the radial nerve in the spiral groove.

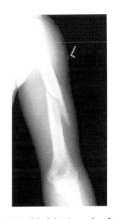

Fig.13.14. A spiral mid-shaft fracture of the humerus

CLASSIFICATION

A descriptive classification e.g. transverse, oblique, spiral, segmental, related to the part of the shaft involved will suffice for management purposes e.g. *"This is a spiral fracture of the left humerus in the middle one-third"*

MECHANISMS OF INJURY

Direct violence accounts for most of the fractures: direct blow or fall on the arm occurring in various circumstances, including road traffic accidents, sporting or construction site accidents. However, indirect forces such as are generated in falls on the outstretched hand can also cause fractures. Missile injuries are the commonest cause of open fractures.

DIAGNOSIS

This is usually easy. The history is often useful. Physical examination reveals bruises along the medial aspect of the arm and elbow; this is a characteristic sign. The shoulder and elbow areas should be examined to exclude associated injuries. Radial nerve function (wrist and finger extension) must be tested for. X-ray examination must also include the elbow and shoulder regions to exclude associated fractures. The possibility of a pathological fracture e.g. through a bone cyst or metastasis, should be borne in mind while examining the X-rays.

TREATMENT

- **Closed Reduction and Immobilisation.** Closed reduction is achievable in 95% of cases.

- **Gravity traction** in a *collar-and-cuff sling alone,* a *U-slab, hanging cast* or *functional cast-brace, supported with a collar-and-cuff sling.* Gravity traction has the weakness of being applicable only to the mobile patient. The patient must be advised not to rest the arm on anything before the achievement of reduction as this will nullify gravity and guarantee failure of this method of treatment. Other methods of treatment have to be used for patients who for one reason or the other (usually associated injuries, debilitating disease or old age) cannot be mobilised to allow gravity to act on the erect arm.

- **Use of external fixator.** High-energy comminuted or segmental fractures may need to be treated with external fixators

- **Open Reduction and Internal Fixation.** Indications for operative treatment include failure of non-operative methods of treatment, young age of patient, segmental fractures, bilateral humeral fractures, polytrauma and severe open fractures, especially if caused by missiles or if associated with major arterial injury. Fixation devices include the *plate and screws* (Figs.13.15 & 16) and *intramedullary nail.*

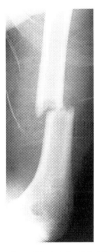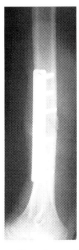

**Figs.13.15 & 16. Plate fixation of
a fracture of the humeral shaft.**

Exercises are an essential part of treatment. All free joints of the upper limb must be exercised actively from the start.

Treatment of Open Fractures

All wounds must be explored, if necessary, by extended skin incisions, and generously washed. Debridement is usually indicated. Prophylactic antibiotics should be given. *External fixation* may be indicated. After the danger of infection has been eliminated, definitive treatment is similar to that applied to closed fractures.

Treatment of Pathological Fractures

These are best treated with an intramedullary nail avoiding opening the fracture site for fear of spreading a malignant disease. Plate and screws can also be used. Union takes place without difficulty in most cases.

COMPLICATIONS

Radial nerve palsy is seen in 2 - 12% of cases. The palsy is usually a neurapraxia and is best treated by observation and exercise. Some surgeons recommend exploration if recovery does not occur by 6-8 weeks.

Delayed union (failure of union at 8 weeks) is common with transverse middle-third fractures. Distraction e.g. with a U-slab or a hanging cast predisposes to this. Further immobilisation usually allows union to occur.

Non-union (no union at 12 weeks) may follow delayed union. Treatment is by bone grafting and internal fixation with a plate or an intramedullary nail.

Shoulder and/or elbow stiffness may be associated if sufficient care is not been taken to prevent it by early exercise.

FRACTURES OF THE DISTAL HUMERUS

Fig.13.17. shows the normal anatomy of distal end of the humerus. The lateral trochlear ridge is the key landmark in analysing humeral condylar fractures.

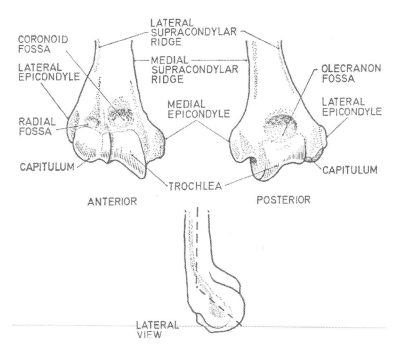

Fig.13.17. Normal anatomy of distal end of the humerus

SUPRACONDYLAR FRACTURES OF THE HUMERUS IN CHILDREN

A supracondylar fracture occurs at about the level of the beginning of the supracondylar ridges. Most supracondylar fractures occur in children, aged 6 to 15 years. Two types are classically recognised – *extension* and *flexion types*.

EXTENSION-TYPE SUPRACONDYLAR FRACTURE (FIG.13.18)

This is by far the more common type, accounting for about 95% of all supracondylar fractures. They are notorious for their:

- liability to injury of the brachial artery or median nerve by the sharp anterior end of the proximal fragment, which usually projects into the antecubital fossa and
- associated massive swelling of the elbow due to associated soft-tissue injury.

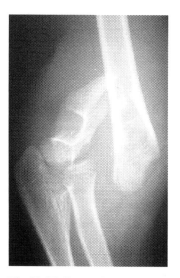

Fig.13.18. Extension type supracondylar humeral fracture in a 4-year-old boy.

Both of these predispose to neurovascular injury, which explains why, among many rural populations in Africa and India, these fractures constitute an important cause of amputation for gangrene secondary to unenlightened initial treatment by the traditional bonesetters.

MECHANISMS OF INJURY

The usual mechanism is an indirect force transmitted to the supracondylar area in a fall on the outstretched hand with the elbow bent. Falls from heights are also common. Direct force from hits with a stick or similar object can also cause the fracture.

DIAGNOSIS

The history of the causative injury is important because its magnitude is a pointer to the severity of associated soft-tissue injury. Pain, deformity (backward bend at the fracture site), swelling and loss of function are the usual features. The pulse should be checked in view of possible brachial artery injury; so also should *anterior interrosseus nerve function* (the pointing index finger sign): ask the child to make a fist – he can but the index finger remains straight due to paralysis of its flexors.

The lateral X-ray view is more informative than the AP: the distal fragment is displaced and tilted posteriorly. The AP view will show a grossly displaced fracture but may not show an undisplaced one.

TREATMENT

This consists of reduction, immobilisation and exercise. There are a number of methods of achieving these:

- **Closed manipulative reduction**
  Closed reduction by traction, counter-traction and manipulation is the first treatment option for a displaced fracture. If successful, an above-elbow POP backslab with the forearm in neutral is applied. If unsuccessful after three attempts, another method of treatment such as traction or open reduction should be considered.

- **Passive traction treatment**
  Reduction can be achieved by continuous skin traction with the elbow flexed to 90 degrees (Dunlop traction) or straight (Fig.13.20). The usual indication for this method of treatment is failure of manipulative reduction. Vigilant monitoring is necessary with this method as pressure sores can result from tight bandages at various points of excessive pressure. After reduction, immobilisation is achieved with an above-elbow P.O.P. backslab. Some surgeons use skeletal traction via a Kirschner wire inserted through the olecranon process. This method should be seen as a reserve one.

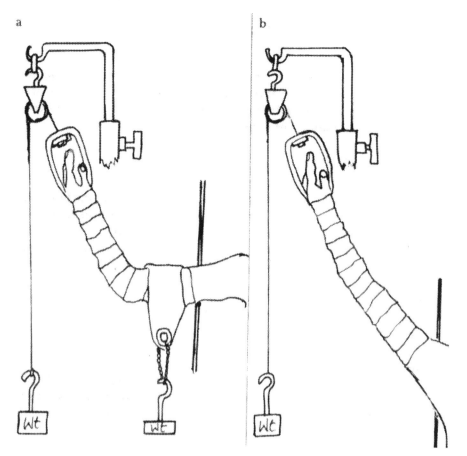

Fig.13.19. Reduction of supracondylar fractures by skin traction
a.   **Dunlop traction with the elbow bent**
b.   **Dunlop traction with elbow in full extension**

- **Closed Reduction and Percutaneous Pinning**
  This method is used in grossly unstable fractures and also if forearm fractures are present in the same limb. Kirschner wires or other suitable pin may be used (Fig.13.20). An image intensifier and powered tools are essential for this option.

- **Open Reduction and Internal Fixation(ORIF)**
  This method is available but is not recommended to the beginner in view of the real danger of injury to the median nerve and brachial artery during this procedure.

- **Exercises**
  Active finger exercises are necessary from the start and pendulum shoulder exercises can be started at one week. Elbow exercises are started as soon as immobilisation is discontinued at 4 weeks. Forced passive exercises must not be done.

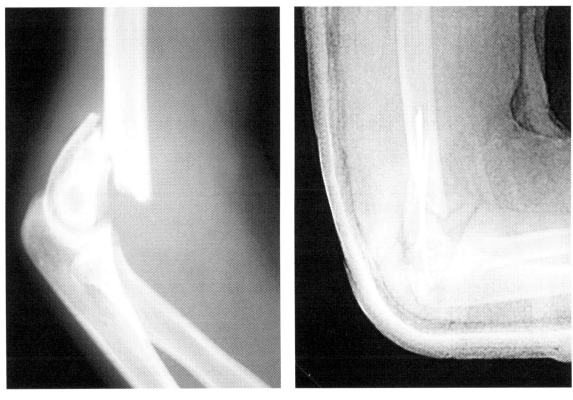

Fig.13.20a&b. Closed Reduction and percutaneous pinning

FLEXION-TYPE SUPRACONDYLAR FRACTURE (FIG.13.21)

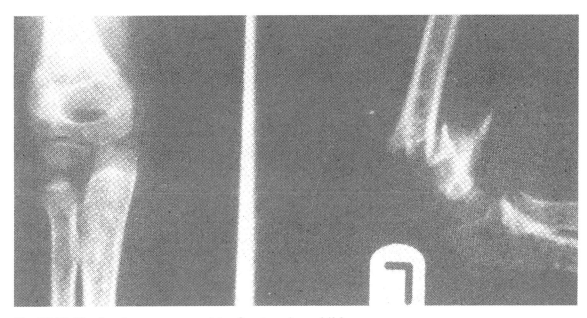

Fig. 13.21. Flexion-type supracondylar fracture in a child.

In common with the extension type, the flexion type is seen mainly in children. It is a rare injury, accounting for less than 5% of all supracondylar fractures. It can result directly from a hit on the distal humerus in the posterior to anterior direction or from transmitted force during a fall on the hand with the elbow fully extended.

Clinically, there is pain, swelling and deformity. The normal prominence of the point of the elbow (the olecranon) is absent. X-rays show the fracture line which is largely transverse on the AP view but oblique on the lateral.

Treatment is usually by reduction by traction, countertraction and straightening of the elbow to correct the anterior displacement and angulation. Since the anterior capsule and the collateral ligaments are usually intact, immobilisation with the elbow in full extension is stable; this is best achieved with a POP *front slab*.

Admission for one or two days for controlled elevation and neurological observation is advisable. The P.O.P. is removed at 3 weeks after which gradual active flexion of the elbow is encouraged.

Open reduction and percutaneous pinning can be carried out if closed reduction fails because of muscle interposition.

SUPRACONDYLAR FRACTURES IN ADULTS

Supracondylar fractures do occur in adults but are rare after the age of 20. The fracture tends to occur more proximally than in children. The clinical and X-ray features are similar. Closed reduction is carried out along lines similar to those described above but the adult elbow is much bigger and so much more difficult to manipulate. However, if operative treatment becomes necessary, the choice of internal devices is wider as considerations based on the need to protect the growth plates from damage do not apply.

COMPLICATIONS OF SUPRACONDYLAR HUMERAL FRACTURES

Early

Neurovascular injury is usually of the median nerve (anterior interosseus branch) (See above) and the brachial artery. Mild injury will probably recover with the treatment of the fracture. More serious injury requiring exploration is rare. Vascular surgical opinion should be sought if vascular compromise is suspected.

Gangrene of the arm was common in Nigeria following uninformed treatment by the so-called native/traditional doctors. Above-elbow amputation is the treatment.

Volkmann's ischaemia is a more specific complication of supracondylar fractures of the extension type. This has been discussed in more detail in Chapter 5.

Late

- *Myositis ossificans* may occur in susceptible individuals.
- *Elbow stiffness* can occur in the absence of myositis ossificans.
- *Mal-union* is a common complication arising from poor reduction of a fracture. Corrective osteotomy may be required towards the end of skeletal growth - at about 12 years of age.

FRACTURES OF THE HUMERAL CONDYLES

FRACTURE OF THE LATERAL CONDYLE

MECHANISMS AND CLASSIFICATION

This classical childhood fracture includes the capitulum and the lateral epicondyle. It usually arises from a fall on the hand in which the radial head or the lateral articular portion of the ulna is rammed against the lateral humeral condyle, causing a fracture. Direct forces on the posterior aspect of a flexed elbow can also cause it.

Diagnosis

Clinically the angle between the longitudinal axis of the humerus and that of the ulna, termed the carrying angle, is usually lost (normal 10 degrees). There is pain, swelling and tenderness, mainly on the lateral aspect of the elbow. The lateral condyle can be moved independently of the rest of the humerus but this should not be attempted for fear of displacing an undisplaced fracture. X-rays will show the fracture line. It should be noted that in the growing bone, a seemingly tiny flake of bone broken off the condyle may represent a sizeable osteocartilaginous fragment (Fig.13.22).

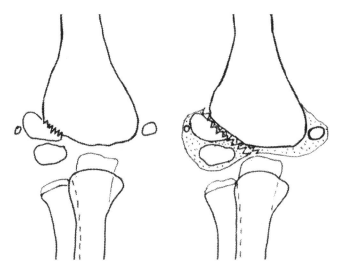

Fig.13.22. A seemingly tiny flake of bone broken off the condyle may represent a sizeable osteocartilaginous fragment

Treatment

An undisplaced fracture should be treated by immobilisation in an above-elbow P.O.P cast with the elbow slightly flexed, the forearm pronated and the wrist slightly flexed to relax the wrist flexors. A displaced fracture is best treated by open reduction and internal fixation, which offers the best chance of restoring a smooth articular surface (Fig.13.23).

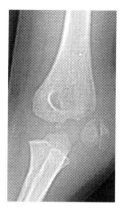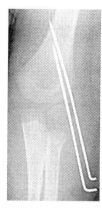

Fig.13.23a&b. Fracture of the lateral humeral condyle in a child: open reduction and K-wire fixation was necessary in the case shown here. Note the abnormal vertical orientation of the epiphyseal plate in the pre-reduction film.

Complications

Mal-union. This occurs mainly with non-operative treatment. The lateral condylar fragment is prone to displacing proximally and this can cause cubitus valgus with possible tardy (delayed) ulnar nerve palsy.

Non-Union sometimes occurs and can also cause cubitus valgus and tardy ulnar palsy.

FRACTURE OF THE MEDIAL CONDYLE

MECHANISMS AND CLASSIFICATION

A medial condylar fracture includes the trochlear and medial epichondyle. It is less frequently fractured than the lateral condyle. The mechanism is a fall on the arm in which the head of the radius or the trochlear surface of the ulna hits against the medial condyle, fracturing it. Direct forces can also cause the fracture.

Diagnosis

The patient complains of pain, swelling and inability to bend the elbow. A specific finding is tenderness on the medial aspect of the elbow. Ulnar nerve function must be tested for. X-rays are vital in confirming the fracture type.

Treatment

An undisplaced fracture should be treated by immobilisation in an above-elbow POP cast with the elbow slightly flexed, the forearm pronated and the wrist slightly flexed to relax the wrist flexors.

A displaced fracture is best treated by open reduction and internal fixation, which offers the best chance of restoring a smooth articular surface.

Complications

Mal-union can occur with resulting *cubitus varus*. Associated joint incongruity results in *post-traumatic osteoarthritis*.

Late ulnar nerve palsy may occur if the groove is roughened as a result of the fracture.

FRACTURE OF THE MEDIAL EPICONDYLE

Mechanism of injury

The medial epicondyle begins to ossify at the age of 5 and fuses to the rest of the bone from the age of 16. However, this fusion does not occur in some adults and this must be borne in mind. X-ray the other elbow for comparison! Most medial epicondylar fractures are avulsion fractures. The usual mechanism is avulsion during a posterior dislocation of the elbow. In many cases, the epicondylar fragment is carried into the elbow joint and remains there even after reduction has occurred spontaneously or by manipulation. In adults, direct blows are an important mechanism and part of the medial condyle may be included in the epicondylar fragment.

Diagnosis

The diagnosis is easier if the elbow is still dislocated. If not, the specific finding is local tenderness. A neurological examination should be carried out to exclude ulnar nerve entrapment. On AP X-ray, the epicondyle is seen lying distally near the joint line (due to pull of the wrist flexors). On the lateral view, the epicondyle may be seen lying in the joint.

Treatment

An undisplaced or a minimally displaced fracture can be treated with a crepe bandage and a sling for support. With a fragment trapped in the joint, manipulation may fail and open reduction and fixation of the fragment to its place should be carried out. The ulnar nerve should be safeguarded during this operation.

There is no consensus on how best a displaced fracture should be treated. Some surgeons advocate open reduction and internal fixation, in order to prevent non-union; others have shown that no significant ill-effect results from the non-union. The author identifies with the latter group, believing that any operative treatment that does not have a distinct advantage over non-operative methods should not be used and certainly cannot be advocated for the developing countries with limited resources.

T AND Y- SHAPED CONDYLAR FRACTURES

T- and Y-shaped condylar fractures, unlike those described so far, occur mainly in adults. They are serious injuries because they are intra-articular and inherently unstable. Fortunately, they are rare. Most of the fractures are considered to result from the splitting wedge-like action of the proximal ulnar articular surface on the trochlear of the humerus during a fall on the hand. Some probably result from a similar action of the lower end of the humerus against the ulnar articular surface. Direct blows from various objects can also be responsible.

Diagnosis

Pain, swelling and bruising is severe. Specific physical findings are the ability to separate the condyles fairly easily by digital pressure and the ability to push the ulna proximally (telescoping) between the condyles. These manoeuvres are however very painful and are best avoided. X-rays are vital; they show details of the fractures without which a rational treatment cannot be carried out.

Treatment

Available treatment options include the following:

- Simple above-elbow cast immobilisation for two weeks followed by mobilisaton exercises is indicated for undisplaced fractures.

- **Manipulative reduction followed by immobilisation for 3 weeks**

- **Treatment by early motion**
  This is used for the highly comminuted type of fracture. In essence, the fracture is ignored, the arm is placed in a collar-and-cuff sling only and movement of the elbow is encouraged from the start. The shoulder, wrist and fingers are also exercised from the start. This is otherwise called the 'bag of bones' technique. It is found that the fragments align reasonably well due to the effect of gravity and active movements and that the final range of movements is satisfactory.

- **Open Reduction and Internal Fixation**
  There are many surgeons who believe that this is the best way to treat these fractures.

Complications

These include possible immediate *nerve injury* to neighbouring nerves - ulnar, median or radial nerve. *Mal-union* and *post-traumatic osteoarthritis* also occur.

Further reading

Konstantinos Kazakos, Stamatis Paraschou, Nikolaos G Lasanianos, Dionysios Verettas and **Dimitrios N Lyras.** A humeral shaft fracture complicated with anterior shoulder dislocation in a young male treated with modified Intramedullary nailing prior to reduction: a case report. *Cases Journal,* **2**:9075 doi:10.1186/1757-1626-2-9075, 2009.

CHAPTER 14

INJURIES OF THE ELBOW AND FOREARM

DISLOCATIONS OF THE ELBOW

In incidence, dislocations of the elbow come third among all the major dislocations - after those of the shoulder, patella and and finger joints. It is more frequent in children than in adults, presumably because the joint is less stable in the former group due to incompletely developed coronoid and olecranon processes.

CLASSIFICATION

Dislocations of both the radius and ulna
Posterior
Anterior
Lateral
Medial
Divergent

Dislocation of the radius alone
Anterior
Posterior
Lateral

Dislocation of the ulna alone
Anterior
Posterior

Comment: Posterior and lateral dislocations are common, accounting for up to 90% of all elbow dislocations. All the other varieties, including isolated dislocations of either the radius or the ulna are rare.

POSTERIOR DISLOCATION OF THE ELBOW (FIG.14.1)

MECHANISM OF INJURY

The usual mechanism is a fall on the outstretched hand with the arm in extension and abduction. Posterior elbow dislocation involves extensive tearing of surrounding soft tissues, which accounts for the characteristic elbow swelling and for certain complications such as myositis ossificans and elbow stiffness.

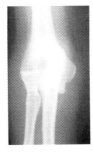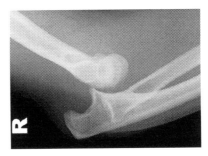

Fig.14.1a&b. Posterior dislocation of the elbow – AP and lateral views

DIAGNOSIS

Clinical diagnosis is easier in early presentation when massive swelling has not yet set in. The patient usually holds the elbow in flexion, the forearm is shortened, the antecubital fossa is full due to the presence of the humeral condyles there, the olecranon process is unduly prominent and the normal equidistant relationship of the olecranon to the humeral epicondyles is distorted. The neurovascular status must also be ascertained.

X-rays confirm the diagnosis, showing the position of the proximal ulna and radius (posterior, postero-lateral, or posteromedial) as well as associated fractures, if present.

TREATMENT

Reduction can be effected under general or intravenous anaesthesia by pulling on the slightly flexed elbow against counter-traction, correcting lateral or medial displacement with one hand and finally returning the coronoid process to its place with further traction, flexion and local finger pressure. Open reduction is resorted to if closed reduction fails (after three attempts), usually due to associated fractures of the distal humerus. Such fractures are best treated by ORIF.

Immobilisation in a collar-and-cuff sling with the elbow flexed beyond 90 degrees usually suffices. Hospital admission for controlled elevation of the arm or for monitoring of the stability/instability of the elbow is advised in children. Immobilisation should not normally exceed 2-3 weeks as disabling stiffness of the elbow joint is a real threat in this injury. Active movement of the shoulder, wrist and finger joints must be started immediately while active exercises of the elbow are encouraged as soon as immobilisation is discontinued.

ANTERIOR DISLOCATION OF THE ELBOW

Two types of this injury are distinguished. Both occur secondary to a blow to the posterior aspect of a flexed elbow.

Type I. A true anterior dislocation in which the olecranon finally comes to lie on the anterior aspect of the distal humerus. This type is very rare.

Type II. A fracture-dislocation in which an anterior dislocation of the elbow has been made possible by a fracture of the olecranon (*Hume fracture*) (Fig.14.2). This type is also rare.

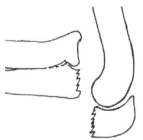

Fig.14.2. Type II anterior dislocation of the elbow (the Hume fracture-dislocation).

Clinically, the forearm appears lengthened and is held in supination with the elbow in full extension. The antecubital fossa is full and massive elbow swelling may be present. In Type I injury, the usually prominent point of the olecranon is absent.

X-rays show the type of dislocation in a given case and are essential for correct treatment. In Type I dislocation, traction and backward pressure on the proximal forearm usually easily achieve reduction. In Type II injury, open reduction and internal fixation of the olecranon fracture effects reduction of the dislocation and is the best method of treatment.

THE PULLED ELBOW

The pulled elbow is a subluxation of the radial head in a small child occasioned by the entrapment of the head in the orbicular ligament. The mechanism is a pull of the child's arm, usually by a parent, in an attempt to lift him or her over an obstacle. The child cries out in pain, there is local tenderness over the radial head and rotation of the forearm is painful and almost impossible. The X-rays appear normal. Reduction should be carried out under a general anaesthetic - by forcible supination and then flexion of the elbow. This is followed by rest in a sling for a few days.

LATERAL DISLOCATION OF THE ELBOW

In this variety, the radial head and the trochlear notch are displaced laterally so that the latter comes to articulate with capitulotrochlear sulcus of the humerus. In this position, some elbow flexion and extension are still possible and as there is no evidence of posterior or anterior dislocation, the unwary may be fooled. X-rays will give out the diagnosis. Longitudinal traction and direct medialward pressure on the radial head can achieve reduction.

MEDIAL DISLOCATION OF THE ELBOW

The shift of the proximal radius and ulna here is opposite to the seen in the lateral variety. Similarly, some flexion and extension are possible. Reduction can be achieved by direct thumb pressure on the medial aspect of the joint.

DIVERGENT DISLOCATION OF THE ELBOW

This rare injury is described as "divergent" because the radius and ulna are made to go in opposite directions by the lower end of the humerus which becomes wedged between them.

Clinically, the anteroposterior type resembles the usual posterior dislocation, except that the radial head can be felt anteriorly in the antecubital fossa. Closed reduction is usually not difficult; this is followed by immobilisation of the elbow in flexion with the forearm in supination – for one to two weeks, followed by mobilisation.

ISOLATED DISLOCATION OF THE RADIAL HEAD

Usually, dislocation of the radial head is associated with fractures of the proximal ulna (*Montaggia fracture-dislocation*). Isolated dislocation is a rare injury, which has been reported mainly in children. The radial head may finally come to lie anteriorly, posteriorly or laterally.

The dislocation can be reduced by direct pressure with the forearm in supination. Immobilisation is effected in a P.O.P. backslab with the elbow in neutral rotation and flexed to 90 degrees - for 2-3 weeks. If reduction is unstable, open reduction and internal fixation using Kirschner wires may be considered. However, the choice is a bad one because soft-tissue dissection around the radial neck may injure the posterior interosseous nerve or predispose to further instability of the radial head.

The surgeon should remember the existence of a congenital type of dislocation of the radial head. Even if there is concomitant trauma, the X-ray gives away this condition: the radial head is dome-shaped, instead of being socket-shaped - from lack of pressure from the capitulum.

ISOLATED DISLOCATION OF THE ULNA

This injury does occur. The proximal ulna may come to rest posteriorly or anteriorly. Diagnosis and treatment should follow lines described earlier in this section for a similar injury of the radius.

UNREDUCED/LATE-DIAGNOSED ELBOW DISLOCATION

Rare in the developed countries, this situation is quite common in Africa, India and other developing countries. Several weeks, months or even years after "successful treatment" by the so-called native doctor, a patient, usually a child, may present with this diagnosis. The elbow is totally stiff (straight) and X-rays may show either complete dislocation or incomplete reduction showing as a sideways displacement of the olecranon process.

Treatment will depend on how old the dislocation is. Up to 6 weeks after injury, manipulative reduction can still be attempted. Between 6 and 12 weeks, the so-called sham reduction can be attempted: under general anaesthesia, the elbow is manipulated into some flexion and exercises are encouraged. A reasonable range of movements is obtained in some patients by this method. Some authors have reported good results with open reduction followed by temporary K-wire stabilisation in children. Elbow arthroplasty could be considered in older patients.

COMPLICATIONS OF ELBOW DISLOCATION

- *Neurovascular injury.* Injury to neighbouring blood vessels (*brachial artery*) and nerves (*median, ulnar, anterior interosseus and radial*) is rare. Nerve injury is usually a neurapraxia, which recovers spontaneously.

- *Compartment syndrome:* this may result from associated massive swelling. This must be looked out for and dealt with if present.

- *Radial head fracture:* reduction of the dislocation takes precedence. if a satisfactory reduction of the radial head fracture does not occur at the same time, most surgeons advocate early excision of the radial head. This topic is further treated under fractures of the radial head.

- *Condylar fractures of the humerus.:* posterior dislocation may be associated with lateral or medial humeral condylar fracture. Such a dislocation tends to be unstable after reduction. Internal fixation of the condyles may be necessary to restore stability.

- *Recurrent dislocation.* This is usually due to loose fracture fragments in the joint or to torn capsule and collateral ligaments. The loose bodies need to be removed and damage to ligaments needs to be repaired.

- *Myositis ossificans (Heterotopic calcification)* is a common complication following elbow dislocations, especially with associated fractures of neighbouring bones. It shows up at about 3-4 weeks after injury. Prophylactic Indomethacin given for 6 weeks, when not contraindicated, may reduce the incidence of myositis ossificans.

FRACTURES OF THE RADIAL HEAD

About 5-10% of elbow dislocations are associated with a radial head fracture. This fracture is common in adults but rare in children. Four types of radial head fractures are recognised, based on the Mason classification (Fig.14.3):

Type I :   Undisplaced or minimally displaced fracture (less than 2 mm).
Type II: Displaced fracture (marginal or segmental) greater than 2 mm or 30 degrees of angulation.
Type III: Comminuted fracture involving the whole head.

Type IV: Fracture of the radial head associated with dislocation of the elbow (usually posterior).

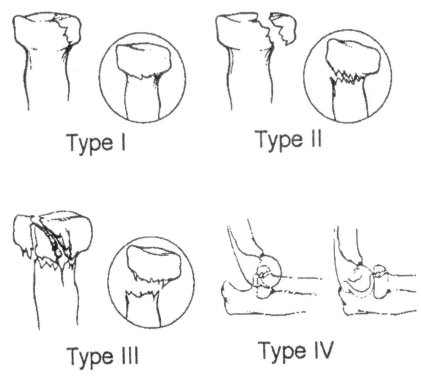

Fig.14.3. The Mason classification of radial head fractures (Broberg & Morrey, 1987).

DIAGNOSIS

The fractures occur when the radial head strikes against the capitulum. This can happen in falls on the outstretched hand with the elbow in valgus strain. Direct hits can also be responsible. The description of the fall may aid diagnosis. There is localised tenderness over the radial head and there is limitation of pronation, supination and particularly extension. Some undisplaced fractures fail to show up on X-rays, leading to diagnostic mistakes. This should be borne in mind; special views or a CT scan may be necessary.

TREATMENT

The treatment depends on the severity of the injury. Undisplaced fractures do well in a collar-and-cuff sling for 3-4 weeks. Mason Type II fractures involving less than one-quarter of the articular surface may also be similarly treated. Mason Type II fractures involving more than one-quarter of the articular surface are best treated by open reduction and screw fixation.

Mason Type III comminuted fractures are treated differently by different surgeons. Conservative management, open reduction and internal fixation, simple excision, excision and prosthetic replacement, and temporary stabilisation with a hinged external fixator have all been used.

Mason Type IV injury: the elbow dislocation is first reduced, followed by ORIF or excision plus or minus prosthetic replacement of the radial head.

COMPLICATIONS

These include:

- *Elbow dislocation* following this injury has been mentioned above.
- Tear and disruption of the interosseous membrane and dislocation of the distal radioulnar joint. This injury complex is called the *Essex-Lopresti fracture-dislocation*.
- *Myositis ossificans* and *elbow joint stiffness* also occur.

Contentious issues in the management of radial head injuries include the need (or otherwise) for *aspiration of the elbow* and the *timing of excision of the radial head*, if indicated. Some surgeons favour early aspiration claiming that it relieves pain, which can be considerable in the more severe fractures. It is the author's view that this issue needs not be overflogged as there is no significant difference in the outcome using the two methods. If joint aspiration is chosen, it must be done under strictly aseptic conditions. Regarding the timing of radial head excision when indicated, the choice is between early and delayed.

FRACTURE OF THE RADIAL NECK

This occurs more commonly in children than adults. As with fracture of the radial head, the mechanism of injury is often a fall on the outstretched hand with the elbow in extension and forearm in pronation. Clinically, there is localised tenderness and painful limitation of rotation. X-rays reveal the finer features of the fracture.

An undisplaced fracture is rested in a collar-and-cuff sling for 3-4 weeks, followed by exercises. In a child, fracture displaced up to 30 degrees is accepted. In an adult, a displaced fracture is reduced by longitudinal traction on the forearm and local digital pressure on the radial head to correct the deformities and immobilised as above. For grossly displaced fractures, closed reduction is virtually impossible and open reduction and internal fixation or excision of the fragments is advised.

FRACTURES OF THE CORONOID

These are usually caused by forced hyperextension of the elbow and are seen in 10-30% of elbow dislocations. Because of the important role of the coronoid in elbow stability, they can lead to significant elbow instability.

Three types are distinguished:

Type I: Fracture of intra-articular tip of the coronoid process (stable)
Type II: Fracture involving <50% of the coronoid (may be unstable)
Type III: Fracture involving >50% of the coronoid (unstable injury)

Type I injury is treated in the same way as elbow dislocation, with early mobilisation unless symptoms of a loose body develop. Type II is treated as Type I, if stable and by ORIF, if unstable. Type III injury is treated by ORIF. External fixation may be required for a grossly comminuted fracture; fragment excision is not advised.

FRACTURES OF THE OLECRANON

CLASSIFICATION AND MECHANISMS

The Colton classification distinguishes the following types:

Type I. *Undisplaced fracture.* This is usually a transverse fracture commonly due to a violent contraction of the triceps. The olecranon fragment may be large or small.

Type II. *Displaced fracture.* This can also be due to a violent contraction of the triceps and the olecranon fragment may be large or small. It may also be due to direct violence in a posterior to anterior direction, in which case the distal fragment together with the proximal radius may displace anteriorly, giving rise to an anterior fracture-dislocation of the elbow (*Hume fracture*). A minimally displaced comminuted fracture may result from a direct blow or fall on the point of the elbow.

Type III. Oblique and transverse fractures from indirect trauma

Type IV. Comminuted fractures from direct trauma

Type V. Fracture-dislocations from severe trauma

Diagnosis

Fractures of the olecranon can be diagnosed easily. There is usually a tell-tale bruise on the elbow, localised tenderness and limitation of elbow movements, especially extension. X-rays elucidate the nature of a given fracture. In a child, the epiphyseal growth plate must be borne in mind. Similarly, the existence of such abnormalities as the bifid olecranon epiphysis and the patella cubiti should also be remembered. In general, the severity of the injury and the physical findings should tally with the X-ray findings.

Treatment (Fig.14.4)

The treatment depends on the type of fracture and the age of the patient.

- *For an undisplaced transverse fracture:* above-elbow P.O.P. or fibre-glass cast is suitable. Immobilisation is retained for 3 - 4 weeks.

- *For a displaced transverse fracture:* (a) ORIF by tension-band wiring (b) fixation with a hook plate (c) fixation with a single screw.

- *Small fragment excision* may be indicated in a young patient with a fracture involving less than one-third of the articular surface.

- *Major fragment excision plus repair of the triceps* is indicated for a comminuted fracture;

alternatively, early exercises is commenced with the aim of regaining as much motion as possible.

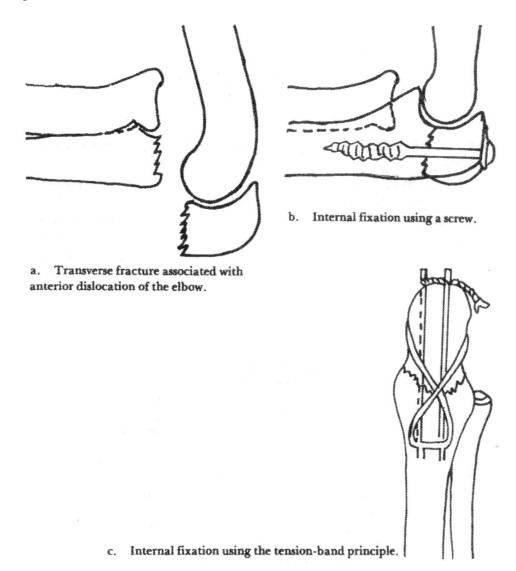

b. Internal fixation using a screw.

a. Transverse fracture associated with anterior dislocation of the elbow.

c. Internal fixation using the tension-band principle.

Fig.14.4. Methods of Treatment of olecranon fractures: figure-of-8 tension-band wiring and screw fixation

COMPLICATIONS

The main complications are:

- *stiffness, especially restricted elbow extension.* This can be prevented or minimised by instituting early exercises irrespective of the method of treatment adopted.
- *Decreased power of extension* may result from triceps tendon elongation.
- *Non-union* is reported in about 5% of cases.
- *Metal prominence or protrusion.* is the most common complication of operative treatment.

THE SIDE-SWIPE FRACTURE-DISLOCATION OF THE ELBOW

Classically, this injury consists of comminuted fractures of the proximal ulna and radius, fractures of the distal end of the humerus and anterior dislocation of the elbow. It is called a sideswipe injury because it is classically sustained when a car driver's elbow sticking out of the car is struck by another car. The "bag of bones" technique is probably the best treatment option. Elbow arthroplasty could be considered later.

FRACTURES OF THE RADIUS AND ULNA

A brief revision of the anatomy of the forearm, especially that of the radius and ulna and the relationship between them, will significantly facilitate the understanding of this topic and make it more interesting. The proximal and distal radioulnar joints, which are essential for the rotational movements (supination and pronation) of the forearm, are liable to be disrupted in isolated fracture of either bone. The aim of treatment, be it surgical or non-surgical, is to restore and maintain the anatomical relationships between the radius and ulna so that the functions of pronation and supination of the forearm are not compromised.

FRACTURES OF BOTH THE RADIUS AND THE ULNA

MECHANISMS OF INJURY

These fractures are seen in both children and adults. Direct injury to the forearm is perhaps the commonest cause of fractures of both bones. These fractures occur at the same level and may be *two-fragment* or *comminuted*, *open or closed*, depending on the injuring force and the circumstances. Road traffic accidents, blows from sticks, and rough plays at school are sources of direct injury. Indirect injuries such as twisting forces transmitted to the bones during falls on the outstretched hand are also frequent causes of these fractures but the bones tend to fracture at different levels in this mechanism. Gunshot injuries are a special type of direct injury, which cause a lot of associated soft-tissue injury. These are fortunately rare.

CLASSIFICATIONS

Descriptive classification

The descriptive classification discussed in Chapter 9 is normally used for radial and ulnar fractures. The diaphysis (shaft) is divided into thirds – *proximal, middle and distal thirds* and the fractures occurring in them are further described according to their nature. A sample description will run as follows: "This is a fracture of the right radius and ulna in the middle one-third. The radial fracture is transverse and undisplaced; the ulnar fracture is also transverse but grossly displaced".

The **AO classification** is reproduced here but has been shown to have a high degree of inter-observer variability.

Type A   Simple fracture, diaphyseal
      A1 Ulna simple, radius intact
      A2 Radius simple, ulna intact
      A3 Radius and ulna, simple

Type B   Wedge fracture, diaphyseal
      B1 Ulna wedge, radius intact
      B2 Radius wedge, ulna intact
      B3 Wedge of radius or ulna, simple or wedge of other

Type C   Complex fracture, diaphyseal
      C1 Ulna complex, simple or wedge of radius
      C2 Radius complex, simple or wedge of ulna
      C1 Complex of both radius and ulna

DIAGNOSIS

The patient, if mobile, usually walks in holding the injured arm with the normal one. There is a wound if the fractures are compound. Pain is severe and aggravated by any movement at the fracture sites. Signs of possible vascular or nerve damage should be sought. Swelling is also present. Ideally the forearm should be splinted with a suitable splint and analgesics should be given before the patient is sent for X-rays.

X-rays show the characteristics of the fractures. Greenstick fractures are common in children. In adults, gross deformities - overlapping, angulation and rotation - are common. A segmental fracture of either bone may also occur.

NON-OPERATIVE TREATMENT

Non-surgical treatment should be tried initially in all cases except in compound fractures in which a wound toilet necessarily has to be carried out immediately.

Children. Closed reduction is easily achieved in a child with greenstick fractures where the deformity consists only of angulation. Reduction is usually stable and moderate angulatory deformities correct with healing and further growth at the rate of about one degree per month, so, a 30-degrees of angulation in a 5-year-old child need not be manipulated.

Adults. Manipulative reduction is less successful in adults but should be tried before resorting to surgery.

Maintenance of reduction is achieved with a long arm P.O.P. fibreglass/polythene cast with the elbow at 90 degrees and forearm in full supination for proximal one-third fractures, mid-supination for middle one-third fractures and full pronation for distal one-third fractures. This is to counter the pull of pronator teres.

The cast should be split to avoid excessive tightness. Immobilisation is retained for 4 weeks in children with spiral or long oblique fractures or for 6 weeks for short oblique and transverse fractures. In adults, immobilisation should be maintained for 6 weeks for spiral or long oblique fractures and 12 weeks for short oblique or transverse fractures.

During immobilisation, shoulder and finger joints exercises are encouraged. Also, check X-rays should be done weekly during the first 2 weeks as late slips are quite common. After the removal of the cast, elbow and forearm movements are regained by physiotherapy. Children naturally regain movements more quickly than adults.

OPERATIVE TREATMENT

The accurate reduction required to ensure good to excellent functional results following concomitant radial and ulnar fractures is seldom achieved by closed reduction. Poor functional results due to mal-union, delayed union, non-union and disruptions of the radioulnar joints have led many surgeons to opt for ORIF. On the other hand, poor facilities in the developing countries make ORIF of these fractures difficult and sometimes unwise.

The operative options available are:

(a) *Compression plating* of each fracture via a separate incision is favoured in both adults and children.
(b) *Intra-medullary nailing* e.g. using Nantes nails, is currently popular for children's fractures.

COMPLICATIONS

Excessive forearm swelling arising per se or as a result of tight casts can cause *Volkmann's ischaemia*. The other complications include *mal-union, delayed union, non-union* and *cross-union*. Restriction of forearm rotation could result from injury to or malalignment of the radioulnar joints or from cross-union. *Nerve injury* is more frequently caused by surgery than by the fractures themselves.

MONTEGGIA FRACTURE-DISLOCATION

In 1814, Monteggia described an injury complex consisting of a fracture of the ulna in the proximal one-third and an anterior dislocation of the radial head. Since then similar injuries consisting of proximal ulnar fractures and dislocations of the radial head in directions other than the anterior direction have been described and Bado has provided a classification encompassing various so-called Montaggia fractures:

BADO CLASSIFICATION OF MONTEGGIA FRACTURES

Type I.   Proximal ulnar fracture, *angulated anteriorly*, with anterior dislocation of the radial head. This is the classical Monteggia fracture-dislocation and constitutes about 60% of all Monteggia-type lesions.

Type II. Proximal ulnar fracture *angulated posteriorly*, with posterior or posterolateral dislocation of the radial head (15%)

Type III. Proximal ulnar fracture, with lateral or anterolateral dislocation of the radial head (20%).

Type IV. Proximal ulnar and radial fracture, with anterior dislocation of the radial head (5%).

DIAGNOSIS

In spite of well-defined characteristics, missed and late diagnosis continue to be recorded. A high index of suspicion needs to be applied to increase the rate of immediate diagnosis. Common to all the types are pain, tenderness and marked inability to carry out any elbow movements. Specific signs are the position of the radial head and the angulation of the ulnar fracture which varies, depending on the type of lesion. Posterior interosseus nerve palsy may occur, so its functions should be tested before and after surgery. X-rays are essential to elucidate the type of lesion and therefore aid manipulative reduction.

TREATMENT

Closed reduction is almost always successful in children; traction and supination of the forearm are the key manoeuvres. It may be unsuccessful in adults. For good functional recovery, it is important that both the ulnar fracture and the dislocated radial head are reduced. Immobilisation is achieved with an above-elbow P.O.P. cast with the forearm in full supination. Clinical union can be expected in 6 weeks in a child and 12 in an adult.

Open reduction and internal fixation by compression plating is indicated if closed reduction is unsuccessful. Closed reduction may, however, be unsuccessful in some children and most adults. Sometimes, the radial head is unstable after reduction. If so, it should be stabilised with a Kirschner wire for 2-3 weeks. Immobilisation in plaster after internal fixation is still advised. The elbow should be in 90-100 degrees of flexion and the forearm in mid-supination.

Complications

These are the same as occur in fractures of both forearm bones. Full recovery of a posterior interosseous nerve palsy usually occurs.

OTHER FRACTURES OF THE ULNAR SHAFT

The *nightstick fracture* is an example of a fracture of the proximal ulna from a direct blow, so-called because it was first described in victims of police night-stick beatings. If undisplaced (which is usually the case), such a fracture can be adequately treated in an above-elbow cast with the elbow flexed beyond 90 degrees and the forearm in mid-supination, but the possibility of late slip should be borne in mind. Other isolated ulnar shaft fractures can be treated in the same way Displaced fractures are probably best treated by ORIF or intramedullary nailing, especially if there is associated radioulnar joint disruption.

ISOLATED FRACTURES OF THE RADIAL SHAFT

An isolated fracture can occur at any point on the shaft but one of the best known examples is the so-called Galeazzi fracture-dislocation.

GALEAZZI FRACTURE-DISLOCATION

This is an injury complex comprising a fracture of the radius in the distal one-third and a dislocation of the *distal radio-ulnar joint (DRUJ)*. This occurs more frequently than the Montaggia fracture dislocation.

DIAGNOSIS

The usual history is that of a fall on the outstretched hand. There is pain, swelling and tenderness in the distal one-third of the forearm and the patient is unable to supinate the hand. X-rays show a displaced and angulated transverse or short oblique fracture of the radius in the distal one-third and a dislocation of the distal radioulnar joint.

TREATMENT

The most important consideration in the treatment of this injury is the need to obtain a satisfactory reduction of the dislocated inferior radioulnar joint in order to ensure recovery of forearm rotation. Happily, this usually occurs spontaneously with the reduction of the radial fracture (Fig.14.5).

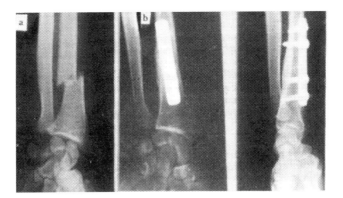

Fig.14.5. Galeazzi fracture-dislocation in an adult

Closed manipulative reduction of the radial fracture should always be attempted. It is often successful in children but less so in adults. A reduced fracture should be immobilised in a long arm cast with the forearm in full supination to stabilise the DRUJ.

Open reduction and internal fixation by compression plating is resorted to if closed reduction fails. Stability of the reduced DRUJ should always be tested. Occasionally, a K-wire through the joint for 4-6 weeks may be required to maintain reduction. An untreated or badly treated Galeazzi lesion may be complicated by wrist pain. In this situation, excision of the ulnar head may give relief.

TREATMENT OF OPEN FRACTURES

Occasionally, fractures of the radius and ulna are open but as the "compounding" is usually from within rather than without, wound contamination is minimal. Gustilo types I, II and IIIA fractures require primary wound toilet and debridement, prophylactic broad-spectrum antibiotics and internal fixation by compression plating. The more severe injury, Types IIIB or IIIC can be treated by internal or external fixation depending on the condition of the soft tissues and whether or not there is bone loss. External fixation is best achieved with an external fixator although only about two-thirds of the patients have good to excellent results.

COMPLICATIONS OF RADIAL AND ULNAR FRACTURES

- *Compounding* has just been mentioned.

- *Nerve injuries* may occur. The posterior interosseus nerve gets injured in 20% of Monteggia fracture-dislocations. Injury to other nerves is rare. *Vascular injuries may also occur.*

- *Volkmann-type muscle ischaemia* can result from excessive forearm swelling arising per se or exacerbated by tight plaster casts.

- *Other complications* include *mal-union, delayed union, non-union* and *cross-union (3%).* Restriction of forearm rotation could result from injury or mal-alignment of the radio-ulnar joints or cross-union.

DISTAL RADIAL FRACTURES (DRFS)

These are fractures occurring about 4-5 cm from the wrist joint line. They have a bimodal age distribution: (a) in the young in whom they result from high energy injuries such as road traffic and sporting accidents and (b) in the elderly in whom they result from trivial accidents such falls at home or in the street. They form a wide spectrum of fractures ranging from the simple fractures requiring minimal management to the complex multifragmental ones posing serious management problems.

About 50% of distal radial fractures are associated with significant soft-tissue injuries, including injuries to the scapholunate ligament, the lunotriquetral ligament and the triangular fibrocartilage complex (TFCC). The best-known distal radial fractures have eponyms – Colles', Smith's, Barton's and chauffeur's fractures.

CLASSIFICATIONS

Descriptive classifications

Distal radial fractures can be classified descriptively as

- *open or closed*
- *extra-articular* or *intra-articular*

- *displaced or undisplaced*
- *angulated or unangulated*
- *comminuted or uncomminuted*

Frykman's classification is one of the more simple and popular amongst the more complicated classifications (Fig.14.6):

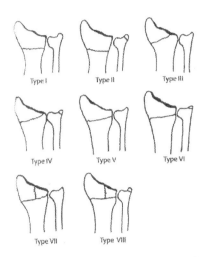

Fig.14.6. Frykman's classification of distal radial fractures (Frykman, 1967).

Type I	Extra-articular fracture without a fracture of the ulnar styloid
Type II	Extra-articular fracture with a fracture of the ulnar styloid
Type III	Radiocarpal joint fracture without a fracture of the ulnar styloid
Type IV	Radiocarpal joint fracture with a fracture of the ulnar styloid
Type V	Radioulnar joint fracture without a fracture of the ulnar styloid
Type VI	Radioulnar joint fracture with a fracture of the ulnar styloid
Type VII	Radiocarpal and radioulnar joint fracture without a fracture of the ulnar styloid
Type III	Radiocarpal and radioulnar joint fracture with a fracture of the ulnar styloid

COLLES' FRACTURE

Colles' fracture was accurately described by Professor Colles of Dublin in 1814, long before the advent of X-rays. Characterised by the diner-fork deformity, it is a fracture of the distal radius about 2.5 cm from the wrist joint line, with dorsal displacement of the distal fragment and an avulsion fracture of the ulnar styloid.

MECHANISMS OF INJURY

Colles' fracture is usually a low energy injury generated by falls on the outstretched hand with the forearm pronated but high energy injuries and direct forces can also cause it.

DIAGNOSIS

The usual patient is past the age of 50 and female. There is a history of fall on the outstretched hand or of a more severe injury. The patient complains of pain, deformity and inability to move the hand at the wrist. Physical examination reveals a characteristic dinner-fork deformity (Fig.14.7). There are also localised bruising, swelling and tenderness as well as an inability to effect active movements at the wrist and finger without undue pain.

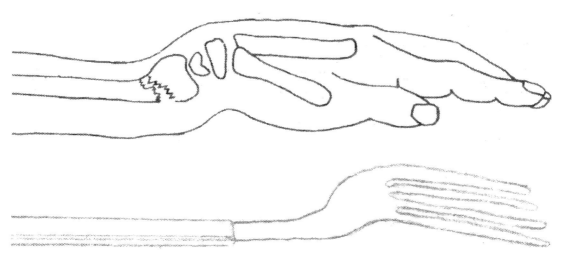

Fig.14.7. Colles' fracture. The dinner-fork deformity is a characteristic feature.

Routine X-ray findings are usually classical. The AP view shows a predominantly transverse fracture of the radius about 2.5cm from the wrist joint line. There is evidence of *impaction, supination, radial displacement* and *radial angulation* of the distal fragment. On the lateral view, the distal fragment is also *dorsally displaced* and *dorsally angulated.* These two features are mainly responsible for the classic dinner-fork deformity. Evidence of its impaction can also be seen and an avulsion fracture of the ulnar styloid may be present.

CT and MRI scans are superfluous for the diagnosis of Colles' fracture. However, the former can be used to assess the degree of displacement and the disposition of intra-articular fragments whilst the latter can be used to assess intra-articular ligamentous injuries. *Wrist arthroscopy* is being increasingly used to diagnose and treat intra-articular injuries.

TREATMENT

The aim of treatment is to achieve as accurate a reduction of displaced fractures as possible because this is correlated with good function. The fracture type/pattern determines the treatment method.

Undisplaced extra-articular and intra-articular fractures

These do well with cast immobilisation. Traditionally, the cast is kept on for 6 weeks but recent studies have shown no difference in results between one and three weeks of cast immobilisation.

However, if early cast removal is opted for, it is wise to apply some form of splintage e.g. a removable Futuro or similar splint to bring the total "immobilisation" period to 6 weeks.

Displaced extra-articular and intra-articular fractures (Fig.14.8)

These need to be reduced. Reduction can be achieved in most cases by closed manipulation. If this fails, other methods of reduction have to be used. The main difficulty lies with immobilisation after reduction. Applicable methods of immobilisation include *casting, external fixation, internal fixation* or a combination of these methods.

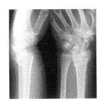 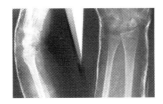 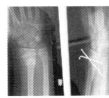

| Fig.14.8. A Colles' fracture in an elderly patient | Fig.14.9a. Same fracture treated by closed reduction and cast immobilisation. | Fig.14.9b. A Colles' fracture in a child treated by K-wire fixation. |

Late displacement of the reduced fractures occurs in some patients. In view of this, check X-rays should be done at the end of the first and second weeks. A re-displaced fracture should be re-reduced.

COMPLICATIONS OF COLLES' FRACTURE

- **Mal-union** is common
- **Delayed attrition rupture of extensor indicis proprius tendon** is sometimes seen in undisplaced fractures

SMITH'S FRACTURE (Fig.14.10)

This is a transverse fracture of the distal radius about 2.5cm from the wrist joint line with volar (anterior) displacement of the distal fragment. It is a rare injury which usually results from a fall on a flexed wrist. The clinical appearance is the reverse of that of Colles' fracture. It is thus a true opposite of Colles' fracture. Three types are recognised:

Type I   Extra-articular
Type II   The fracture line enters the dorsal rim of the articular surface
Type III The fracture line enters the middle of the radiocarpal articular surface. This type is equivalent to a *volar Barton's fracture.*

Diagnosis is by physical and radiological examination. Treatment is by manipulative reduction and cast immobilisation. If closed reduction is unsuccessful, ORIF with a volar locking plate can be carried out.

BARTON'S FRACTURE (Fig.14.10)

This is an anterior marginal fracture of the distal radius with anterior subluxation of the wrist joint. The distal radial fragment comes off with the rest of the hand which may displaced volarly (*volar Barton's*) or dorsally (*dorsal Barton's*).

The appearance and mechanisms of injury are similar to those of Smith's fracture but it is important to note that here we are dealing with an intra-articular fracture here, which is intrinsically much more difficult to treat. Closed reduction by traction, supination and dorsiflexion may be successful but it is usually unstable. Therefore, most surgeons opt for open reduction and internal fixation with a plate as with Smith's fracture.

BARTON'S FRACTURE (Fig.14.10)

Also called "Backfire fracture" and "Hutchison fracture", this is a significant marginal fracture of the radial styloid. It is called a *chauffeur's fracture* because it was common in the 1930s when drivers were prone to the injury from the crank as the cars back-fired.

An undisplaced fracture is treated with a Colles-type cast for about 6 weeks or by percutaneous screw fixation. A displaced fracture requires accurate open reduction and internal fixation using or two screws in order to restore a smooth articular surface.

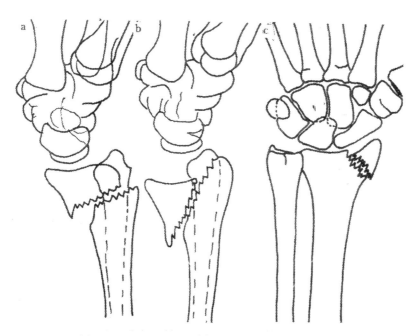

Fig.14.10. (a) Smith's fracture (b) Barton's fracture (volar variety) (c) Chaffeur's fracture.

COMMINUTED DISTAL RADIAL FRACTURES

DRFs in the elderly are often comminuted because of predisposing osteoporosis. They are best fixed with a locking plate (Fig.14.11).

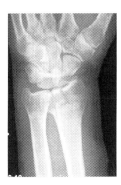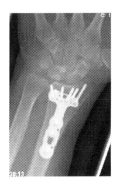

Fig.14.11a&b. Volar locking plate fixation of a comminuted distal radial fracture in an elderly patient.

DISTAL RADIAL FRACTURES IN CHILDREN

These were mentioned in Chapter 10. They are very common injuries, constituting about 10% of all new fractures seen in an average Fracture Clinic. About 90% of these fractures occur in boys aged 5 to 13 years and result from "falls on the out-stretched hand" during running, sports and climbing. Associated distal ulnar fractures are common.

FRACTURE TYPES

Physeal (Growth plate) injuries.

These involve the growth plate and are classified according to the Salter-Harris classification (please check this up in Chapter 10). Most are Type II injuries but other grades of injury are also seen. Significantly displaced fractures should be reduced by closed manipulation and cast immobilisation for 4-6 weeks. There may be indications for open reduction and K-wire fixation.

Metaphyseal injuries

- *Buckle fractures* are compression fractures of one cortex. This shows as a cortical crumple on X-ray.

- *Green-stick fractures* are tension fractures of one cortex. On X-ray, the fracture is seen to be hinging on the opposite cortex.

- *Complete fractures* are usually seen in the older age group or in high-energy injuries. The ulna is usually also fractured at the same level. A dinner-fork deformity similar to the one seen in the classic Colles' fracture is present. Displacement of the radial fracture less than 25% of medio-lateral contact and 50% of dorso-volar contact is considered acceptable. If more, reduction is necessary. Closed reduction is usually achievable and cast immobilisation should be for at least 6 weeks. The cast should be below elbow for fractures within 2.5cm of the wrist joint line and above elbow for more proximal fractures, in which re-displacement is possible from elbow joint movements. A check X-ray in a week is advised to check for redisplacement. Some surgeons use K-wires as insurance against this complication. Fractures irreducible by the closed method should be treated by open surgery and K-wire fixation.

ACUTE INSTABILITY OF THE DISTAL RADIOULNAR JOINT (DRUJ)

This can occur with the following injuries:

- distal radial fractures
- radial sigmoid notch injuries
- distal ulnar shaft fractures
- basilar ulnar styloid fractures
- articular ulnar dome fractures
- forearm fractures e.g. Galeazzi and Essex-Lopresti injuries.

With the exception of forearm fractures, the above injuries can cause TFCC injury. With distal radial fractures, 25 degrees of dorsal angulation and 5 mm of shortening are predictive of DRUJ instability and possible TFCC injury. Acute instability with dislocation or subluxation can be both volar and dorsal in direction. Treatment is by closed reduction under image intensification during which stability can be assessed. If stable reduction is achieved, the wrist is immobilised in an above elbow cast, with the forearm in supination for a dorsal dislocation or pronation for a volar dislocation – for 6 weeks. If instability persists, open reduction is carried out, with clearance of interposing soft tissues followed by pinning and cast immobilisation for 6 weeks.

FRACTURES OF THE DISTAL END OF THE ULNA

Isolated fractures of the distal end of the ulna are rare. Usually they occur in association with distal radial fractures. They may take the form of fracture above the wrist or of avulsion fracture of the ulnar styloid as seen in a classical Colles' fracture

COMPLICATIONS OF DISTAL RADIAL FRACTURES

Median nerve compression in the carpal tunnel may occur acutely or late. Surgical decompression may be necessary.

Mal-union secondary to an initially poorly reduced fracture or to a late slip is the commonest complication. If gross, wrist pain may be severe enough to justify corrective osteotomy of the distal radius.

Non-union. The radial fracture always unites but an associated ulnar styloid fracture may not. This may cause local tenderness for sometime.

An unreduced distal radioulnar joint disruption may result in disabling pain. This may be relieved by excision of the ulnar head (*Darrach's operation*).

Stiffness of the shoulder joint and the fingers used to occur commonly until surgeons realised the need to exercise these joints from the start.

Delayed rupture of the extensor pollicis longus tendon (about 6 weeks after the fracture) is a frequently mentioned attrition injury in connection with Colles' fracture but the point has been emphasised that this complication is more characteristic of an undisplaced distal radial fracture than of a displaced fracture, which Colles' fracture really is (Helal, Chen and Iwegbu, 1982).

Sudeck's atrophy is seen in about 25% of cases.

Further reading

Bado JL. The Monteggia Lesion. *Clin Orthop 50:* 71-86, 1967.

Broberg MA and Morrey BF. Results of treatment of fracture-dislocations to the elbow. *Clin Orthop* 216: 109, 1987.

Cohn MS and Hastings HII. Acute Elbow Dislocation: Evaluation And Management. *J Am Acad Orthop Surg:* 15-23, 1998.

Egol KA, Koval KJ and Zuckerman JD, eds. *Handbook of Fractures, 4ʰ edition.* Lippincott Williams & Wilkins, 2010.

Frykman G. Fracture Of The Distal Radius, Including Sequelae – Shoulder-Hand-Finger Syndrome, Disturbance In The Distal Radioulnar Joint And Impairment Of Nerve Function: A Clinical And Experimental Study. *Acta orthop Scand 108(Suppl):* 1, 1967.

Helal B, Chen SC and Iwegbu G. Rupture Of The Extensor Pollicis Longus Tendon In Undisplaced Colles'-Type Fracture. *The Hand 14(1): 41, 1982.*

Hume AC. Anterior Dislocation Of The Head Of The Radius Associated With Undisplaced Fracture Of The Olecranon In Children. *J Bone Joint Surg 39B:* 508-512, 1957.

Mason ML. Some Observations On Fractures Of The Head Of The Radius With A Review Of One Hundred Cases. *Br J Surg 42:* 123-132, 1954.

McFarland B. Congenital Dislocation Of The Head Of The Radius. *Br J Surg 24:* 4q-49, 1936.

Moed BR, Kellam JF, Foster RJ et al. Immediate Internal Fixation of Open Fractures Of The Diaphysis Of The Forearm. *J Bone Joint Surg.* 68A: 1008, 1986.

O'Driscoll SW. Classification And Evaluation of Recurrent Instability Of The Elbow. *Clin Orthop* 370: 34-43, 2000.

Parasa RB and Maffulli N. Surgical Management Of Radial Head Fractures. *J R Coll Surg Edin* 46: 76-85, 2001.

Reckling FW. Unstable Fracture-Dislocations of The Forearm (Monteggia and Galeazzi Lesions). *J Bone Joint Surg.* 64A: 857, 1982.

Viola RW and Hastings H II. Treatment Of Ectopic Ossification About The Elbow. *Clin Orthop* 370: 65-86, 2000.

Wei SY, Born CT, Abene A et al. Diaphyseal Forearm Fractures Treated With And Without Bone Graft. *J Trauma 46:* 1045-1048, 1999.

Distal radial fractures

Sun JS, Chang CH, Wu CC et al. Extra-articular deformity in distal radial fractures treated by external fixation.*Can J Surg 44(4):* 289-294, 2001.

Trumble TE, Culp R, Hanel DP et al. Intra-Articular Fractures Of The Distal Aspect Of The Radius. *J Bone Joint Surg 80A:* 582-600, 1998.

Tumia N, Wardlaw D, Hallett J et al. Aberdeen Colles' Fracture Brace As A Treatment For Colles' Fracture. A Multicentre, Prospective, Randomised Controlled Trial. *J Bone Jt Surg 85B:* 78-82, 2003.

Walton NP, Brammar TJ, Hutchinson J et al. Treatment of unstable distal radial fractures by intrafocal, intramedullary K-wires. *Injury 32(5):* 383-9, 2001.

Williams RL, Haddad FS and Lavy CB. Current management of fractures of distal radius and ulna. *Br J Hosp Med 55(6):* 320-328, 1996.

CHAPTER 15

FRACTURES AND DISLOCATIONS OF THE WRIST (CARPUS)

Of the 8 bones that make up the wrist (carpus), only two, the scaphoid and the lunate, are relatively frequently fractured or dislocated. Accurate diagnosis requires good quality X-ray pictures and special views. The MRI is a marvellous additional investigative tool.

FRACTURES OF THE SCAPHOID

Scaphoid fractures are seen in all groups but young men appear to be more frequently affected than other age groups. They account for about 75% of all carpal fractures. Although the scaphoid can be fractured at any point, most fractures occur in the middle third labelled the "waist". The usual mechanism is forced dorsiflexion and radial deviation of the wrist. A scaphoid fracture may be undisplaced or displaced.

DIAGNOSIS

The diagnosis of a fresh fracture relies heavily on the history and physical findings, as most fresh fractures do not show up even on special scaphoid X-ray views. There is usually a complaint of pain on the radial aspect of the wrist. *Tenderness in the anatomical "snuff-box" is a characteristic physical finding.*

TREATMENT

Most doctors opt to err on the side of caution by assuming that the presence of tenderness in the anatomical snuff-box is equal to a fractured scaphoid until proven otherwise, even if the X-ray does not show a fracture. A "scaphoid" plaster of Paris cast (Fig.15.1) is applied and retained for 10-14 days, when check X-rays will normally reveal a fracture, if there is one.

An undisplaced fracture is treated with a new scaphoid cast for 4-10 more weeks. The period of immobilisation is determined by the physical findings at 6, 9 and 12 weeks, from the date of fracture. Ninety per cent of fractures will unite with immobilisation for 6-12 weeks. Continued tenderness suggests that the fracture is yet to unite. X-ray monitoring of healing is unreliable as a fracture line may be hidden by positioning or may be visible for sometime after clinical union. If cast immobilisation is considered necessary for more than 12 weeks, alternative treatment option should be considered as disabling stiffness could result from such prolonged immobilisation.

A displaced fracture may be reduced by manipulation, in which case it can be treated in a scaphoid cast as outlined above. Open reduction and internal fixation with a percutaneous small screw is advocated by some surgeons as a way of avoiding prolonged cast immobilisation and non-union. However, it has been shown that there are no significant differences in the functional outcome between cast immobilisation and operative treatment.

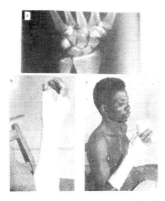

Fig.15.1. Fracture of the scaphoid: a patient in a sca- phoid cast should be able to hold a cup of water.

COMPLICATIONS

- *Avascular necrosis of the proximal fragment* following fractures in the proximal or middle thirds is the most important complication. It is seen in 5-16% of cases. If symptomatic, the avascular portion can be excised and replaced with a silicone rubber prosthesis.

- *Non-union* is the next. It is seen in 5-10% of cases. Symptomatic cases are treated with bone grafting and screw-fixation.

These complications are linked to the anatomy of the blood supply to the bone. Firstly, 80% of its surface is covered by articular cartilage, which limits the area available for vascular penetration. Secondly, the blood supply to the bone comes from distally to proximally.

- *Other complications* include: *Concomitant Colles' fracture*, which is common; other carpal bones may also be fractured along. *Associated dislocation* of the lunate or of the whole carpus may occur. *Sudeck's atrophy* and *Post-traumatic osteoarthritis of the wrist joint* may also occur.

FRACTURES OF THE LUNATE

The dorsal horn, volar horn or body may be fractured as a result of falls on the palm or direct injury. The blood supply is from both intraosseous and extraosseous sources coming from both dorsal and volar directions but the bone, like the scaphoid, is also prone to avascular necrosis (Kienbock's disease).

Diagnosis in the acute stage requires a high index of suspicion. Like scaphoid fractures, the fracture line may not show on initial X-rays.

Treatment. If physical signs are impressive, a cast should be applied for 3 – 4 weeks.

Complications.

Avascular necrosis of the lunate (*Kienbock's disease)* is the most important complication. Cast immobilisation or relief of compression on the lunate with an external fixator has been advocated for early disease whilst surgery is recommended for advanced disease.

FRACTURES OF OTHER CARPAL BONES

Fractures of the trapezium may involve the body or trapezial ridge and the fracture line could extend into the trapeziometacarpal joint. Special views are often required to see the fractures e.g. carpal tunnel views are necessary to show fractures of the ridge. Undisplaced fractures are treated in a below-elbow cast for 4–6 weeks. Displaced ones may require ORIF.

Fractures of trapezoid, capitate, hamate, triquetrum and pisiform do occur but are quite rare. In most cases they occur in association with other injuries around the wrist joint. In the acute stage, cast immobilisation for 4 -6 weeks usually suffices.

CARPAL INSTABILITY

The proximal row, formed by the scaphoid, lunate and triquetrum (+ pisiform) forms intercalated segments with the distal row consisting of the trapezium, trapezoid, capitate and hamate. There are no muscle or tendon attachments. The scaphoid is considered to function as the slider-crank control that links motion at the radiocarpal and intercarpal joints. Fractures of the carpal bones are associated with injuries to various carpal ligaments which may cause instability of the carpus.

Three patterns of carpal instability are distinguished:

- Radiocarpal
- Transverse and
- Axial

Pure radiocarpal dislocations are rare; dorsal and volar dislocations at this level are associated with Barton's fracture. Transverse dislocations are of particular interest and include the better-known lunate and perilunate dislocations which predispose to *dorsiflexion* and *volar flexion intercalated segmental instability* (DISI and VISI).

DISI, the most common form of carpal instability, is usually associated with an injury to the scapholunate ligament, which allows the lunate to extend with the triquetrum.

On the other hand, disruption of the lunotriquetral ligament causes VISI by allowing the lunate to flex with the scaphoid.

VOLAR DISLOCATION OF THE LUNATE AND PERILUNATE DISLOCATION OF THE CARPUS

Diagnosis

These are the commonest of all carpal dislocations. They are usually secondary to a fall on an extended hand. In *volar lunate dislocation*, the lunate pops out into the volar aspect of the wrist like a bean seed from its pod whilst the carpus remains aligned with the radius. Although the history and the location of a subcutaneous bony lump in front of the wrist may suggest the diagnosis, *volar lunate dislocation* cannot be accurately diagnosed without a good X-ray examination.

In *perilunate dislocation of the carpus (Fig.15.2)*, the lunate remains in alignment with the radius while the rest of the carpus together with the hand dislocate dorsally (usually) or volarly (rare). The characteristic deformities are diagnostic but, again, good X-rays are essential.

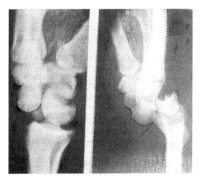

Fig.15.2. Perilunate dislocation of the carpus. The dorsal variety (left) is more common but the author has come across a few of the volar variety (right).

The most informative X-ray view for the two dislocations is a *true lateral view*. On this view, in **lunate dislocation**, the lunate is seen to occupy an anterior position, with its crescentic (concave) surface facing anteriorly and distally, with the scaphoid and triquetrum remaining in alignment with the radius. In **perilunate dislocation of the carpus**, the latter is seen to lie dorsal or volar in relation to the lunate. The normal *scapholunate angle* is 30-60 degrees. With DISI, this angle exceeds 70 degrees. With VISI, it is <30 degrees and the volar flexion of the lunate results in a capitolunate angle of >20 degrees.

In the *AP view*, the usual contours of the carpus are distorted, with parts of the lunate overlapping with other bones. The *Terry Thomas sign* is seen on this view: the scapholunate diastasis is > 3mm (Terry Thomas was a famous comedian with a huge gap between his incisors). Also in this view, there is a "double cortical ring" of the scaphoid produced by the overlay of the distal pole of the scaphoid which is in excessive flexion.

Unfortunately, many X-ray departments consistently fail to provide true APs and laterals unless when prevailed upon and as the trainee surgeon usually does not know the importance of true projections in this injury, the injury is often missed. Arthrography, CT scan, MRI scan, a bone scan and wrist arthroscopy may have diagnostic roles.

Treatment

Closed manipulation usually succeeds in a fresh injury. With *volar lunate dislocation*, the hand is supinated, traction is applied to it against countertraction and the thumbs are then used to press in the lunate. The reduction can usually be felt with the thumbs. With *perilunate dislocation*, reduction is achieved by traction and thumb pressure. In both cases, immobilisation is achieved with a below-elbow POP cast applied with the wrist in 45 degrees of flexion. A check X-ray is taken and if the position is satisfactory the cast is retained for 4-6 weeks. Elevation is essential in the first 1-2 weeks to contain swelling which can be severe in this injury. Open reduction is indicated if closed manipulation fails to effect reduction.

Late presentation and missed diagnosis are common. This obviously makes treatment difficult. Massive swelling, a constant feature, makes closed manipulation unlikely to succeed in these cases. It also hampers open reduction and skin closure afterwards. High elevation and active finger exercises should be carried out before open reduction is attempted in such cases. Open reduction may fail, especially in dislocations older than 4 weeks. In such a case, excision of the lunate may be considered.

Complications

Median nerve compression is a common immediate complication. Early reduction normally solves the problem. A dislocated lunate may undergo *avascular necrosis*. This is called *Kienbock's disease*. Such a lunate may be excised and replaced with a silicone rubber implant.

Associated fractures: Other carpal bones, especially the scaphoid may be fractured concomitantly. *Post-traumatic osteoarthritis* is common if a dislocation is missed or if an avascular lunate is not excised. *Persistent subluxation of the scapholunate joint* is another well-recognised complication.

TRANS-SCAPHOID DISLOCATION OF THE LUNATE

A scaphoid fracture is sometimes associated with a volar lunate dislocation, the proximal scaphoid fragment is carried along anteriorly by the lunate. The priority is to first reduce the lunate. After this, the scaphoid fracture is treated like an uncomplicated scaphoid injury. Internal fixation may have to be done if instability persists.

DISLOCATIONS OF OTHER CARPAL BONES

These injuries are rare and usually occur in association with other injuries around the wrist joint.

INJURIES TO THE THUMB METACARPAL

Green and O'Brien have classified thumb metacarpal base fractures into four types as follows:

Type I: avulsion of the volar lip and subluxation of the carpometacarpal (CM) joint (Bennett's fracture).

Type II: comminuted fracture of the base of the metacarpal, involving the CM joint (Rolando fracture).

Type III: extra-articular fractures of the metacarpal base.

Type IV: epiphyseal injuries (children).

Fracture-dislocation of the carpometacarpal joint of the thumb (Bennett's fracture) (Fig.15.3).

This is a marginal fracture of the base of the first metacarpal with dislocation of the larger radial fragment. The injury was first described by Edward Bennett in 1882. Subtle points about this entity should be noted, namely:

- It is an intra-articular fracture

- The carpo-metacarpal joint in question here is the trapezio-metacarpal joint.

- The 'marginal' (small) fragment of the fracture is medial and volar in position; it remains attached to the trapezium by the anterior oblique ligament and is often undisplaced.

- It is the larger metacarpal fragment that dislocates and slides (telescopes) proximally, radially and dorsally, thanks to the pull of the abductor pollicis longus. There is a comminuted variety of this fracture. If the fracture lines take a T or Y shape, the injury is called a *Rolando's fracture* (described in 1910).

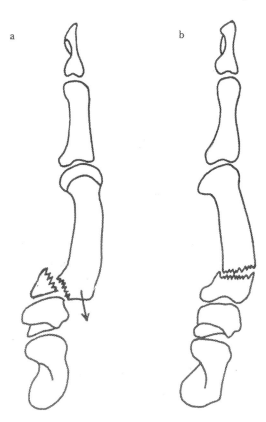

Fig.15.3a and b. Fractures at the base of the thumb. (a). Bennett's fracture-dislocation: this is an intra-articular fracture, which should not be confused with a fracture through the base of the 1ˢᵗ metacarpal (b), which is extra-articular.

Closed reduction under image intensification should always be attempted first. Traction is exerted on the thumb against countertraction. The thumb is then abducted, and at the same time, pressure is applied to the base of the thumb metacarpal, both in an effort to reduce the subluxation. A below-elbow P.O.P cast is then applied reaching distally the knuckles of the four fingers and the IP joint of the thumb. As the plaster sets, traction, abduction and thumb pressure to the base are maintained. The plaster is moulded around the base of the thumb. A check X-ray is done to ensure that good reduction is maintained.

Very often, reduction is imperfect or a slip may be seen on a subsequent check X-ray. Consequently, many surgeons go for closed reduction and percutaneous K-wire fixation as the first option. One or two K-wires may be put through the fracture or fixation can be achieved by passing it through the 2ⁿᵈ metacarpal (Fig.15.3) Occasionally, the above methods are unsuccessful and open reduction and internal fixation with a K-wire or small screw is resorted to. Immobilisation in a cast for 3-4 weeks should be used whether or not internal fixation has been carried out. The Rolando fracture is rare and usually requires ORIF.

Mal-union and *secondary osteoarthritis* are the commonest complications.

Fracture across the base of the thumb metacarpal.

This must be distinguished from a Bennett's fracture; the CM joint is not involved here. Closed reduction may be successful, otherwise open reduction and internal fixation should be carried out.

Fractures of the shaft of the thumb metacarpal

These are rare. Undisplaced fractures can be treated by splintage with an Aluminium splint. Displaced fractures are best treated by ORIF.

DISLOCATIONS OF THE THUMB

At the Base

This may occur at the trapezio-metacarpal or at the scapho-trapezial joint. Reduction is by traction and thumb pressure to the base of the thumb. Immobilisation in a scaphoid-type cast is required for 3 weeks. Function is regained by active exercises.

At the MP Joint

Dislocation. In most cases the dislocation is in the posterior direction. Manipulative reduction often succeeds. Failure is usually due to buttonholing of the capsule by the metacarpal head. In this case, open reduction through a lateral approach should be done.

Rupture of the ulnar collateral ligaments. This is called the *Gamekeeper's thumb* in English Literature. It is caused by forced abduction of the thumb at the MP joint. The origin or insertion of the ligament may be avulsed. There is pain and tenderness at the *medial aspect* of the MP joint. Conservative treatment by reduction and immobilisation in a scaphoid-type cast for 3 weeks is used in mild injuries with minimal subluxation. More severe injuries with more instability are best treated by surgical repair plus cast immobilisation.

Rupture of the lateral collateral ligament also occurs but is very rare. Management should follow similar lines.

At the IP joint

Posterior dislocation is the more frequent type. Reduction and immobilisation should follow lines similar to those described for MP joint dislocation.

INJURIES OF THE FINGERS

Metacarpal Fractures

These may occur at the base, in the shaft or at the neck. The neck is the weakest and most frequently fractured site. Displacement is usually minimal in these fractures because of the supporting role of neighbouring metacarpals and soft tissues. Physical examination should include an assessment of the alignment of the affected finger or fingers. In full flexion, each of the fingers should point to the scaphoid; this does not happen if there is significant rotation. Possible associated injury to the tendons and neurovascular structures should also be searched for. AP and oblique X-rays are essential for assessment of possible rotational deformity.

Isolated undisplaced or minimally displaced fractures will usually do well with crepe bandage only. Fractures involving two or all of the four metacarpals may require splintage in a front slab extending to the knuckles.

Displaced fractures are more problematic. Ideally, any angulatory or rotatory deformity or overlapping should be corrected so that the palmar arch may be preserved. Open reduction and internal fixation with miniature plates and screws best treat uncomminuted fractures. Stabilisation with cross Kirschner wires applied percutaneously is sometimes successful. Any immobilisation involving the MP and IP joints must be such that the MP joint is put into 90degree of flexion and the IP joint is kept straight (180 degree) or only very slightly flexed (5 degree). The reason for this is explained below.

Fracture of the neck of the 5th metacarpal deserves special mention because of its relatively frequent occurrence. Classically sustained as a result of punch-ups, it is common among lovers of alcohol and other pugilistic groups, especially adolescent males, it is otherwise called *"Boxer's fracture"*. However, the history usually given in A & E and fracture clinics is that of punching the wall in anger.

The metacarpal breaks at the neck and the smaller distal fragment angulates anteriorly. Up to 70 degrees of angulation is well tolerated. Manipulation is advocated for rotational deformity or lateral angulation. It is generally possible to reduce this fracture under local anaesthesia (injection of 1-ml of 0.5-2% lignocaine into the fracture haematoma) but maintenance of reduction in a cast is seldom successful. Percutaneous K-wire fixation is the preferred option.

Phalangeal Fractures and Dislocations

The three phalanges of each finger may be fractured at any point, the proximal and middle thirds being more frequently involved than the distal. The fracture line may be transverse, oblique or spiral. Comminuted fractures also occur.

Management will depend on the fracture in question. Certain methods of treatment may be mentioned as follows: *"Neighbour" or intermittent strapping* for about 3 weeks is useful in undisplaced fractures. The *Aluminium and foam splint* is useful following stable reduction of some fractures. The *rolled bandage* is a useful splint for certain fractures of the proximal and middle phalanges. Certain fractures are best treated by *internal fixation (K-wire or screw)*.

Intra-articular fractures may involve the MP or the IP joints. These are serious injuries because they often cause finger stiffness. They should be assessed carefully both clinically and radiographically. If a collateral ligament injury is associated, a surgical repair may give a better result than conservative treatment.

If the marginal fragment of the fracture is sizeable, internal fixation may provide the only chance of restoring a good articular surface. A comminuted intra-articular fracture is probably best managed with early exercise.

Whatever treatment method is adopted, the surgeon must continuously remind himself that he is involved in a race against stiffness and that the race period is roughly 3 weeks.

Finger dislocations or subluxations are frequent at the IP joints and may occur at the MP joints also. They may be associated with fractures as mentioned above or with tendon injuries. In general, reduction should be effected urgently. The danger of development of disabling stiffness is as real here as with intra-articular fractures.

SOME CLASSICAL FINGER INJURIES

The Mallet Finger

This results from avulsion of the extensor tendon from its insertion into the dorsum of the base of the distal phalanx. Sometimes a tiny piece of bone is pulled along. The distal phalanx goes into flexion at the DIP joint and cannot be actively extended. Treatment with a *mallet finger splint* is effective if instituted within a few hours of injury and maintained for about 6 weeks. The mallet splint hyperextends the finger at the distal inter-phalangeal (DIP) joint. The classical splint is made from plastic but one can be improvised from P.O.P. Some surgeons prefer early surgical repair. This is not easy to justify in most cases as the result of conservative treatment is satisfactory and disability in untreated cases is slight. Appropriate tendon repairs or arthrodesis of the DIP joint can used to treat late cases.

The Boutonniere Finger

This really means a "button-hole" finger. Secondary to a rupture of the central slip of the extensor tendon over the proximal interphalangeal (PIP) joint, the head of the proximal phalanx button-holes through the gap in the tendon, allowing the combined tendons of the lumbricals and the interossei to slip anteriorly, thereby becoming flexors (instead of extensors) of the finger at the PIP joint; hyperextension of the DIP joint occurs at the same time. Urgent reduction and repair of the ruptured tendon should be carried out. The result of suture is hardly good.

WOUNDS OF THE HAND

Puncture, Incised or Lacerated wounds

These are common. The danger lies in *possible associated injuries* to tendons, nerves and blood vessels and in *possible infection* of the wound. A careful clinic examination is imperative. Any doubt about the nature and extent of the injury must be clarified by *surgical exploration.*

FLEXOR TENDON CUTS

Most of the tendons arise from muscles arising from the elbow and forearm. Cuts can occur at any level, between their origins and their insertions into the bones of the hand.

Repair of cut flexor tendons

Primary repair gives the best results. Various suture techniques e.g. Bunnell, Kessler, Lambert etc are available. It is important that the blood supply is preserved. The annular pulleys A2 and A4 over the shafts of the proximal and middle phalanges respectively; they prevent the tendons from bow-stringing and must be preserved. *Delayed repair* is also attended with good results. *Tendon graft* is indicated when there is tendon loss.

On the basis of results of primary repair, the following 5 zones of the hand have been delineated (Fig.15.4):

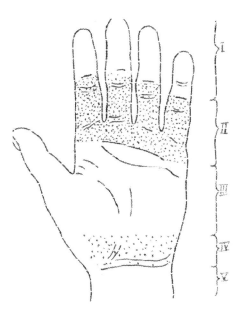

Fig.15.4. The five flexor tendon zones.

Zone I. This includes the area from the insertion of the superficialis tendon to the base of the middle phalanx to the tip of the finger. Here, there is only the profundus tendon. When cut in this zone, the proximal stump may retract considerably but the result of primary suture is generally satisfactory.

Zone II is the area between the distal skin crease and the level of insertion of the superficialis tendon of each finger. In this zone, the superficialis and profundus tendons lie together in a common tight fibro-osseous tunnel. Because of the disastrous result of tendon repair in this zone in the past, the zone was nicknamed *no man's land* by Bunnell. The concept of no man's land does not apply in a pure sense now since some expert hand surgeons have shown that good results can be obtained after primary repair in this zone. However, non-experts continue to get bad results and beginners are warned not to attempt any form of repair in this zone. If confronted with an injury in this zone, the non-expert who has no immediate access to a hand surgeon should carry out a conscientious wound toilet, if necessary, close the skin, give prophylactic antibiotics, institute high elevation for 48 hours in order to prevent oedema and then refer the patient as soon as possible.

Zone III lies between the distal edge of the carpal tunnel to the distal palmar crease. Considerable retraction of cut tendons can also occur here. If the ends can be found, primary repair also has a good prognosis, as in Zone 1. The other consideration is that the profundus and superficialis, lying closely together in this zone, get severed together. If, for any reason, one of them has to be sacrificed, it should be the superficialis.

Zone IV is formed by the carpal tunnel.

Zone V is between the musculotendinous junction and the proximal edge of the carpal tunnel. When the tendons are cut at this site, retraction of the ends can be considerable and may continue for sometime after the cut. The wound should be explored as early as possible and cut tendons should be identified and repaired primarily. The result of such repair is generally good.

The Thumb. In general, primary repair can be carried out on the thumb flexors.

Practical Tips

1. The state of the wound is an important consideration when primary repair is contemplated, as wound infection will militate against good results. Whatever the surgeon decides to do should be done quickly. Delay makes bad results and infection more likely.

2. Suture should be done under tourniquet. The 'lead hand' should be used, if available.

3. The tendons should be correctly identified before suture. Pulling on the distal stump will usually show where a given tendon is going. This is particularly important in zones 1 and 2.

4. Immobilisation must ensure that there is no tension on the suture line. Flexion at various joints usually ensures this. Immobilisation should be limited to the finger(s).

5. High elevation of the hand after operation is imperative, so also is the administration of prophylactic antibiotics.

EXTENSOR TENDONS

The extensor area is also divided into zones as follows:

Zone I: distal to the central slip of the PIP joint
Zone II: MP joint to the central slip
Zone III: distal to the extensor retinaculum
Zone IV: under the extensor retinaculum
Zone V: in the forearm

Accordingly, the mallet and boutonniere finger injuries discussed earlier are injuries in Zone I and II respectively. In general, extensor tendon cuts are easier to treat than flexor tendon cuts. This is explained by their anatomy.

- They are joined to one another and so retraction following a division hardly occurs so that finding the stumps is easier.
- They have short sheaths, so adhesion is a lesser problem with them than with flexor tendons.

Primary repair should be attempted in all extensor tendon cuts if there are no contra-indications. The issue of immobilisation following such a repair is controversial. The traditional recommendation is splintage with the wrist 40 degrees of extension and the fingers in slight flexion at the MP joints for 3 weeks. Now, dynamic splintage with a volar slab or plastic with an outrigger allowing passive finger extension is favoured.

NERVE CUTS

Various agents can cut any of the nerves innervating the hand. Their management should be carried out along lines outlined in the section on "Peripheral Nerve Injuries".

MULTIPLE INJURIES OF THE HAND

The main sources of the injuries are industrial and road traffic accidents. In a given case there may be fractures and joint injuries, injury to skin, muscles, tendons, nerves and blood vessels or even amputation of digits. Such an injury is an *acute surgical emergency*. Alarming haemorrhage is a common feature. Management is very difficult and is certainly not a job for the novice. However, no qualified doctor, no matter how young in the profession, has an excuse for being unable to give satisfactory initial management. This initial management involves:

1. A cool and collected approach and avoidance of panic.
2. Arrest of haemorrhage. The most effective emergency measures are high elevation of the whole arm and pressure bandage.
3. Taking blood for grouping and cross-matching and institution of an I.V. drip.
4. Giving parenteral prophylactic broad-spectrum antibiotics and anti-tetanus measures.
5. Wherever possible, getting a good history of the injury, which should include finding out the patient's dominant hand and occupation.
6. Taking X-rays to determine any bone or joint involvement.
7. Carrying out a generous primary wound wash and judicious debridement under tourniquet.
8. Splinting the hand in the *optimum position* to lessen the chances of disabling stiffness later.
9. Instituting high elevation of the hand and continuing other general measures post-operation.
10. Referring the patient to more senior colleagues as soon as it is safe to do so.

Where manpower and adequate facilities are available, definitive treatment can and is in fact best carried out at the time of initial inspection, toilet and debridement of the wound. With a tourniquet on, the separate injuries can be examined accurately. In general, fractures should be stabilised first before tendon and nerve injuries are tackled. In vascular injuries, anastomotic repairs are seldom indicated as the rich collateral circulation in the hand make ischaemia following ligations rare. Post-operatively, the hand must be immobilised in the *optimum position.

Immobilisation of the hand following injury: the optimum position

The bitter experience with hand stiffness has taught doctors the importance of immobilising the injured hand in the *optimum position*, rather than in any other position. *The optimum position of immobilisation of the hand can be defined as that position which, should stiffness result, offers the best chance of retaining or regaining useful hand function.* This position should be borne in mind anytime the hand is being immobilised following injury.

The term "optimum position of function", was used in the past but has been dropped because it was realised that it does not describe what it was intended to do, for example, in the straight position (which most fingers assume when they become stiff from injury) the fingers can perform the function of slapping with the palm, so, the straight position is a position of function even though stiff and straight finger joints are otherwise undesirable.

The optimum position for the various joints of the hand (and wrist) are as follows:

Wrist joint: neutral position
Thumb: the abducted position, in opposition to the fingers
Fingers: (a) MP Joints: 90degrees of flexion
(b) PIP & DIP Joints: 180degrees (straight)

The rationale of these positions is as follows:

Thumb. Most of the functions of the thumb require thumb abduction. Contracture of the adductor pollicis will militate against this by bringing the thumb into the palm. Abduction of the thumb is the most effective prophylaxis of adductor muscle contracture.

Fingers. Contracture at the joints are caused mainly by collateral ligament contracture. The collateral ligaments of the MP joints are taut (and so, longer) in flexion while those of the IP joints are taut in extension. Contracture in the taut state is better than in the lax state.

How about an optimum period of immobilisation following hand injuries? This is difficult to set. However, experience shows that an unacceptable amount of stiffness sets in after about 3 weeks of immobilisation. On the other hand, most injuries, accidental or surgical, are know to stabilise by 3 weeks. Accordingly, three weeks can be considered to be the optimum period.

Further reading

Ashkenadze DM and Ruby L. Metacarpal Fractures And Dislocations. *Orthop Clin of N Am 23:* 19-33, 1992.

Ip WY and Chow SP. Results Of Dynamic Splintage Following Extensor Tendon Repair. *J Hand Surg, 22B:* 283-287, 1997.

Jupiter JB. Hand fractures: assessment and concepts of surgical management. In:*AO Principles of Fracture Management* Ruedi TP and Murphy WM, eds. Thieme, Stuttgart. New York, 2000.

Leddy JP: Flexor Tendons: Acute Injuries. In Green DP (ed): *Operative hand surgery, 3rd ed.* New York. Churchill Livingstone, pp1823-1852, 1993.

CHAPTER 16

FRACTURES OF THE SPINE AND PELVIS

INTRODUCTION

Fig.16.1 has been put up again in order to remind ourselves of the basic anatomy of the spine (vertebral column), which forms the basic structure of the trunk. It consists of five regions – cervical (7 vertebrae), thoracic (12 vertebrae), lumbar (5 vertebrae), sacral (5 vertebrae) and coccygeal (4-5 vertebrae). The sacral vertebrae are fused to form the sacrum and the coccygeal vertebrae are fused to form the coccyx. A typical vertebra (Fig.16.2) e.g. C6, T2 or L1 consists of a *body, two pedicles two transverse processes, two laminae and one spinous process.* Each transverse process bears a *superior* and an *inferior articular facet* for articulation with its upper and lower neighbour respectively.

Compared with the limb bones, significant injuries of the spine are less frequent but their incidence is exaggerated in people's minds because of their association with possible injury to the spinal cord and roots with the attendant serious effects. Mobility is the key factor in spinal injuries: the more mobile parts (the cervical, thoracolumbar and lumbar) are more prone to injury than the more rigid thoracic, sacral and coccygeal regions.

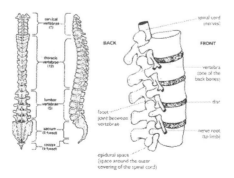

Fig.16.1. The spine. The spine is made up of 33-34 vertebrae grouped into five parts – cervical, thoracic, lumbar, sacrum and coccyx.

273

SPINAL FUNCTION AND THE CONCEPT OF STABILITY/INSTABILITY

The most important function of the spine is the protection of the spinal cord and associated neural elements. To be able to perform this function, the spine must be structurally stable and the significance of any given injury to the spine is judged by the extent to which it affects its stability.

Stability of the spine is provided by bony and soft-tissue (ligamentous) elements

- **The bony elements** are the vertebral body, the neural arch (pedicle and lamina), the spinous process, the transverse and accessory processes and the facet joints.

- **The soft-tissue elements** are the anterior and posterior longitudinal ligaments, the annulus fibrosus and intervertebral disc, the ligamentum flavum (yellow ligament), interspinous, supraspinous and intertransverse ligaments and other connective tissue elements.

- **A stable injury**, be it a fracture or a dislocation or both, may be defined as one which, during the healing period, is unlikely to move or displace enough to cause neurological damage. In general, a stable injury rarely causes neurological damage and does not need to be immobilised

- **An unstable injury** is one, which is likely to move or displace sufficiently to cause neurological damage during the healing period. An unstable injury often causes neurological damage and needs to be immobilised – by non-surgical or surgical methods.

The three column concept of spinal stability (Fig.16.2)

Denis (1983) proposed the 3-column concept of spinal stability. He divided the above-enumerated bony and soft-tissue structures into *three columns – anterior, middle and posterior* as follows:

- *Anterior column* consisting of the anterior longitudinal ligament, the anterior portion of the annulus fibrosus and the anterior half of the vertebral body

- *Middle column* consisting of the posterior portion of the vertebral body, the posterior portion of the annulus and the posterior longitudinal ligament

- *Posterior column* consisting of the pedicles, facets, laminae and the posterior ligament complex (ligamentum flavum, interspinous ligament, supraspinous ligament and the facet joint capsule).

An unstable injury is one with a two-column failure or middle-column failure.

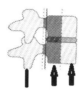

Fig.16.2. The three column concept of spinal stability (Denis, 1983). Even though originally formulated for thoraco-lumbar injuries, this classification is applicable to the lower cervical spine (C3-C7), the anatomy of which is broadly similar. In injury, these columns may fail individually or in combination.

FRACTURES AND DISLOCATIONS OF THE CERVICAL SPINE

The cervical spine can be divided into two parts – upper and lower – on the basis of anatomy and function. The upper cervical spine has been structured to permit *nodding* (occiput/atlas) and *shaking* (atlas/axis) *of the head*. The 3-column theory of stability applies to the lower cervical spine: C3-C7.

FIRST AID AND ATLS

Anybody suspected of having sustained a cervical spinal injury must be handled with extreme care, as it is easy to cause neurological damage in a patient who had luckily escaped such injury in an accident. First apply the ATLS principles – ABCDE. Ensure that the airways are patent, the patient is breathing, not bleeding to death and has good circulation. After this, the minimum first aid measure is to immobilise the neck. This is best carried out by trained paramedics but if they are not available, a *cervical collar* can be improvised from rolled newspapers or magazines or strips of a carton box and tied round the neck with a handkerchief, scarf or muffler (Fig.16.3). The patient should then be transported expeditiously and safely to a hospital with facilities for effective diagnosis and treatment of spinal injuries. The "DE" part of ATLS aid is completed in the hospital.

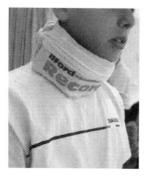

Fig.16.3. First-aid in cervical spine injuries: a cervical collar can be improvised from rolled newspapers or magazine or strips of carton box and tied round the neck with a handkerchief, scarf or muffler.

MECHANISMS OF INJURY

Various mechanisms apply here. The injuring forces are usually indirect - flexion-rotation, compression, extension, forward flexion and lateral flexion. Direct forces from direct blows/hits or from missiles e.g. bullets are rare. The resulting injury could be a fracture, a dislocation or both. Also, violent contraction of spinal muscles in the region can cause avulsion fractures of the various processes, especially the spinous process.

Diagnosis

A diagnosis can be made on the basis of a good history and physical findings. Lack of sophisticated diagnostic facilities is not a good excuse for inability to make a reasonable diagnosis of a C-spine injury.

Physical examination

This should be carried out systemically as follows:

Brief general examination should include all the systems. The pulse, BP, heart sounds and the respiratory status must be recorded, at least. A low BP is normal in a quadriplegic patient, as the injury in effect constitutes a sympathectomy of the trunk and lower limbs. Associated injuries e.g. rib fractures, should be noted.

Local examination (Status localis). This should include:

Inspection. The way the patient holds their head may be indicative of a neck injury and should be noted. Any abrasion, laceration, bruises or swelling in the neck is also noted. In a male, sustained penile erection is indicative of a severe cervical cord injury.

Palpation. This will confirm any local symptoms or signs present. It must be gentle. The interspinous distances should be determined to see if there is any increase, which will be indicative of posterior ligamentous disruption.

Movement. Any movement of the neck must be done gently and must be stopped if it causes pain.

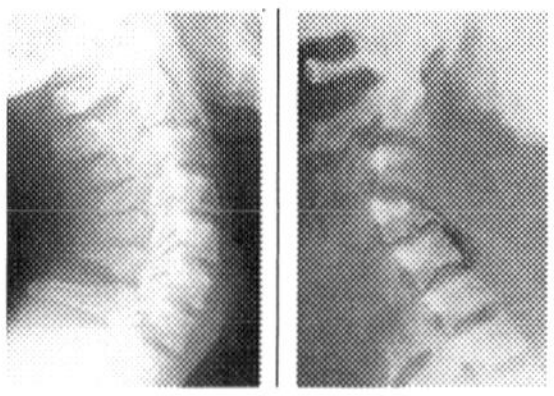

Radiological examination (Fig.16.4)

Radiological examination is imperative and the whole seven cervical vertebrae and T1 must be included on the film. AP, lateral, oblique and "open mouth" views, at least should be taken; a systemic examination is essential.

Fig.16.4. X-ray Diagnosis of cervical spine injuries: The lateral view is the most informative; all the seven cervical vertebrae and T1 must be visualised. The normal curvatures are broken at C3/C4 in the second picture as a result of a C4 fracture.

- An *open-mouth view* will show fractures of the odontoid as well as a lateral overhang of C1 burst fracture (Jefferson's fracture).

276

Special X-ray views

- When a dislocation is suspected but is not seen on an X-ray, **flexion and extension lateral views** should be taken. Bending of the neck must be done with care and under medical supervision. *Tomographic films* may help.

CT scan

- may reveal subtle fractures of the occipital condyles, C 1 ring and the odontoid process
- 3D sagittal and coronal reconstructions help in visualising dislocations, subluxations as well as the assessment of fracture fragment size and bony impingement into the spinal canal.

MRI scan

- may be required to show more precisely the state of the intervertebral discs, ligaments and the contents of the spinal canal.

Neurological examination

A significant fraction of patients with spinal fractures and dislocation have neurological injury. Sixty per cent of spinal cord injuries involve the cervical spine. All patients with neck injury must at least be asked to actively move the limbs to exclude possible motor deficit. If the history of the injury and the physical findings produce evidence of neurological injury, then a full neurological examination must be carried out. It consists of examination of sensory, motor and reflex functions.

Sensory function. This can be done by light finger touch, pinprick and light pressure. A knowledge of the dermatomes and myotomes of the upper limbs (Chapter 12) is helpful in this examination. Particular attention is paid to a search for evidence of sacral sparing by testing the sacrally innervated areas (the peri-anal, anal, scrotal or labial skin and the sole of the toes.) Presence of sensation in these areas indicates preservation of the lateral columns of the spinal cord, in which case, recovery of motor function may be possible.

Similarly, evidence of anterior or dorsal column sparing and of a Brown-Sequard lesion is also sought. Thus, from the findings of sensory examination alone it can be decided whether a lesion is that of a root or the cord and whether it is complete or incomplete.

Motor function. Motor functions are tested for cord segments. A patient with a lesion higher than C4 is likely to die from respiratory paralysis before reaching the hospital but one with a lower lesion may survive. A knowledge of the root innervation of movements of the upper limbs is helpful. After establishing the motor level of the injury, evidence of sacral motor sparing is sought by testing for voluntary muscle function of the anal sphincter (by rectal examination) and the toe flexor muscles. It is important not to mistake the flexor withdrawal reflex for voluntary toe muscle contraction.

Reflex function. The *bulbocavernosus reflex* is positive if, on squeezing the glans penis or the clitoris, the anal sphincter contracts on a gloved finger put into the anus. It is absent only when spinal shock is present. Its return (about 24 hours after the injury) signifies the end of the spinal shock.

Absence of sensory and motor function after the expiration of spinal shock signifies a complete and irreversible cord damage.

Spinal shock. For the first 24 hours or so after a spinal cord injury, the cord is in shock (*'spinal shock'*) and cannot mediate any reflex activity. After the expiration of this period, the bulbocavernous and anal reflexes return

TYPES OF POSSIBLE NEUROLOGICAL DAMAGE

- **Spinal shock**
  In spinal shock, all cord function, including reflex function ceases. The *bulbocavernosus reflex* is easily tested and found to be absent i.e. on squeezing the glans penis or the clitoris, the anal sphincter *does not* contract on a gloved finger put into the anus. Its return (about 24 hours after the injury) signifies the end of the spinal shock. Absence of sensory and motor function after the expiration of spinal shock signifies a complete and irreversible cord damage.

- **Cord concussion**
  The cord is "bruised", so to say, not badly hurt. There is flaccid motor paralysis, sensory loss and visceral paralysis below the level of the cord lesion. However, the lesion is functional rather than anatomical. Recovery begins in a few hours and is complete eventually.

- **Root transaction**
  In this lesion, motor paralysis, sensory loss and visceral paralysis occur in the distribution of damaged root. However, unlike with cord damage, the motor fibres of an affected root can regenerate, being a peripheral nerve; also, residual motor paralysis is permanently flaccid.

- **Complete cord damage**
  In a complete lesion, there is complete motor paralysis, sensory loss and visceral paralysis below the level of the cord lesion. Motor paralysis is at first flaccid, then becomes spastic with increased muscle tone and tendon reflexes after some days or weeks. Clonus may be present too. The triad of features of an upper motor neurone lesion - 3**H**s: **H**ypertonia, **H**ypertrophy and **H**yper-reflexia - is thus completed. Flexor spasms and contractures may develop later but the sensory loss never recovers.

- **Central cord syndrome**
  This syndrome is the commonest amongst the partial cord lesions. It usually results from a hyperextension injury in the older patient with cervical spondylosis or from a flexion injury in the younger patient. The corticospinal and spinothalamic tracts are injured whilst the sacral tracts, which are situated on the periphery of the cord, are spared (*sacral sparing*). Consequently, the following features manifest:

  - lower motor neurone (flaccid) paralysis of the upper limbs
  - upper motor neurone (spastic) paralysis of the lower limbs
  - spared peri-anal sensation and
  - spared bladder control

The prognosis is good in up to 50% of cases and the patient can be expected to regain reasonable sensory and motor function in the lower limbs and trunk; in the upper limb similar recovery occurs except in the hand. Bowel and bladder control can also be expected to be regained.

- **The anterior cord syndrome**
  This syndrome which usually results from a hyperflexion injury with resulting burst fracture which compresses the anterior spinal artery and spinal cord. Motor paralysis and sensory loss are complete. Only the dorsal tracts (medial and lateral) which transmit pain, temperature, light and deep touch sensations are spared (*dorsal column sparing*). However, in practice, only sensation to deep pressure is spared (trunk and lower limbs). The prognosis is good if there is evidence of progressive recovery in the first 24 hours.

- **The posterior cord syndrome**
  This is perhaps the rarest of all the syndromes. Only the dorsal tracks are damaged, with consequent loss of deep pressure sensation, deep pain sensation and proprioception. Motor power and pain and temperature sensations are retained.

- **Brown-Sequard syndrome**
  This is less common in cervical than in thoracic cord injuries. Either the lateral or the medial half of the cord is damaged resulting in ipsilateral motor paralysis and loss of proprioception and contralateral loss of pain and temperature sensation. The prognosis for partial recovery is good and most of the patients regain bowel and bladder function and are able to walk.

- **Cauda equina syndrome**
  This is caused by multilevel lumbosacral root compression within the lumbar spinal canal. The clinical signs include saddle anaesthesia, bilateral radicular pain, numbness, weakness, hyporeflexia or areflexia and loss of voluntary bladder and bowel function.

GRADING OF SPINAL CORD INJURY

The most popular is that proposed by Frankel:

Grade A. Absent motor and sensory function
Grade B. Absent motor function; sensation present
Grade C. Motor function present but not useful(2/5 or 3/5); sensation present
Grade D. Motor function present and useful (4/5); sensation present
Grade E. Normal motor function and sensory function

SURGICAL Treatment OF SPINAL CORD INJURY

It is right to say that there is no curative surgical treatment for established and complete spinal cord injury. However, incomplete lesions in a situation involving spinal column instability will definitely benefit from surgical stabilisation by a competent spinal surgeon.

MEDICAL Treatment OF SPINAL CORD INJURY

There is medical treatment for reversible spinal cord injury:

- Corticosteroids given in high doses, starting within 4 hours of a reversible cord lesion, is known to limit cord damage. They have no benefit if started more than 8 hours post-injury. They are said to work by their anti-inflammatory action, which limits tissue oedema. Currently, Methylprednisolone is the preferred steroid. An initial intravenous bolus doze of 30 mg/kg body weight is given, followed by a continuous intravenous infusion of 5.4 mg/kg body weight/hour for about 48 hours. Alternatively, Dexamethasone can be given intravenously as Dexamethasone phosphate: 10 mg initially, then 4 mg by intramuscular injection every 6 hours as required for 2-10 days.

- Experimental drugs currently used include Nalozone, an opiate receptor antagonist and GMI gangliosides.

DISLOCATIONS OF THE CERVICAL SPINE

OCCIPUT/C1 DISLOCATION

Dislocation at the occiput/C1 level can occur as a result of a violent twisting force to the head. All the ligamentous connections between the occiput and C1 rupture may be severed, allowing a dislocation to one side or the other. Most patients with the injury die from a high cord damage. In those who survive, the injury remains unstable and immediate immobilisation is necessary. This can be achieved with a halo-body cast, a Minerva jacket, skull traction or surgical fusion with bone-grafting.

C1 - C2 DISLOCATIONS

There are four main types of dislocations at the C1-C2 level – anterior dislocation with rupture of the transverse ligament, anterior dislocation with fracture of the base of the odontoid peg, posterior dislocation and rotatory subluxation.

Some of these injuries are likely to be fatal because there is a good chance that an intact odontoid peg will injure the spinal cord, causing a high cord injury. Determining cervical stability clinically and with conventional X-rays or CT scan is important.

Treatment options include skull traction, halo-jacket, halo-body cast and posterior fusion of C1 to C2.

C3 – C7 DISLOCATIONS

These injuries usually result from flexion-rotation forces. The posterior ligament complex ruptures, the intervertebral disc is disrupted and the facet joints dislocate or sublux. This injury is best seen on lateral X-rays, CT and MRI scans (Fig.16.5).

Facet joint dislocations could be unilateral or bilateral. In a *unilateral facet dislocation*, the chin of the patient is turned to the side opposite to the side of the dislocation. The lateral X-ray shows the vertebral body 25% subluxed anteriorly. The injury may not be apparent on this view but will be so on left and right oblique views which show the facet joints clearly. There is a radiculopathy in 75% of patients though only 10% have spinal cord injury. In *bilateral facet dislocation*, there is a 50% or more anterior displacement of the vertebral body. Associated spinal cord injury is common but the author has treated a number of patients with 100% displacement but no neurological deficit; the dislocations were successfully reduced by skull traction.

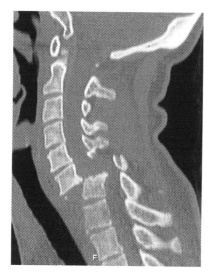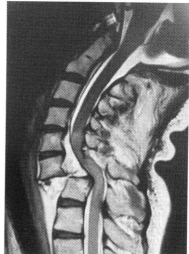

Fig.16.5a&b. CT and MRI scan of the C-spine showing a fracture-dislocation at C6/C7. The spinal cord was injured and the patient was quadriplegic.

The key issues in treatment are the questions of stability and whether or not neurological damage is present. An MRI scan is the best tool because it shows the soft tissues well. Management options include reduction e.g. by skull traction, followed by immobilisation e.g. a halo-jacket contraption.

FRACTURES OF THE UPPER CERVICAL SPINE (C1-C2)

FRACTURE OF THE NEURAL ARCH OF C1 (JEFFERSON'S FRACTURE)

This fracture occurs at the weakest points of the ring of the atlas - the junctions between the posterior arches and the lateral masses. It is usually due to axial compression such as can occur from a weight falling on the head, the head striking the roof of a car in an accident or a fall on the heels from a height. The injuring structures are the occipital condyles. There is usually no encroachment of the spinal canal, so neurological damage is rare. However, when there is neurological injury, it is usually fatal because of the high level. The injury is best diagnosed with a CT scan.

Treatment. Treatment is best administered in a dedicated Spinal Unit. A stable fracture can be treated with a hard collar for 6 weeks. An unstable fracture can be treated in a number of ways. Immobilisation in a halo-body jacket for about 3 months is probably the best option. Other treatment options include skull traction and use of a Minerva jacket.

FRACTURES OF THE ODONTOID PEG

The odontoid may be fractured at its tip, middle or base. This is the basis of the Anderson and D'Alonzo classification. Rotational or shearing forces are probably responsible for these fractures.

Anderson and D'Alonzo classification

Type I: Fracture of tip
Type II: Fracture of middle part, at the junction of the body and the neck
Type III: Fracture of base

Stability or lack of it is determined indirectly by the **atlanto-dens interval (ADI)**, the distance between the anterior aspect of the odontoid and the posterior ring of the atlas, which should not be >3mm. A bigger gap suggests a transverse ligament rupture and possible instability. A CT scan may show a bone avulsion by the ligament and an MRI scan can show the ligament directly.

Treatment. Type I fractures usually settle with neck collar stabilisation for a short period – 4-6 weeks. Types II and III fractures require immobilisation in a halo-jacket for about 3 months. Type III fractures usually heal well; Type II has up to 50% non-union rate.

Comment. The possibility of congenital anomalies of the odontoid (complete absence, hypoplasia, persistent os odontoideum) should be borne in mind. Tomograms or CT scanning may be required. The key to diagnosis is the spatial relationship between the anterior surface of the odontoid peg and the posterior surface of the anterior arch of the atlas - *the atlanto-dens interval (ADI).*

FRACTURE OF THE PEDICLE OR LATERAL PILLAR OF C2 (HANGMAN'S FRACTURE)

There are two mechanisms by which this fracture can come about. In the first mechanism, there is a hyperextension force accompanied by distraction of the neck. After the fracture has occurred the neck continues to be distracted, leading to death from cord damage - *Hangman's fracture.* In the second mechanism, hyperextension is accompanied by compression. The same fracture occurs but injury to the cord is rare. Some surgeons treat this injury with a cervical collar but it is probably safer to treat it with a halo-body jacket for about 12 weeks. Posterior or anterior C2-C3 discectomy followed by fusion may be indicated in some patients.

FRACTURES OF THE LOWER CERVICAL SPINE (C3-C7)

Anterior wedge fracture. This rare fracture results from a pure flexion force. It involves only the anterior column and is stable, requiring only a neck collar for treatment.

Split fracture. This results from a compression force of moderate magnitude. Usually the lower cervical vertebrae are involved. The fractures are also stable; the neck should be immobilised in a cervical collar until neck movement becomes pain-free.

Burst fracture. This also results from powerful compression forces, resulting in 'bursting' of the vertebral bodies. In everyday life, the injury is commonly seen in swimming pool diving accidents. Even though essentially stable, burst fractures have a high potential for injuring the spinal cord because of the tendency of the vertebral fragments to be pushed backwards (retropulsed) into the spinal canal. Highly comminuted burst fractures are called teardrop fractures; they are usually associated with *quadriplegia.*

Treatment is by continuous skull traction for 6 weeks, after which a collar is worn until interbody fusion occurs, usually within another 6-12 weeks. Check X-rays - normal lateral and flexion and extension laterals - are taken at 12 weeks from the injury. The collar is discarded if clinically there is no neck pain and if X-ray show evidence of interbody fusion. Surgical fusion may be indicated if non-union results.

Avulsion fractures of the cervical spine

Resisted violent contractions of cervical muscles may cause avulsion fractures of the processes, especially the spinous processes. Avulsion of the spinous process of C7 is one of the better known examples and is called the "clay-shoveller's" fracture because it was common among labourers who used to use the shovel a lot.

WHIPLASH INJURIES OF THE NECK

This is usually seen in road traffic accidents. In the classical case, it occurs in an occupant of a stationary vehicle, usually a car that has been hit from the rear by another vehicle at a road junction or roundabout. On impact, the neck of the occupant hyperextends and then returns to the neutral or slightly flexed position.

The commonest symptoms are neck pain (88-100% of patients) and stiffness. Other complaints include occipital headaches, shoulder and arm pain, interscapular pain, paraesthesia and weakness in one or both arms, vertigo, concentration and memory loss. There may also be complaints of dysphagia, or of visual or auditory deficits. Possible neurological deficit ranges from transient numbness or hyperaesthesia or paraparesis to full-blown quadri- or para-plegia. Complaint of low back pain is also common.

Immediate X-rays may show loss of the usual lordosis of the cervical spine from spasm of the paraspinal muscles. An MRI scan may be indicated only if the history and a proper physical examination point to possible root compression.

Treatment. This very much depends on the time the patient presents post-injury. In general, less than a quarter of patients present acutely to the orthopaedic surgeon, who usually sees them in connection with compensation claims. Those presenting acutely to the Accident and Emergency departments may benefit from *soft collars* and *analgesics.* Supervised physiotherapy is almost always helpful.

Despite the protection accredited to them, seat belts have not been shown by many studies to be of much benefit; it has been suggested in some quarters that mandatory seatbelt wearing has possibly increased the incidence of *whiplash associated disorders (WAD)*.

The Quebec task force on whiplash injuries has graded WAD as follows:

- Grade I: complaint of neck pain, stiffness or tenderness.
- Grade II: neck complaints with musculoskeletal signs of localisedtenderness and decreased range of movement.
- Grade III: neck complaints and objective neurological signs.
- Grade IV: neck complaints and fracture or dislocation.

Multidisciplinary team evaluation is recommended for patients who have not been able to return to their normal work 6-12 weeks post-injury. *Surgery* (discectomy; anterior fusion) may be indicated in the occasional patient with disc protrusion and severe root signs. The prognosis in whiplash injuries is guarded. Compensation claims tend to muddle the waters.

FRACTURES AND DISLOCATION OF THE THORACO-LUMBAR SPINE

FIRST AID

As mentioned earlier in this Chapter, it is vital to institute first-aid measures in any patient with suspected thoracolumbar injury. Basically, the spine should be immobilised to avoid further damage. Inflatable splints are available to paramedics working in the context of the Ambulance services. Where this is not available, the patient can be immobilised on a *long spinal board* or *wooden plank* and *a cervical collar* can be improvised too (Fig.16.4. above). The patient should then be transported expeditiously and safely to a hospital with facilities for effective diagnosis and treatment of spinal injuries.

MECHANISMS OF INJURY

Thoracolumbar injuries can arise from the following mechanisms:

- Flexion
- Flexion-rotation
- Extension
- Compression

Most **thoracic spine injuries** result from hyperflexion. Anterior wedge fractures are common in elderly ladies with osteoporosis. They are usually stable but may progressively lead to kyphotic deformity, especially if more than one vertebra is involved. Severe injuries in young people tend to involve T11 and T12, which are "unsplinted" by the ribs and carry a high risk of spinal cord injury, which, unfortunately, tend to be complete.

Most severe thoracolumbar fractures and dislocations arise from *indirect trauma*. Injuring forces can be predominantly flexion, extension, rotational, shear, compression and distraction forces. Avulsion fractures result from violent muscle contractions. *Direct trauma* can result from direct blows or hits from solid objects such as a stick, from falls on sharp or blunt solid structures or from missiles such as bullets. Although some of the resulting injuries may be unstable, most are stable and associated spinal cord injury is uncommon.

DIAGNOSIS

A diagnosis can be made on the basis of a good history and physical findings. Lack of sophisticated diagnostic facilities is not a good excuse for inability to make a reasonable diagnosis of a thoracolumbar injury.

History

It is important to obtain a history of the accident that has caused the injury. Falls of heavy objects on the back are characteristic. In road traffic accidents enquiry should be made about whether a seat belt was worn or not. Sometimes trivial injury like that caused by lifting a relatively small object in the stooping position or sneezing can be the cause of a thoracolumbar injury. This is more likely to occur in spines weakened by disease such as osteoporosis, osteomalacia or metastatic deposits. The past medical history (known malignancy, coeliac disease, and menopause) may point to a possible contributing factor.

Physical examination

A brief general and local examination examination should be carried out along established lines of "looking", "feeling" and "moving". Both must be systematic.

Radiological examination

Conventional *AP, lateral and oblique views* should be done routinely; other views may be indicated. The *CT scan* is probably the most important single investigative modality. Most surgeons consider it an essential investigation before any operative intervention can be undertaken. It demonstrates bony impingement on the neural canal and helps in the assessment of stability. An *MRI scan* may demonstrate more precisely the state of the intervertebral disc, local ligaments, the spinal cord and neural elements.

Neurological examination

If neurological injury is suspected from the history and physical findings, a full neurological examination must be carried out along the same lines.

A sensory test should be carried out according to the dermatomes. Motor function is easier to test especially with the co-operation of the patient. After the expiration of the period of spinal shock (24 hours or so after the injury), the cremasteric and bulbocavernous reflexes return. If sensory and motor paralysis still persist, the cord lesion is complete and irreversible. The deep tendon reflexes are intact (and exaggerated) in a complete cord lesion; in a root lesion i.e. cauda equina lesion, they are absent and motor paralysis is flaccid.

MANAGEMENT OF INDIVIDUAL INJURIES

The issue of management often revolves around two factors:

- Is the injury *stable or unstable?* and
- Is there a *neurological deficit?*

The *3-column theory of stability* discussed under cervical spine injuries was actually formulated by Denis for thoracolumbar spinal injuries. As a reminder, the 3 columns are the *anterior, middle and posterior. An unstable injury is one with any two-column or middle-column failure.*

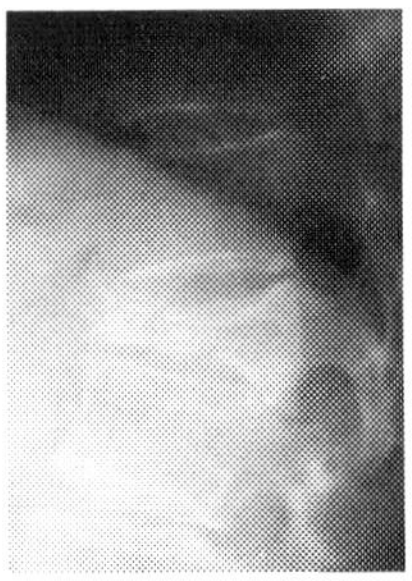

Anterior Wedge Compression Fractures (Fig.16.6)

These result from flexion injuries. If loss of anterior column height is less the 50%, the injury is considered to be stable and it is treated by a short period of bed rest (1-2 weeks) and analgesics followed by gradual mobilisation in a hyperextension brace for 3 months.

Height collapse more than 50% is best regarded as potentially unstable. Treatment options include longer bedrest (for 3-4 weeks) and surgical stabilisation.

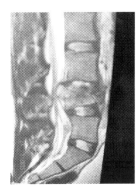

Fig.16.6. Conventional *lateral view* **showing anterior wedge fractures of L1. The height collapse is more than 50%, so the injury is potentially unstable.**

Burst Fractures

These result from hyperflexion injuries with or without axial compression causing anterior body compression fracture with or without disruption of the posterior elements. If the posterior ligament complex is intact, the injury may be considered stable. Most of them are probably unstable and bony fragments may be pushed backwards to cause cord/root damage (Fig.16.7).

Treatment is non-operative, with a hyperextension brace, or operative. Surgical stabilisation is advocated even for complete neurological deficit to facilitate nursing care and rehabilitation.

Fig.16.7. Burst fracture of L4 with retropulsed fragments compressing the spinal cord.

Fracture-Dislocations

These involve disruption of the three columns by a combination of anterior compression, distraction and rotation. They are highly unstable and associated with significant neurological deficit, dural tears and intra-abdominal injuries and should be treated by both anterior and posterior stabilisation.

Chance Fracture

The classical Chance fracture passes through a vertebral body from front to back, like a thin knife through soft butter, leaving the affected vertebra "intact". It is usually stable and can be treated by extension bracing. However, an injury passing through soft tissues – intervertebral disc and ligaments - from front to back has since been recognised. This latter injury may not heal with bracing and operative treatment by posterior reduction and stabilisation is recommended.

Posterior Column Injuries

These are extension injuries with an anterior vertebral body avulsion fracture and fractures of the posterior column, including the spinous process, lamina and occasionally pedicles. They are best demonstrated on oblique films. They are usually stable and will heal with brace or cast immobilisation for 6-12 weeks.

COMPLICATIONS OF THORACOLUMBAR INJURIES

- The immediate complication is neurological injury.

- Early complications include *bed sores* and *intolerance of bracing* as well as *surgical complications,* including possible vascular and neurological injury and infection.

- The main late complication is *increasing deformity from chronic instability,* which in turn results from failure of healing by bony fusion, *pseudarthrosis, chronic pain* at the site of the injury and *progressive neurological deficit.* A lumbar corset may be helpful. Pain from instability can be successfully treated by fusion.

THE MANAGEMENT OF PARAPLEGIC AND QUADRIPLEGIC PATIENTS

Definitions

Paraplegia: occurs in spinal cord injuries from T1/T2 to L1/L2 vertebral level. The brachial plexus having escaped, the arms are neurologically normal. The paralysis is that of all motor and sensory and reflex function involving the trunk below the injury level and both lower limbs. With regard to reflex function, there is areflexia (absence of reflexes) in lower motor neurone and hyper-reflexia in upper motor neurone lesions. **Quadriplegia:** there is paralysis of the upper limbs (usually incompletely), the whole trunk and both lower limbs.

The Aims of Management

The aims are to achieve the *total rehabilitation of the patient - physical, mental and occupational.* The achievement of this aim is not easy even in medical centres with the best of facilities. Under-staffed and under-equipped general hospitals are not the best place to rehabilitate paraplegic and quadriplegic patients, except if there are no better alternatives.

The problem and methods of tackling them

The bulk of the work of management lies in preventing and treating the complications of paralysis. In the main, these complications arise from

1. *the anaesthetic skin*
2. *partially denervated bladder and rectum*
3. *denervated muscles* and
4. *immobilised joints.*

Concretely, measures need to be instituted to prevent:

- *horrifying bedsores*
- *intractable skin, urinary and respiratory tract infections*
- *possible burns* from hot water bottles or hot drinks
- *rock-stiff joints* and
- *other preventable complications* seen on the wards.

Other problems have to do with *the patient's psyche*, the way he or she now sees themselves vis-à-vis their family, friends and the entire environment. The methods of tackling these problems are complex but have been worked out. To be successful, team work is essential, with the physician, nurse, physiotherapist, occupational therapist and the patient's relatives and friends contributing in equal measure.

"CLEARING THE SPINE"

Clearing the spine means excluding spinal injury in a patient brought to the hospital with multiple trauma. In many hospitals in the developed countries, a multi-disciplinary team, usually termed the **Trauma Team,** is charged with the compulsory duty of initially managing such a patient. Clearing the spine is considered **a must-do** in **a multiple trauma patient** because of the real possibility that the injuring forces that have caused him or her multiple injuries could easily have also caused a cervical or other spinal fracture, which may, in turn, have caused spinal cord injury or may do so if doctors and other hospital staff handling the patient are not aware that such an injury is present in the patient. Clearing the spine is the job of the orthopaedic and radiology members of the Trauma Team, who must be available to do the job 24/7.

Clearing the spine is based on:

- A good history-taking, which may point to possible spinal injury.
- A careful and competent physical examination, which may elicit tenderness and pain in the spinal column or the presence of neurological deficit.
- Radiological imaging (XRs and CT) based on physical findings. Patients who are *corpus menti*, not intoxicated and with normal physical findings do not have to have X-rays or CT scans.

It goes without saying that a reasonable level of knowledge and clinical acumen in spinal anatomy and injuries are needed to be able to "clear the spine".

FRACTURES OF THE PELVIS

Introduction

Fractures of the pelvis constitute about 3% of all fractures but occupy a special place in surgical practice because of their capacity to cause immediately life-threatening or delayed life-crippling complications. Most patients are victims of road traffic accidents or falls from high heights.

- The pelvis can be considered to be a *bony ring* composed by the two halves of the pelvis, the sacrococcygeal spine, the two sacro-iliac joints and the symphysis pubis. The ring lies on the horizontal plane and can be squashed in the anterior-posterior and lateral to lateral directions. It can be divided into an anterior segment (made up of the pubis and the ischium) and a posterior segment (made of the ilii and the sacrum) by a line joining the posterior borders of the acetabulum (Fig.16.8). .

- Any given fracture can be considered mainly with regard to its effect on the *stability of the ring*: (1) Fractures or dislocations that go through the ring at only one point are stable injuries as far as the ring as a whole is concerned and hardly require active treatment. (2) Those breaking the ring at two or more points are potentially unstable fractures, prone to complications and generally requiring active treatment. The stability of the pelvis is heavily dependent on the posterior structures – the ilii, sacrum and the sacroiliac joints.

- **Pelvic fractures are notorious for their serious complications requiring emergency treatment before the fractures themselves are treated:**

  1. *Severe haemorrhage.* is a real danger in pelvic fractures because (a) the iliac bone is rich in marrow vessels and (b) the iliac vessels lie very close to the bone and both are liable to injury by pelvic fractures
  2. *Urinary bladder and urethra injuries* are common because of the proximity of these delicate organs to the pelvis.

A patient with a suspected pelvic fracture must be assessed with the mentioned complications in mind and action must be taken quickly if they are present.

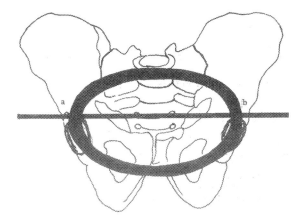

Fig.16.8. The pelvic ring.

CLASSIFICATION (Fig.16.9)

The classification proposed by Burgess et al (1990) recognises four patterns of injury: - *lateral compression* (LC), *antero-posterior compression* (APC), *vertical shear* (VS) and *combined mechanism* (CM).

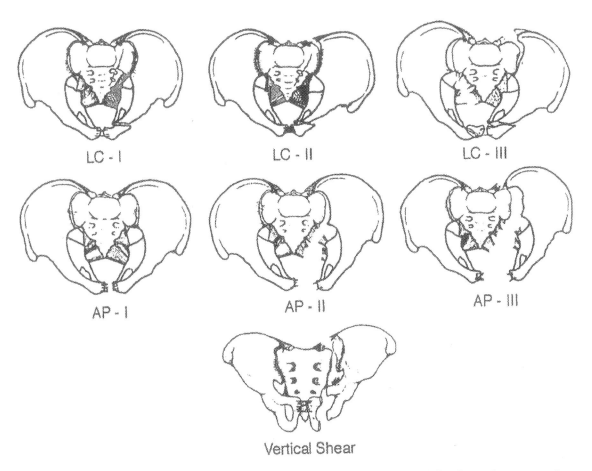

Fig.16.9. Young-Burgess classification of pelvic injuries. Abbreviations: LC = lateral compression; AP = antero-posterior compression (VS = vertical shear)

LC injuries. The injuring force is from the side and the severity (Types I-III) is determined by the presence or absence of disruption of the posterior sacroiliac structures. Acetabular fractures are commonly associated.

LC-I :   anterior transverse fracture (pubic rami), but there is no posterior instability but a crush fracture of the sacrum may be present.

LC-II: medial displacement of the anterior hemipelvis is associated with a fracture of the iliac wing, or disruption or fracture of the sacroiliac joint, producing posterior instability. Anteriorly, there is a transverse fracture of the pubic rami.

LC-III: the deforming force opens up the pelvis on the contralateral side to produce a windswept pelvis.

APC injuries. These result from direct anterior or posterior trauma and are divided into three subtypes, depending on the degree of displacement:

APC-I: minimal displaced pubic rami fractures or mild symphysis pubis diastasis (less than 2cm).

APC-II: the pelvis opens like a book and the anterior sacroiliac, sacrospinous and sacrotuberous ligaments are disrupted.

APC-III: all the sacroiliac structures, including the posterior ligaments are disrupted.

APC-II and APC-III injuries represent the *Malgaigne* injuries and are commonly associated with significant haemorrhage.

VS injuries. These result from falls from a height. A fracture goes through the pubic rami and the posterior pelvis, displacing the hemipelvis vertically (Fig.16.2).

CM injuries. These result from a combination of injuring forces e.g. LC/VS or LC/APC.

DIAGNOSIS AND TREATMENT OF ASSOCIATED LIFE-THREATENING INJURIES

Haemorrhage. is a real possibility in pelvic fractures because (a) the iliac bone is rich in marrow vessels and (b) the iliac vessels lie very close to the bone and both liable to injury by pelvic fractures. If there is apparent bleeding or signs of shock, this must be tackled immediately along established lines. If adequate fluid/blood replacement does not succeed in controlling shock, then bleeding is continuing. From the orthopaedic point of view, if there is pelvic disruption, a significant fraction of the bleeding should be presumed to be coming from *gaping marrow vessels* which require immediate fracture reduction and compression for control. The quickest and most effective way of achieving this is by the application of an **external fixator** (Fig.16.10), which, in experienced hands can be done in about 20 minutes in the resuscitation room. The stabilisation of any posterior instability can be left till later.

Other sources of internal bleeding include abdominal vessels, the symptoms and signs of which could be lower abdominal pain, abdominal distension and rigidity, bruises and expanding ecchymosis over the anterior abdominal wall, the flanks, the perineum and proximal thigh. The other source of haemorrhage is pelvis vessels. The help of the general surgeon, vascular surgeon and the radiologist should be sought to deal with these problems.

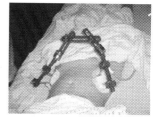

Genito-urinary injuries are common. Injuries to the urinary bladder, urethra and vagina may require urgent treatment. Urgent help from a urological colleague must be sought.

Fig.16.10. The external fixator is used to control haemorrhage from pelvic fractures and can be a life saver.

DIAGNOSIS OF PELVIC FRACTURES

A patient with a pelvic fracture is usually in considerable pain and must be examined with care. Physical signs may include bruises, swelling, deformity, tenderness and crepitus. Pressing on the symphysis pubis, exerting pressure on the iliac crests and compressing the pelvic ring in a side-to-side direction will elicit pain at corresponding points. Testing for hip joint movements must be carried out to exclude acetabular fractures.

Conventional X-rays are the main diagnostic tool. The standard views are the *anteroposterior, the pelvic inlet* (60 degree caudad) and *the pelvic outlet* (45 degree cephalad) (Fig.16.11). It is thought that 90% of all pelvic injuries can be diagnosed on an AP film alone; adding of inlet and outlet views brings this figure up to 94%.

CT scan, especially with 3-D reconstruction, gives very valuable information, especially if acetabular injury is suspected. It also shows the posterior portion of the pelvic ring much better than conventional X-rays.

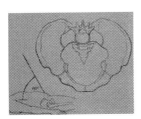 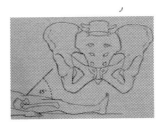

Fig.16.11a&b. X-ray Diagnosis of pelvic fractures: (a) pelvic inlet and (b) outlet views.

TREATMENT OF INDIVIDUAL PELVIC INJURIES

Avulsion Fractures

The common ones are:

- anterior superior iliac spine (avulsed by the sartorius),
- the anterior inferior iliac spine (avulsed by the straight head of the quadriceps)
- the pubis (avulsed by adductor longus)
- the ischium (avulsed by the hamstrings

The usual mechanism is sudden resistance to violent contraction of the corresponding muscles. The injuries are more common in athletic young people before the fusion of the relevant secondary centres of ossification to the main bones.

Rest, analgesics and reassurance usually suffice and most patients are able to start walking within a few days and resume athletic activities within 4 weeks or so. Immobilisation in a hip spica or by open reduction and internal fixation is reserved for the more severe avulsions.

Treatment of single bone injuries

Isolated pubic rami fractures are common in lateral compression injuries (LC1). There is no posterior instability. The patient is treated with bedrest, analgesics and physiotherapy and mobilised on crutches as soon as it is comfortable to do so. Bed rest can be enforced with bilateral skin traction (Fig.16.12). Check X-rays are taken two days into mobilisation to monitor possible displacement of the fractures.

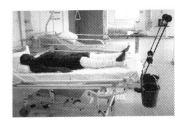

Fig.16.12. Here, bedrest has been enforced with skin traction on an IWOT frame

Treatment of complex injuries

Complex and unstable injuries are caused via various mechanisms and require stabilisation. This may be anterior or posterior stabilisation or both. External fixation (Fig.16.10), Ganz frame, lag screws and ORIF are options. Individual components of the injury are addressed separately along established lines.

POSTOPERATIVE CARE

When used, the *external fixator* is kept in place for varying periods, depending on the injury being treated. If used for pain control e.g. in LC injuries, it is retained for 3-6 weeks; for full or partial stabilisation of anterior ring disruption with intact posterior ring - 8 weeks; for vertically unstable fractures – 12 weeks. Pin-track care is essential and pin-track infection may affect the timing of fixator removal.

Check X-rays are taken 1-2 weeks to monitor possible early loss of reduction or fixation and thereafter 3 monthly for the first year.

COMPLICATIONS

Early complications

1. Haemorrhage has been discussed.
2. Bladder and urethra.
3. Vaginal lacerations should be promptly sutured and prophylactic antibiotics given.
4. **Nerve injury.** The *sciatic nerve* is liable to injury in pelvic fractures in which fracture fragments get displaced posteriorly in the region of the hip joint or in those associated with posterior dislocation of the hip. The *obturator nerve* is also sometimes injured. Expectant symptomatic treatment is adequate in many cases but exploration (of the sciatic nerve) may be indicated.

Late complications

These include infection, DVT, mal-union and non-union.

PROGNOSIS

Long-term pelvic pain, altered sexual activity and disability are common and are related to the severity of the original injury and of residual deformity.

FRACTURES OF THE ACETABULUM

ANATOMY OF THE ACETABULUM (Figs.16.13&14)

The acetabulum is made of an anterior column and a posterior column. The anterior column is the mass of bone stretching downwards from the anterior inferior iliac spine to include the pubis and the anterior half of the acetabulum. The posterior column is the mass of bone stretching downwards from the sciatic notch to the ischial tuberosity, including the posterior half of the acetabulum. The acetabular dome, which is the weight-bearing area, is not a separate entity but consists of portions of both the anterior and posterior columns.

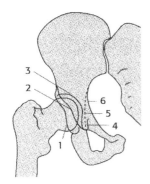

Fig.16.13. The anterior and posterior walls and the roof of the acetabulum:
1: Posterior wall   2: Anterior wall   3: Roof   4: The teardrop
5: ilioischial line (posterior column)   6:Pelvic brim (anterior column).

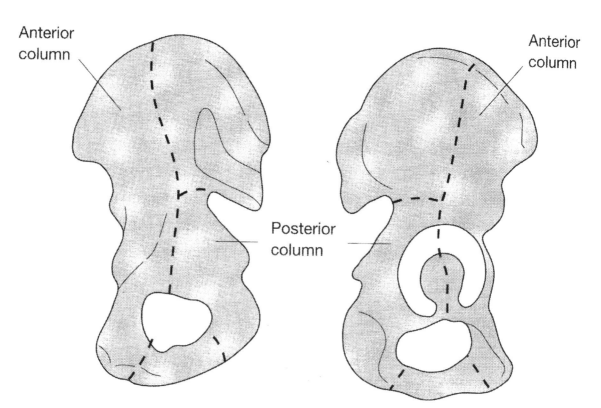

Fig.16.14. Anatomy of the acetabulum showing the anterior and posterior columns.

CLASSIFICATION

Letournel and Judet classification is based on the walls and columns of the acetabulum.

Summary

- *Simple fracture types:* simple fractures are those involving only one wall or column

- *Associated fracture types:* the associated fracture types involve both columns and have more complex fracture patterns such as T-shape fractures

Details

Type A: Partial articular one column fracture
        A1: posterior wall
        A2: posterior column
        A3: anterior wall and/or anterior column

Type B: Partial articular transverse fracture
        B1: Transverse plus posterior wall
        B2: T-types
        B3: Anterior with posterior hemitransverse

Type C: Both column fractures (all articular segments, including the roof, are detached from the remaining segment of the intact ilium – "the floating acetabulum").
        C1: Both column – anterior column fracture extends to the iliac crest (high variety).
        C2: Both column – anterior column fracture extends to the anterior border of the ilium (low variety).
        C3: Both column – anterior column fracture enters the sacro-iliac joint.

MECHANISMS OF INJURY

Various injuring forces, direct and indirect, can cause acetabular fractures. The femoral head is hammered into the acetabulum, causing it to fracture. Its position at the moment of impact determines the various fracture patterns. Low-energy injuries, such as from simple falls, cause isolated and simple fractures whilst high-energy ones, such as result from road traffic accidents, produce the more complex fractures.

DIAGNOSIS

A good history of the causative accident may suggest the mechanism and through this, the fracture sustained. Clinical features include bruises, swelling, tenderness and pain in the affected hip joint area. These features may also be present in other areas of the lower limb, depending on the mechanism of injury in a given patient. In particular, symptoms and signs in the foot (calcaneum), knee and greater trochanter areas are usually of significance. Characteristic signs of acetabular fractures are pain on movement of the hip and limitation of ranges of hip movements.

X-rays (routine AP and lateral plus Judet views) are essential for accurate diagnosis of acetabular fractures. *CT scanning*, especially spiral CT with 3-D reconstruction, provides valuable additional information such as evidence of fragmentation of the anterior or posterior wall.

TREATMENT

Non-operative Treatment

Skeletal traction applied through the distal femur or upper tibia for 8 – 12 weeks could be considered for:

- undisplaced and minimally displaced fractures (<3mm) of the dome.
- low anterior column and low transverse fractures.
- "secondary congruence" displaced fractures of both-column in which comminuted fragments assume a position of congruency around the femoral head.
- when there are medical contra-indications to surgery.
- local soft-tissue problems, such as infection, wounds and bruises may contra-indicate both skeletal traction and surgery.

Operative Treatment

Reconstructive surgery is indicated in unstable fractures resulting in disruption of the ball and socket configuration of the hip joint. The principle of operative treatment is to effect anatomical reduction of the fractures and to achieve a good fixation with lag screws and appropriately contoured pelvic reconstruction plates, acting as neutralisation plates.

Postoperative Care

Supportive therapy includes prophylactic antibiotics and active physiotherapy. Non-weightbearing may be required for the first post-operation week; partial weightbearing is prescribed for 8-12 weeks, depending on the fracture and the stability of the fixation.

COMPLICATIONS

- *Mortality and post-op infection.* There is a 0-2.5% *mortality* associated with acetabular fractures. The *infection* rate following surgery is quoted as 1-5%.
- *Sciatic nerve palsy* occurs in up to 15% (2-6% following surgery).
- *Loss of fracture reduction.* This is often due to inadequate fixation or early weight bearing.
- *Deep vein thrombosis* involving the pelvic or ipsilateral femoral veins may occur within 2-3 weeks of a pelvic fracture.
- *Heterotopic calcification* is often related to the surgical approach used, occurring in almost all extensile approaches. Indomethacin, 25mg twice daily for 4-6 weeks or low-dose radiation reduces the incidence.
- *Avascular necrosis* of the posterior wall and of the femoral head in posterior dislocations is not uncommon (1.6-7.5%).
- *Post-traumatic osteoarthritis* of the hip is common. This may necessitate total hip replacement.

PROGNOSIS

The gold-standard treatment for displaced acetabular fractures is open reduction and internal fixation performed early post-injury in a specialised centre. Poor prognostic factors include advanced patient age, delay to surgery, poor-quality reductions and some fracture patterns. Complications are common in the medium- to long-term and the functional outcome is variable.

Further reading

Bohlman HH. Acute Fractures and Dislocations Of The Cervical Spine. *J Bone Joint Surg. 61A*: 119, 1979.

Malanga GA and Nadler S (eds). *Whiplash.* Hanley and Belfus. Philadelphia, 2002.

Denis F. The Three Column Spine And Its Significance In The Classification Of Acute Thoracolumbar Spinal Injuries. *Spine 9*: 817-831, 1983.

Iwegbu CG. Traumatic Paraplegia In Zaria, Nigeria: The Case For A Centre For Injuries Of The Spine. *Paraplegia 21*: 81, 1983.

N. Briffa, R. Pearce, A. M. Hill, M. Bircher. Outcomes of acetabular fracture fixation with ten years' follow-up. *J Bone Joint Surg Br* 93-B:229-236, 2011.

Burgess AR Eastridge BJ and Young JW et al. Pelvic Ring Disruptions: Effective Classification System And Treatment Protocols. *J Trauma 30*: 848-856, 1990.

Burgess A. Young-Burgess classification of pelvic ring fractures: does it predict mortality, transfusion requirements, and non- orthopaedic injuries? (Invited commentary). *J Orthop Trauma.* 24(10):609, 2010.

John H. Harris Jr., Kevin J. Coupe, Jody S. Lee1, Thea Trotscher. CT-Based Acetabular Fracture Classification. *Am. J. Roentgenol* 185:277-280, 2005.

Letournel E and Judet R (eds): *Fractures of the acetabulum,* 2nd ed, Berlin, Springer-Verlag, 1993.

Pennal GF, Tile M, Waddell JP and Garside H. Pelvic Disruption: Assessment and Classification. *Clin Orthop 151*: 12-21, 1980.

Tile M. *Fractures Of The Pelvis and Acetabulum.* Baltimore: Williams & Wilkins, 1995.

Young JWR, Smith RM and Kellam JF. Mini-Symposium: Pelvic Fractures. *Current Orthopaedics 10*: 1-23, 1996.

CHAPTER 17

DISLOCATIONS OF THE HIP JOINT AND FRACTURES OF THE FEMUR

DISLOCATIONS OF THE HIP JOINT

The first point to make is about dislocations of the hip joint is that this joint is undoubtedly the strongest and the most stable of all the synovial joints of the human body. This stability has been made possible by both bony and soft-tissue structures (ligaments and muscles). Accordingly, only forces of great magnitude such as are generated in road traffics, construction and mine accidents and falls from considerable heights can dislocate the hip.

The second point is the complication of *avascular necrosis of the femoral head* following hip dislocations as a result of the injury to some of the precariously arranged blood vessels to the femoral head (Fig.17.1). Traumatic dislocations of the hip are much more common in adults than in children or the elderly.

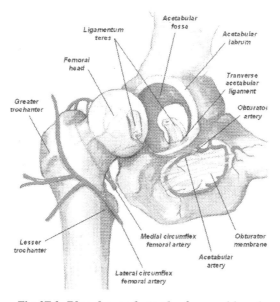

Fig.17.1. Blood supply to the femoral head.

Classification

Three types of hip dislocation are distinguished – *posterior, anterior* and *central* depending on the position of the femoral head in relation to the acetabulum.

POSTERIOR DISLOCATION

Mechanisms of injury

The classical mechanism is a strike on the flexed knee as happens when the knee strikes the dashboard of a car in a head-on collision.

Diagnosis

The history may suggest the injury. The leg on the affected side is shortened and lies adducted, internally rotated and slightly flexed, with the knee resting on the other thigh (Fig.17.2). The patient has severe pain in the hip. On palpation, there is marked tenderness in the hip and the femoral head cannot be felt in its socket; it may be palpable in the buttock. It is important that a systematic general examination of the patient is carried out to rule out associated injuries, which are common.

A routine *AP X-ray* shows the femoral head out of the acetabulum, usually riding high behind the ilium (Fig.17.2). *Oblique views* are needed to show associated fractures of the acetabulum or femoral head. It is important that the femoral shaft is visualised on X-ray as many surgeons have been caught out by an associated femoral shaft fracture. After reduction, a *CT scan* can be carried out to check out possible femoral head or acetabular rim fracture as well as intra-articular fragments.

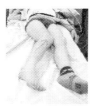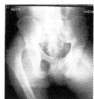

Fig.17.2a&b. The attitude of the affected leg in posterior dislocation of the hip (internal rotation) and X-ray picture showing the femoral head riding high and lying against the side of the iliac bone.

Treatment

Early reduction is imperative. This is best carried out under general anaesthesia with good muscle relaxation but can also be done under intravenous sedation.

There are a number of methods of reduction of posterior dislocation. Allis and Stimson's methods are described here.

- **Allis manoeuvre**

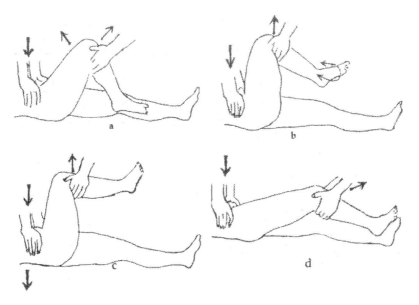

Fig.17.3a-d. Allis manoeuvre

The patient should be laid on a low table but the floor is probably better. An assistant steadies the pelvis by pressing on the anterior superior iliac spines with his palms while the surgeon pulls vertically on the leg, bent to 90degree at both the hip and knee joints. This is usually sufficient to effect reduction although, sometimes, rotatory movement may be needed to disengage the femoral head from entangling soft tissues. Re-entry of the femoral head into the acetabulum can be clearly felt and sometimes heard.

- **Stimson's manoeuvre**

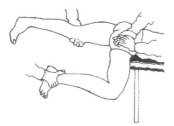

Fig.17.4. Stimson's manoeuvre

Like his manoeuvre for the reduction of shoulder joint dislocation, this one also partly uses the action of gravity. The patient is laid prone with his hips lying at the level of the bottom edge of a low operation table. The good leg is held straight, and supported by an assistant who also holds the affected leg flexed to 90 degrees at both the hip and knee joints. The surgeon then reduces the dislocation by pressing the femoral head down with both palms.

Post-reduction management

The leg is immobilised with skin traction with 5kg weight for about 4 weeks to rest the traumatised soft tissues and aid their healing. Graduated weight-bearing is then allowed.

Open reduction

Open reduction is indicated if closed reduction fails or if there is an associated femoral head or acetabular fracture needing open reduction and internal fixation.

ANTERIOR DISLOCATION

Types of anterior dislocation

Anterior dislocations of the hip are uncommon, accounting for about 10% of all hip dislocations. Four subtypes are distinguished, depending on where the femoral head comes to lie or the presence or otherwise of a femoral head fracture:

- Obturator
- Iliac
- Pubic
- Anterior dislocation with fracture of the femoral head

Mechanisms of injury

The usual mechanism is forced abduction, external rotation and extension of the hip.

Diagnosis

The limb is held abducted and externally rotated, with the hip slightly flexed. It looks longer than it's opposite. X-rays show the femoral head out of the acetabulum, usually in the obturator but sometimes in the pubic or iliac position. Rarely, an associated fracture of the femoral head may be present.

Treatment

Anterior dislocation is best reduced under general anaesthesia with good muscle relaxation. The reduction methods are as follows:

- ***Allis manoeuvre.*** The patient lies supine. An assistant stabilises the pelvis and the surgeon applies longitudinal traction on the thigh *which is adducted and internally rotated at the same time* to achieve reduction.
- *Stimson's gravity method* described for posterior dislocation can also be used here.
- *Post-reduction treatment* is the same as for posterior dislocation.

CENTRAL DISLOCATIONS

Central dislocations are the rarest types of hip dislocation, accounting for only about 5% of cases. The name is a misnomer as it is actually a comminuted fracture of the acetabulum. The acetabular fracture may be that of the inner wall only, a partial acetabular dome fracture or a comminuted fracture of the dome. It is the loss of the integrity of the acetabular floor that permits the femoral head to enter the pelvic cavity.

Mechanisms of injury

The mechanism of injury is either a direct hit on the greater trochanter as in a sideways fall or on indirect force transmitted to the acetabulum during a fall on the foot or a strike on the bent knee with the hip in abduction.

Diagnosis

Physical signs include evidence of injury e.g. bruise, at the point of application of the injuring force. An AP X-ray clearly shows the injury but a CT scan, especially one with 3-D reconstruction provides very useful information (Fig.17.5).

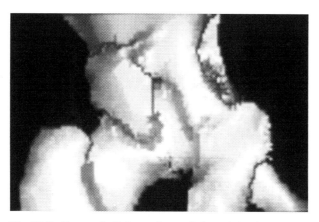

Fig.17.5. Central dislocation of the right hip. Conventional X-rays are the main diagnostic tools but a CT scan, especially with 3D reconstruction, gives a more picturesque information.

Treatment

Treatment aims to achieve a good reduction but this is seldom achieved in practice. There are a number of treatment methods:

1. Forcibly pull out the femoral head with a sudden and forced adduction of the hip bent to 110 degree or so.
2. Employ lateral traction via a trochanteric screw
3. Open reduction and internal fixation of the acetabular fragments. Post-traumatic osteoarthritis usually supervenes and the patient will eventually need a total hip replacement (or hip arthrodesis).

COMPLICATIONS OF HIP DISLOCATIONS

- *Sciatic nerve injury.* This occurs in about 15% (2%-40%) of posterior dislocations. Recovery should take place within one year. If this does not occur, exploration is indicated.

- *Vascular injury.* The femoral vessels are at risk in anterior dislocations so, their function must be checked.

- *Associated fractures* are common and numerous – acetabular rim or floor; femoral head and neck; femoral shaft.

- *Myositis ossificans (Ectopic ossification)* occurs in apparently susceptible individuals.

- *Recurrent dislocations* are rare.

- *Osteoarthritis of the hip* is common following dislocations complicated by acetabular floor fractures or ANFH. Severe osteoarthritis can be treatment with hip replacement.

- ***Avascular necrosis of the femoral head (ANFH).*** This may occur in about 15% of cases, with risk increasing with time to reduction. It is the most serious of all the complications of hip dislocations. The principles of treatment of early disease are to prevent collapse and aid revascularisation. These can be achieved by protecting the hip from weight-bearing for up to 2 years (a near-impossible task even in a cooperative adult). Operative treatment options include core decompression and bone-grafting (Fig.17.6)

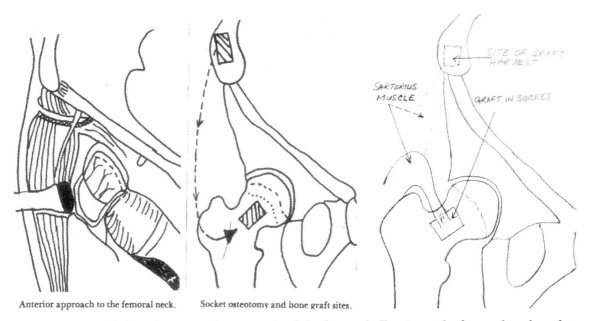

Anterior approach to the femoral neck.   Socket osteotomy and bone graft sites.

Fig.17.6a-c. Post-dislocation avascular necrosis of the femoral : Treatment by femoral neck socket osteotomy plus bone grafting (a) – anterior approach to the femoral neck (b) free bone graft from the iliac crest into a socket in femoral neck (c) - Sartorius muscle pedicled bone graft (Iwegbu, 1982; 1991).

LATE UNDIAGNOSED HIP DISLOCATIONS

These are seen in parts of the developing world. The main cause is initial trial of the so-called native treatment. Up to 10 cases may be seen in an Orthopaedic Department in one year; the story is monotonously the same. Most of the dislocations are posterior, followed by central. The post-dislocation period ranges from 3 months to well over 15 years. Treatment options include traction, arthrodesis and Girdlestone procedure.

FRACTURES OF THE FEMORAL HEAD

As isolated injuries, these fractures are rare. Usually they are associated with fractures of the pelvis, especially the acetabulum, and dislocations of the hip. Confirmation of the diagnosis requires special oblique views and CT scanning of the hip joint. The general principle of treatment is that small fragments not interfering with hip movements should be ignored. Medium-sized fragments on a non-weight-bearing surface should also be ignored, if not causing mechanical obstruction. Large fragments should be screwed back routinely. If most of the head has been broken off or if avascular necrosis supervenes, arthroplasty (or arthrodesis) will have to be considered.

FRACTURES OF NECK OF FEMUR

INTRODUCTION

There is a pattern of occurrence in these fractures relating to *age, sex, geography*. In Europe, these fractures are most commonly seen among postmenopausal and elderly women. This high incidence has been related to post-menopausal oestrogen deficiency and to nutritional factors, among others. In countries with younger populations e.g. in Africa, the incidence is lower. Generally, femoral neck fractures are rare in children.

The first point to make concerns *terminology*. Conceptually, it is better to stick to the terms *"intracapsular"* and *"extracapsular"*, rather than *"fracture neck of femur - #NOF"* as randomly used to denote femoral neck **and** intertrochanteric fractures. The clinical value of using the terms "intracapsular" and "extracapsular" is this: *intracapsular fractures* can be complicated by *non-union* and *avascular necrosis of the femoral head* (because of the peculiarities of the blood supply in the region of the neck mentioned earlier), whereas *extracapsular fractures* are rarely attended with these serious complications. Please note that basal cervical fractures, like intertrochanteric fractures, are extracapsular and have the same prognosis.

MECHANISMS OF INJURY

Three mechanisms are usually identified:

- *Cyclical loading.* In old patients with osteoporosis or osteomalacia, cyclical loading is capable of producing *trabecular fractures*. These stress fractures weaken the bone and make it liable to *complete fractures* on application of torsional forces to the area as obtains even in a minor tripping incident. Secondary tumour deposits in the femoral neck also predispose to fractures.

- *Direct force.* A fall generating a direct blow on the greater trochanter can occasion a femoral neck fracture.
- *The lateral rotation forces* can also cause proximal femoral fractures.

GRADING OF FEMORAL NECK FRACTURES (Fig.17.7)

Garden's X-ray grading or staging of femoral neck fractures (1971) remains the most popular because it is precise and useful for planning treatment and for prognostication.

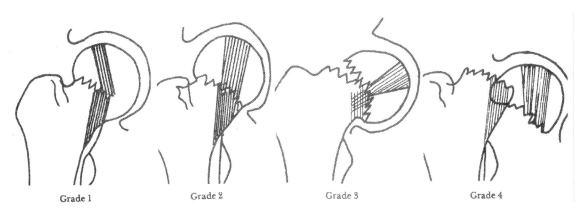

Grade 1   Grade 2   Grade 3   Grade 4

Fig.17.7. Garden's classification of femoral neck fractures:
Grade I. An incomplete fracture involving mainly the superior aspect of the neck (also called *impacted or abducted fracture*).
Grade II. Complete but undisplaced fracture
Grade III. Complete fracture with moderate displacement
Grade IV. Complete fracture with complete displacement

DIAGNOSIS

The age, sex, build and nutritional status of the patient may be useful pointers, so also may some knowledge of the circumstances of the accident and the magnitude of the causative force. The patient has hip pain, the limb is short and externally rotated (Fig.17.8). Any attempt to move the leg at the hip causes excruciating pain. X-rays are essential for an accurate diagnosis. The fracture could be subcapital, transcervical or basal cervical.

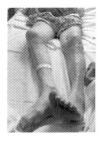

TREATMENT

Fig.17.8. Attitude of the leg following a displaced fracture of the neck of femur

Treatment of Garden I and II fractures

Garden Grade I and II fractures in elderly patients should be treated with 2 or 3 *parallel cannulated screws* (Fig.17.9). X-ray control is required for this procedure. Some surgeons first try mobilising Grade I fracture patients without fixation and go on to fixation if the fracture displaces with weightbearing.

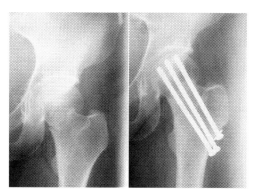

Fig.17.9. Internal fixation of a Garden II fracture using cannulated screws.

Treatment of Grades III and IV fractures (Fig.17.10)

Grades III and IV fractures are much more difficult to treat for obvious reasons: delayed and non-union as well as avascular necrosis of the femoral head are distinct possibilities with them. The treatment options are hemiarthroplasty or total hip replacement, depending on the age and other relevant circumstances surrounding the patient.

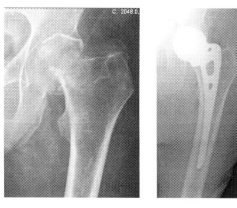

Fig.17.10a&b. Garden grade 4 subcapital fracture in an elderly patient treated with an uncemented prosthesis (Austin Moore).

Basal cervical fractures

Most authors quite rightly group these with trochanteric fractures because they are both extracapsular. However, as far as treatment options are concerned, they get the best of both worlds in that they can be treated by cannulated screw fixation as well as by DHS fixation and even hemiarthroplasty/total hip replacement.

COMPLICATIONS OF FEMORAL NECK FRACTURES

- *Mortality.* This is high (up to 24% in the first 6 months and 29% in the first 12 month) in the elderly. Their age and general ill-health are probably more contributory than the fracture itself.
- *Avascular necrosis of the femoral head* is a common (20-55% within 18 months) and serious complication.
- *Non-union* is related to compromise of the blood supply in the region of the femoral neck and to poor treatment. Its incidence could be as high as 30% if optimal treatment is not given.
- *Associated dislocation of the hip* or *femoral shaft fracture.* These are seen occasionally.

COMPLICATIONS OF TREATMENT

- *Loss of reduction* with coxa vara deformity: this may be due to implant failure (see below) or to bone failure.
- *Implant failure.* Breakage of metallic fixation devices is common, especially in elderly patients with weak bones.
- *Implant penetration* into the hip joint may occur with screws.
- *Bone cement problems.* When bone cement (polymethyl-methacrylate) is used to cement in the prostheses, loosening may occur.
- *Dislocation of prostheses* may occur due to errors in seating them. An incidence of 15 – 30% is quoted. A mortality of 60 – 70% at 12 months is quoted following dislocations of hemiarthroplasties.
- *Other complications* of major surgery include *wound infection, deep vein thrombosis chest infections* and *bed sores* in the elderly.

FRACTURES OF THE FEMORAL NECK IN CHILDREN

True fractures

These are due to severe violence such as are present in road traffic accidents or falls from high heights, especially trees, garden shades and walls. They may be subcapital (which is the same as traumatic separation of the capital epiphysis) or transcervical.

Traumatic Separation of the Epiphysis

The features are similar to those of a subcapital fracture in the adult. Reduction is achieved by skin traction for 2-3 weeks during which the limb is put into internal rotation to realign the fragments. A hip spica is then applied but weight-bearing on the limb should be avoided for about 3 months.

Slipped upper femoral epiphysis (SUFE)

Slipped upper femoral epiphysis is seen in adolescents of characteristic physiognomy: either very tall and thin or very fat, rotund and sexually immature. Commoner in males than females, only about 30% of cases are related to significant trauma.

The diagnosis of an acute slip is more difficult than that of a traumatic separation whose features are more dramatic and clear-cut. The characteristic appearance mentioned above is helpful. The child walks with a limp and there is pain in the groin or knee (referred pain). On examination, the leg is held externally rotated at the hip, a feature which becomes accentuated as the hip is gradually flexed from the horizontal position. Furthermore, internal rotation is restricted.

On an AP X-ray, a tangent to the superior surface of the neck misses the epiphysis, unlike in the normal. A pure lateral view is even more accurate in detecting a small slip. The slip is posteriorly and inferiorly.

The treatment depends on the degree of slip as determined on the X-rays. If the slip is slight (less than one-third of the head diameter), the head is pinned in situ with multiple pins (Moore, Garden, Howse, etc.); cannulated screws can also be used. A slip of more than one-third of the head diameter should be reduced. Closed reduction is difficult and has the potential of causing damage. Open reduction is also difficult and also has the potential of causing damage. It should not be attempted by inexperienced surgeons. The result can be gratifying in experienced hands (Fig.17.11).

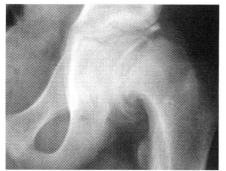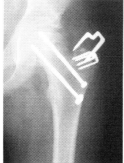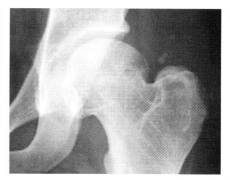

Fig.17.11a-c. Pre-op and post-op X-rays of a severe slipped upper femoral epiphysis treated by open reduction and internal fixation by the author.

Complications include coxa vara, avascular necrosis and secondary osteoarthritis.

TROCHANTERIC FRACTURES (FIG.17.12)

INTRODUCTION

An isolated fracture of the greater or lesser trochanter is a minor injury but an intertrochanteric fracture is not. Like femoral neck fractures, trochanteric fractures are common in Europe, a major fraction of whose population is accounted for by elderly people. In parts of the world with younger populations, these fractures are uncommon. When they do occur, it is the young that are usually affected. They are very rare in children.

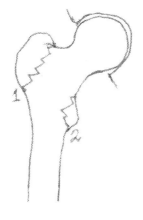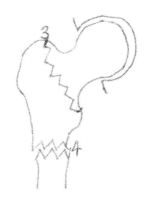

Fig.17.12. Fractures in the trochanteric region of the femur:
1. greater trochanter
2. lesser trochanter
3. intertrochanteric and
4. subtrochanteric fractures.

ISOLATED FRACTURES OF THE GREATER TROCHANTER

Direct blows are the usual mechanism. They may be undisplaced or displaced (by the abductors). Pain can be considerable so, bed rest for a week or so should be described. Following this, the patient should be mobilised starting with partial weight bearing on crutches.

ISOLATED FRACTURES OF THE LESSER TROCHANTER

These are usually seen in young sporty people. The usual mechanism is avulsion by the iliopsoas tendon. They are managed along the same lines as greater trochanter fractures.

INTERTROCHANTERIC FRACTURES

The term 'pertrochanteric' is sometimes used for these fractures but for all practical purposes, the two terms (intertrochanteric and pertrochanteric) are the same. What is really important about these fractures is *the concept of stability* before and after reduction and the features of a given case by which the concept is defined.

CLASSIFICATION

Intertrochanteric fractures can be classified as follows:

A. **By the presence or absence of displacement:**
   - Undisplaced
   - Displaced

B. **By the number of fracture fragments:**
   - 2-part fracture (comprising a head-and-neck and a shaft fragment.
   - 3-part fracture (head-and-neck, shaft and lesser trochanter fragments).
   - 4-part fracture (head-and-neck, shaft, lesser trochanter and greater rochanter fragments.

C. **Intertrochanteric fractures with subtrochanteric extension.**

MECHANISMS OF INJURY

Direct blows to the greater trochanter and forces transmitted to the trochanteric region via the femoral shaft can cause the fractures. In the young forces of great magnitude are required.

DIAGNOSIS

The hip is painful in all cases. With undisplaced fractures, the limb is not shortened or rotated but with displaced ones, it is externally rotated and may be shortened. X-rays will show one of the several variants. In the elderly, the possibility of the fracture being pathological must be borne in mind so that secondary deposits could be looked for. It is important to determine whether or not the fracture is inherently stable before embarking on treatment.

TREATMENT

Non-surgical Treatment

There is hardly a place for non-surgical treatment of intertrochanteric fractures for the following reasons:

- **In young patients:** Treatment by traction, skin or skeletal, is possible but requires at least 3 months. This is unacceptable in economic and psychological terms

- **In elderly patients** with various disabling medical conditions, the prolonged period in bed necessary for the success of the method can cause various complications such as bedsores, limb muscle atrophy, joint stiffness, urinary calculi and depression. This is unacceptable.

Surgical Treatment

Operative treatment is the treatment of choice in both old and young patients. In this method, the patient is placed on the fracture table and the fracture is reduced closed with the help of an image intensifier. Internal fixation of the fracture is then effected with one of the several fixation devices available (Fig.17.13).

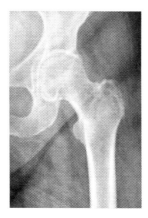 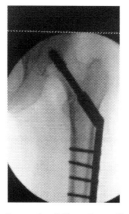

Fig.17.13a&b. The classical surgical fixation of an intertrochanteric fracture is with the Dynamic Hip Screw (DHS).

COMPLICATIONS

The complications of the fracture itself are few:

- *Mortality* is high (up to 30% in the first year) in the elderly in poor health. In hospital mortality is about 15%.

- *Mal-union* (healing in varus or external rotation) is fairly common because reduction is commonly lost during early weight bearing. Varus deformity results in limb shortening. External rotation deformity is common with Ender's nails.

- *Delayed and non-union* are extremely rare.

- *Weakness of hip flexion* is due mainly to iliopsoas weakness secondary to detachment of the lesser trochanter in a comminuted fracture.

The complications of treatment are more serious. Most are due to poor operative technique or implant failure usually occasioned by poor quality bone.

- *Implant failure* - breakage, implant penetration through the femoral head, cutting out (all implants) or backing out (Ender's nails).

- *Collapse of fracture* with development of coxa vara deformity is related to implant failure or cutting out due to poor bone quality.

- *Complications of major surgery.* These are the same as enumerated in the section on femoral neck fractures.

SUBTROCHANTERIC FRACTURES (FIG.17.14)

These are seen in all age groups, except children. In young adults, they often result from injuring forces of considerable magnitude. In the elderly, they require less severe injuring forces and may be related to osteoporosis or secondary deposits in the region.

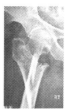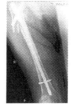

Fig.17.14. Treatment of an unstable subtrochanteric fracture using a proximal femoral nail (PFN).

Complications. *Mal-union, delayed and non-union* are common intrinsic complications. *Bone grafting* at the time of the initial fixation is recommended in fractures with severe medial comminution. *Treatment-related complications* are similar to those mentioned for intertrochanteric fractures.

FRACTURES OF THE FEMORAL SHAFT

INTRODUCTION

The femoral shaft can be defined as the region between the lesser trochanter and the epicondyles. Considerable violence is usually needed to cause femoral shaft fractures and young people are more frequently involved than old people. Traditionally, the femoral shaft is divided into three equal parts - *proximal, middle and distal thirds*. In common with fractures of shafts of other long bones, fractures of the femoral shaft are subject to the deforming actions of attaching muscles and this varies according to the level of the fracture.

AO classification

32-A with subtypes
32-B with subtypes
32-C with subtypes

Irrespective of this classification, in clinical practice, a number of fracture types are distinguished, which are of practical importance for management:

- **A.** Open or Closed
- **B.** Uncomminuted or Comminuted
- **C.** Transverse or Oblique or Spiral

MECHANISMS OF INJURY

Both direct and indirect forces cause these fractures. Direct forces may take the form of hits from or against various objects: comminuted fractures are likely to result. Indirect forces are mainly torsional forces applied at a distance from the fracture site: oblique and spiral fractures are likely to result. Irrespective of the mechanism, considerable violence is usually needed to cause femoral shaft fractures and young people are more frequently involved than old.

DIAGNOSIS

This is usually easy. Severe pain, shortening and deformity are constant features and the patient cannot move the limb. These features can be confirmed objectively. Other local findings are ecchymosis and swelling. A general examination must also be carried out as general complications, especially haemorrhage with possible resultant hypovolaemic shock, and associated injuries are common.

Other associated injuries to look out for include vascular injuries (in 2% of cases), dislocation of the ipsilateral hip, fracture of the ipsilateral femoral neck (2-5%), injuries to ipsilateral knee ligaments (in 7-49% of cases), fracture of the patella, spinal and rib fractures and head injury. X-rays are necessary to define the femoral and other fractures more accurately; their interpretation is usually straightforward. The hip and knee joints must be shown on the films to ensure they are in place.

TREATMENT

Non-surgical and surgical methods of Treatment are available. The choice of method should be based on the site and type of fracture, the age and circumstances of the patient and the level of expertise of the surgeon and the facilities available in a given hospital. In practice, most fractures can be treated by either method, depending on the circumstances.

Non-surgical Treatment

The indications for conservative treatment include fracture in a child, openness (open fracture), fracture comminution, segmental fracture and lack of expertise or facilities for operative treatment. Various methods of conservative treatment are available.

- *Traction only.* In this method, upper tibial skeletal traction (skin traction is used in children and the elderly) with increasing traction weight (from 10 to 15% of the body weight) is used to achieve reduction of the fracture. Angulatory deformity is corrected with the help of a padded sandbag placed under the fracture site. Regular check X-rays are taken to monitor the reduction. Following reduction, the traction weight is reduced to a maintenance value (about 5% of the body weight). Traction is continued until clinical union is achieved.

  Clinical union of the fracture can be expected in 3-4 weeks in a child aged 4 years and in about 8 weeks in an adult. However, the average time in bed is 12 weeks and this is a big disadvantage. Mobilisation is initially partial-weight bearing on crutches, in a hip spica or in a weight-relieving calliper. A certain amount of knee stiffness is to be expected, so knee joint exercises are usually required for several weeks.

- *Initial traction followed by cast bracing.* In this method, reduction and initial immobilisation is achieved by traction as above. This is then followed as from the 4th post-fracture week (when the fracture has become sticky) by cast bracing. Some surgeons advocate a shorter immobilisation period – about 2 weeks. Cast bracing is particularly suitable for fractures in the distal one-third of the shaft but can also be used with modification for fractures in other regions. It can also be used to complement other treatment methods for the purpose of providing additional stability or facilitating knee function or both.

- *Immediate manipulative reduction followed by immobilisation by traction.* It is possible to achieve reduction by manipulation but in practice so many factors can militate against it. These include bulkiness of the thigh, fracture comminution, fracture obliquity, segmentation and soft-tissue interposition. This option is seldom used except in children with thin limbs.

- *Use of the external fixator.* The external fixator may be used in the treatment of certain femoral shaft fractures. The special indications are open fractures, comminution, presence of infection and non-union.

Surgical Treatment

Operative treatment must be considered and used in each case, if it is the optimal treatment and if circumstances permit. A number of operative methods of treatment are available:

Intramedullary nailing (IMN) (Fig.17.15)

Intramedullary nails are currently the gold standard in the treatment of femoral shaft fractures. They are particularly suited to transverse fractures in the proximal and middle one-thirds of the shaft but can be used for fractures in the distal one-third as long as there is enough room for one or two distal locking screws. The nail is inserted by the closed antegrade route under image intensification. Distal femoral fractures can also be treated with a locking nail introduced retrogradely from the knee (Retrograde intra-medullary nailing).

There are *reamed* and *unreamed options* for the insertion of the IM nail but the superiority of reamed over undreamed nails has now been established for most fractures. The femoral canal must be reamed to a diameter 1-1.5 cm greater than the nail diameter. Trainee surgeons unsure of the technique of IM nailing must have competent assistance at hand before embarking on the procedure. *The 3 main technical difficulties are fracture reduction, negotiating the reamer past the fracture site during reaming and inserting the locking screws.*

The old non-locking nails, such as the Kuntscher nail, inserted by the open retrograde route, is still being used in parts of the developing world for various reasons, including financial constraints. It is hoped that this practice will change soon.

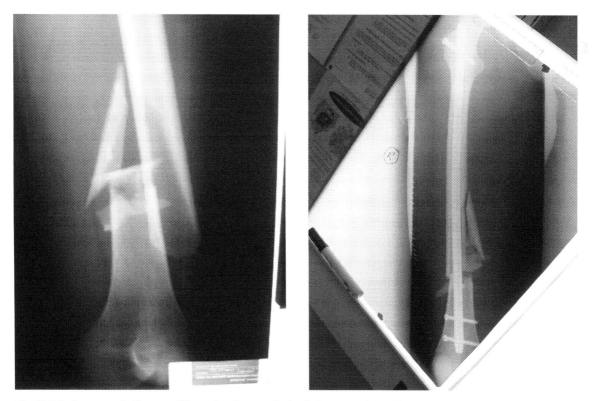

Fig.17.15. Intramedullary nailing of a femoral shaft fracture in a 20-year-old man.

Plating

Enthusiasts of the AO methods used to plate femoral shaft fractures in adults with AO Dynamic Compression Plates (DCP), some with well over 15 screw holes. However, while many surgeons would not mind plating femoral shaft fractures in children, they would mind doing the same in adults. Quite apart from considerations such as infection and weakening of bone by screw holes, IMNs are biomechanically superior to plates and screws. Fractures in children, the presence of an ipsilateral pelvic or acetabular fracture, fractures with associated vascular injury are considered good indications for plating femoral shaft fractures.

COMPLICATIONS

- Shock may accompany significant blood loss.
- Dislocation of the ipsilateral hip.
- Other associated fractures mentioned above.
- Knee injury (ligaments and menisci) complicates 10% of cases.
- Femoral or popliteal artery injury.
- Sciatic nerve injury.
- Fat embolism/Acute respiratory distress syndrome.
- Infection: up to 20% of compound fractures may get infected.
- Complications of healing. Mal-union (angulatory, rotatory or shortening) delayed or non-union may occur.
- Knee joint stiffness is common. It could be due to quadriceps adhesion to the femur at the fracture site, or to stretch of the knee ligaments during traction. Quadriceps-plasty may be required in the former case.

Surgical/post-surgical complications

Nail impaction. Impaction is best avoided by over-reaming by 1-1.5 mm. Disimpaction is often difficult and may result in fracture of the femoral shaft.

Complications due to fixation devices. The various devices (nails, plates and screws) can bend, break or protrude. Accidental bending of an in situ intramedullary nail is a terrible event. If the bending is significant, the nail cannot be removed by conventional methods even when such removal is indicated by the presence of symptoms. This is the strongest case for removing such nails as soon as they have served the purpose for which they were inserted i.e. hold the fracture reduced till solid union.

Advantages and Disadvantages of Operative Treatment

The main advantages are accurate reduction and early mobilisation and discharge from hospital. Most patients will leave hospital within 2 weeks of their injury. The disadvantages include technical difficulties, risk of infection and a need for a second operation to remove the implant (which also carries the above risks).

FEMORAL SHAFT FRACTURES IN CHILDREN

Gallows traction is used in children under 2 years. Older children (3-10 years) are treated with simple skin traction. Skin care is important in these patients; if the crepe bandage is allowed to "bunch" up, it may form constriction bands at various levels and pressure sores and distal limb swelling may result. Following clinical union in about 3 weeks, depending on the age of the patient, a "one-and-half" hip spica is applied and the child is discharged to outpatient follow-up. The spica can usually be removed 4 weeks later. Plating within 7 days of fracture is permissible in the older child aged 7–10, if gross malalignment persists.

Over-lapping of fracture fragments in children. It is classically taught that an overlap of 2cm or so should be allowed in children under 10 years as observation has shown overgrowth (lengthening) where accurate reduction was secured.

SUPRACONDYLAR FRACTURES

The supracondylar region is an area about 5cm long lying just proximal to the femoral condyles. Technically speaking, a part of it forms part of the distal one-third of the femoral shaft. Fractures in this region have a characteristic deformity, namely, posterior displacement and angulation of the distal fragment - due to the action of the gastrecnemii. Most of the difficulties of treatment emanate from this deformity.

FRACTURE TYPES

The fracture may be impacted, undisplaced, displaced or comminuted.

MECHANISMS OF INJURY

Indirect forces (rotational forces, valgus or varus stress with axial loading) are the more common mechanisms. Direct forces e.g. direct hits; may also cause the fracture. In the elderly, osteoporosis and osteomalacia are predisposing factors. In young patients, high-energy violence is needed. Vehicular and sports accidents and falls from heights are common sources of the fractures.

DIAGNOSIS

Local pain and swelling are severe. Deformity is obvious. Distal pulses must be felt as the sharp end of the distal fragment may injure the popliteal vessels. X-rays are necessary to show details of the fracture and help make management decisions.

TREATMENT

Undisplaced or impacted fracture. A long leg non-weight bearing cast is applied with the knee flexed to about 20 degrees. Elevation is instituted for 24-48 hours after which the patient is discharged home to outpatient follow-up.

Displaced uncomminuted fracture. The choice is between surgical and non-surgical treatment. Non-surgical treatment is by upper tibial skeletal traction by means of which reduction and immobilisation can be achieved. This is difficult to attain. If attained, the limb is stabilised by cast bracing after 2-3 weeks of traction.

Operative treatment is by open reduction and internal fixation using a Dynamic Condylar Screw (DCS), an intramedullary nail or an external fixator.

Intramedullary devices inserted via the retrograde route in the intercondylar notch have replaced the Zickel and Ender's nails which used to be inserted through the supracondylar regions. The newer devices have the advantages of easy technique, better stability by allowing load sharing as well as better length and rotation control.

Comminuted fractures are best treated by the traction followed by cast bracing or by cast-bracing. There may also be a place for the external fixator.

OPEN FRACTURES OF THE FEMUR

With open fractures, the danger (as always) is possible infection. Debridement is indicated. The fracture is best treated conservatively but some surgeons carry out immediate open reduction and internal fixation in up to Gustilo-Anderson Grade IIIA injuries.

Complications

Popliteal vessel or nerve injury may occur. Mal-union is common with inadequate conservative treatment. Delayed and non-union may also occur. Treatment of these complications are carried out along established lines.

DISTAL FEMORAL EPIPHYSEAL INJURY

In this injury, the fracture line passes through the distal growth plate. The injury could be any of the Salter-Harris variants. Most can be successfully treated by closed reduction followed by traction or cast immobilisation. But open reduction and internal fixation is indicated if closed reduction is unsuccessful or the knee joint is involved. Growth disturbances may occur later in some cases.

T AND Y SHAPED FRACTURES

These are a combination of intercondylar and supracondylar fractures. They are more serious injuries than supracondylar fractures because of the involvement of the knee joint, with the attendant real risk of stiffness in the short-term and osteoarthritis in the long-term. The probable mechanism is a hammer-type action of the tibial condyles on the femoral condyles during a vertical fall on the foot. Diagnosis is not difficult. Treatment by traction will suffice in most cases, Surgical options include LISS plate or DCS fixation. Stiffness and secondary osteoarthritis due to inaccurate restoration of the articular surface are the main complications.

CONDYLAR FRACTURES

Isolated fractures of the condyles are rare. They result from hyperabduction or hyperadduction forces combined with axial loading. Being intra-articular, they are serious injuries. They may be displaced or undisplaced. Although conservative treatment with traction may effect reduction, open reduction and internal fixation with a DCS is the only reliable method of achieving accurate reduction and maintaining it. With firm fixation, early knee exercises can be started which reduces the chances and degree of knee stiffness.

Further reading

Alonso CG, Curiel MD, Carranza FH et al. Femoral bone mineral density, neck-shaft angle and mean femoral neck width as predictors of hip fracture in men and women. Multicenter Project for Research in Osteoporosis. *Osteoporos Int 11(8):* 714-720, 2000.

Garden RS. Malrotation and Avascular Necrosis in Subcapital Fractures Of The Femur. *J Bone Joint Surg, 53B:* 183-197, 1971.

Helal B and Skevis X. Unrecognised Dislocation Of The Hip In Fractures Of The Femoral Shaft. *J Bone Joint Surg. 49B:* 293, 1967.

Iwegbu CG. The Place of Ender Nails In The Evolution of Methods of Treatment of Trochanteric Fractures Of The Femur. *MChOrth Thesis,* University of Liverpool, 1981.

Iwegbu CG and Patel RJ. Difficulties and Complications Of The Ender Method of Treatment of Trochanteric Fractures Of The Femur. *Injury 13(2):* 116-124, 1981.

Iwegbu CG. Ipsilateral Fracture Of The Head and Neck of Femur With Partial Fusion To The Acetabulum. *Injury 15(2):* 113-115, 1983.

Iwegbu CG, Maude B and Danfulani D. The Zaria Metal Hinge Joint. *E Afr Med J 60(11):* 789, 1983.

Iwegbu CG. Cast-Bracing of Femoral Fractures: Further Experience With The Zaria Metal Hinge Joint. *E Afr Med J 63(4):* 228, 1986.

Iwegbu CG. Foam Slipper in Place of The Walking Heel For Lower Limb Plaster of Paris Casts. *E Afr Med J 67(7):* 507-511, 1990.

Iwegbu CG. Avascular Necrosis of The Femoral Head in Sickle-Cell Disease Part I: Pathology and Principles of Management. *Postgraduate Doctor (Afr) 13(1):* 7-13, 1991.

Iwegbu CG. *Principles and Management of Acute Orthopaedic Trauma.* Authorhouse, 2004.

Moulton A, Agunwa WCR and Hopkins JS. Closed Femoral Fractures: Why Not Simple Traction? *Injury 13(3):* 244, 1981.

Parker MJ, Pryor GA and Thorngren K.G. *Handbook of hip fracture.* Oxford: Butterworth Heinemann, 1997.

Rogmark C, Carlsson A, Johnell I and Sernbo I. A Prospective Randomised Trial Of Internal Fixation Versus Arthroplasty For Displaced Fractures Of The Neck Of Femur. Functional Outcome For 450 Patients At Two Years. *J Bone Joint Surg, 84B:* 183-188, 2002.

Ryder SA, Reynolds F and Bannister GC. Refining the indications for surgery after proximal femoral fracture. *Injury 32(4):* 295-297, 2001.

Rockwood CA, Green DP, Bucholz RW and Heckman JD (eds): *Rockwood and*

Shatzker J. Fractures of the distal femur revisited. *Clinical Orthopaedics: 347;* 43-46, 1998. *Green's Fractures in Adults, Vol 2, 4th ed.* Philadelphia, JB Lippincott, 1996.

Wardlaw D. Cast Bracing in Practice: A Two Year Study in Aberdeen. *Injury 12(3):* 213, 1980.

Wiss DA Gibson T. IM nailing of the femur and tibia: indications and techniques. *Current Orthopaedics* (8): 245-254, 1994.

CHAPTER 18

FRACTURES OF TIBIA AND FIBULA

INTRODUCTION

Fractures of the tibia and fibula are quite common. Although usually considered together, tibial fractures are much more significant then fibular fractures. This is because the tibia is the major weight bearing bone of the leg and also takes part in the formation of both the knee and ankle joints. Fibular fractures of major significance are those occurring at the distal end where the fibula contributes to the formation of the ankle joint. The other points worthy of mention here are:

- The propensity of tibial fractures to being open (compound) because most of its medial border lacks muscular cover.
- The real possibility of development of the compartment syndrome following tibial (and fibular) fractures because of the tight nature of the musculofascial compartments of the leg.

FRACTURES OF THE TIBIAL PLATEAU

Mechanisms of injury

Road traffic accidents, sports injuries and falls from heights are the commonest causes of tibial plateau fractures. The injuring forces are lateral or medial bending forces combined with axial loading.

CLASSIFICATION

The Schatzker classification

Schatzker has classified these fractures into six types as follows (Fig.18.1):

Type I: split fracture of the lateral tibial plateau without articular depression; seen mainly in young adults with strong cancellous bone that resists depression. Account for about 50% of all tibial plateau fractures. Also referred to as "bumper fracture".

Type II: split depressed fracture of the lateral tibial condyle.

Type III: local/isolated depression of the lateral tibial condyle.

Type IV: split fracture of the medial condyle. These account for about 15% of all tibial condylar fractures. Isolated fractures are rare and are probably due to a varus strain and the action of the medial femoral condyle.

Type V: bicondylar fracture with varying degrees of articular depression and displacement of the condyles. Account for 25% of all tibial plateau fractures.

Type VI: bicondylar fracture with metaphyseal/diaphyseal involvement.

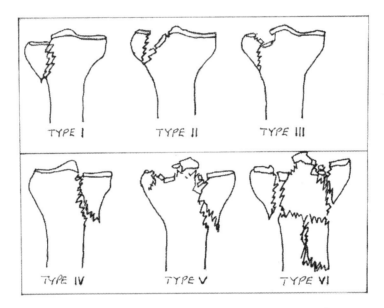

Fig.18.1. The Schatzker classification of tibial plateau fractures

Diagnosis is usually not difficult. The clinical features include knee pain, haemarthrosis, localised soft-tissue swelling, localised tenderness and possible instability due to a displaced fracture or ligamentous injury. When ligamentous (and capsular) rupture is present, joint effusion is absent or minimal because the haemarthrosis drains into the soft tissues. Peripheral pulses and nerve function must be tested. Associated injuries - fracture of the fibular head, injury to the collateral ligaments, the cruciate ligaments or the lateral meniscus are common.

Most of the fractures will show on routine AP and lateral views. Special studies are helpful in the more difficult types of fracture: tomography will show a depressed fracture better; 40 degree internal and external oblique views will show fractures not visible on routine AP views; stress views will demonstrate ligamentous injuries. CT scan, especially with 3D reconstruction, will display nicely the fragments and depressions and is helpful in planning operative treatment.

Treatment. The most important consideration here is that we are dealing with largely intra-articular fractures, which are, by nature, difficult to manage. General treatment includes aspiration of the knee joint when effusion is considerable and initial control of pain with analgesics. The ideal treatment for a given fracture is one which achieves an accurate restoration of the articular surface. The extent to which this ideal situation can be achieved depends on the type of fracture:

NON-OPERATIVE TREATMENT

Immobilisation in a cast

Undepressed and Undisplaced fractures are immobilised in a POP or fibreglass cast. They can, however, displace with weight bearing or other stresses and so the limb must be kept immobilised until this danger no longer exists. This can be achieved with a long-leg cast kept on for about 8 weeks. Quadriceps exercises should be done inside the cast. Full weight-bearing should not be started until after 12 weeks.

Traction and early mobilisation

Most depressed, displaced and comminuted fractures can be treated by skeletal traction. Traction is applied through a Steinman or Denham pin inserted at the level of the tibial tubercle. The advocates of traction (Apley was one the of champions) show good to excellent results and are quick to point out that brilliant reductions achieved with metalwork are sometimes attended by stiff knees. The main advantage of traction is that it allows early exercises, which is generally helpful in intra-articular fractures. Exercises whilst on traction can be carried out using a split or similar bed. A cast brace can be applied after about 2-3 weeks, when the fractures have become "sticky". Exercises should be continued in the brace.

OPERATIVE TREATMENT

The indications for operative treatment include:

- *depression:* "significant" articular depression, i.e. depression greater than 1mm - is considered unacceptable.
- *Instability:* > 10 degrees with the knee extended.
- *Open fractures*
- *Compartment syndrome*
- *Vascular injury*

SURGICAL OPTIONS

- **Percutaneous screw fixation** is suitable for Type I to IV fractures
- **Plate fixation** is also suitable for Type I to IV fractures
- **Open reduction plus bone-grafting and internal fixation (Fig.18.2)**

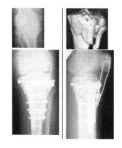

This option is advocated for depressed fracture of either condyle. Most operations are done for depressed and displaced fractures of the lateral tibial condyle. The approach is either anterolateral or anteromedial. The fracture line and depressed articular surface are exposed. A window, centred on the vertical fracture line and about 1.5 cm below the articular surface is opened. Through it the upper table is elevated to restore the depressed articular surface and *corticocancellous bone grafts* from the ipsilateral iliac crest are inserted and

Fig.18.2. ORIF of a Schatzker Type VI fracture

carefully punched in to support the elevated bone. This is further supported with a *buttress plate and screws*. In bicondylar fractures, two plates are usually used. Some surgeons advocate the repair of associated ligamentous ruptures at the same time. Early non-weight bearing joint exercises are instituted.

External fixation

Most authors think that Types V and VI fractures are best managed with a hybrid ring fixator. The Ilizarov frame has also been successfully used in the treatment of these injuries. Articular fragments may be fixed with one or two cannulated cancellous screws. The main advantage of external fixators here is that they allow early mobilisation and weight-bearing.

COMPLICATIONS OF TIBIAL PLATEAU FRACTURES

- *Vascular injury*
- *Nerve injury*
- *Compartment syndrome*
- *Infection* is common in ill-advised surgical intervention, especially in Types IV to VI fractures.
- *Knee stiffness*
- *Malunion/Nonunion*
- *Avascular necrosis/loose bodies*
- *Valgus deformity of the knee* (lateral condyle fractures)
- *Posttraumatic osteoarthritis*

DIAPHYSEAL FRACTURES OF THE TIBIA

Mechanisms of injury

- **Direct forces** are often implicated in diaphyseal fractures. Direct injuring forces can be generated in road traffic accidents, in which transverse, comminuted and displaced fractures are common. Other sources of direct forces include gunshot injuries and bending injuries e.g. ski boot injuries. Associated skin and other soft-tissue injuries are common in direct mechanisms.

- **Indirect forces** may take the form of twisting applied to the foot or ankle or may be angulatory in nature. A twisting force is likely to cause spiral fractures of both the tibia and fibula at different levels.

Classification

Fractures of the tibia have been classified in different ways over the years. *Classifications* have been based on:

- *fracture site* - proximal, middle and distal thirds
- *fracture characteristics* - greenstick, stress, transverse, comminuted, etc

- *fracture stability* - stable and unstable
- *fracture severity* - minor, moderate and major.

Although there is logical thinking behind each classification, the multiplicity of classifications is a recipe for confusion. With minor modifications, the Orthopaedic Trauma Association (OTA) has adopted the AO alphanumeric classification.

The OTA classification.

In this classification, the tibia is divided into 3 parts – proximal, middle and distal. Articular fractures are included in the proximal and distal zones.

- **Extra-articular proximal tibial fractures:**
  Type 42   A (Simple)
               A1 - Spiral
               A2 – Oblique (> 30 degrees)
               A3 – Transverse (>30 degrees)

- **Diaphyseal tibial fractures**
  Type 42:   A - Simple
                B - Wedge
                C - Complex

- **Distal tibial fractures**
  Type 43:   A1 (Simple).
                A2 (Metaphyseal wedge).
                A3 (Metaphyseal complex).

Tscherne and Gotzen have classified soft-tissue injuries associated with closed tibial fractures:

- *Grade 0* - superficial abrasion or contusion caused by fragment pressure from within.
- *Grade 1* - a deep, contaminated contusion from direct trauma.
- *Grade 2* - extensive contusion or crushing of skin or muscle.

Diagnosis

Usually the patient is brought to the A & E by Ambulance or good Samaritans. Ideally, the fractured leg should be splinted at the accident site. A good history of the causative accident may suggest the site and nature of the fractures. There is localised pain, swelling and deformity. A grossly deformed or a compound fracture is obvious. Undue pressure or movement should not be exerted during physical examination. The examiner should, however, check out the following:

- the status of the arterial pulses (dorsalis pedis, posterior tibial)
- exclude compartment syndrome and
- test for possible nerve injuries.

Intravenous analgesics are given to minimise pain in all fractures, bleeding is controlled and a temporary antiseptic dressing is applied in compound fractures. A temporary splint is applied before the patient is sent for X-rays. AP and lateral films usually suffice but 3-D CT scanning, if available, provides beautiful imaging and a better understanding of the fracture, which will aid management planning. An angiogram is necessary if arterial injury is suspected.

Treatment

Tibial fractures come in so many different varieties that it is difficult to be dogmatic about their treatment. This is why so many huge volumes of work have been written on the subject and virtually all the methods of fracture treatment enumerated in the introductory section have been applied to tibial fractures. Although fibular shaft fracture is kept in mind as well, it is the tibial fracture that is given the greater attention. This is because little disability results from "non-active" treatment of fibular shaft fractures.

In summary, treatment consists of:

- immobilisation of undisplaced fractures
- reduction and immobilisation of displaced fractures and
- measures directed at aiding maximum recovery of function.

Other points of general interest worthy of mention here include:

- issues of the technique of fracture reduction
- what degree of accuracy of reduction should be considered acceptable
- post-reduction redisplacement of a fracture
- when can the patient start weight-bearing on the broken leg and
- the optimal period of immobilisation of a given fracture.

Technique of fracture reduction

It is fare to state that most of it is best learnt "on the job", as a single practical experience is more valuable than a thousand words of description and explanation in a book.

Acceptable reduction

Acceptable reduction" may vary from surgeon to surgeon but it can be defined as "reduction compatible with good healing and subsequent good function". Briefly, in an acceptable reduction:

a. Cortical contact is more than 50%
b. Varus/valgus angulation is less than 5 degrees
c. Anterior/posterior angulation is less than 5 degrees
d. Rotational deformity is less than 10 degrees
e. Shortening is less than 1 cm

When can weight-bearing be permitted?

The most important consideration here is the stability of the fracture. With unstable fractures, weight-bearing should not be permitted. With stable fractures, weight bearing can be started gradually as soon as the initial pain and swelling of trauma have subsided. This usually occurs within 2 weeks of injury.

Possibility of redisplacement

Redisplacement of a fracture after an initial acceptable reduction should always be borne in mind. It should be monitored by check X-rays in the initial period of about 3 weeks during which the fracture becomes "sticky".

How long should a tibial shaft fracture be immobilised?

This is related to the stability of the fracture and its speed of healing and therefore varies for different fracture types. Fracture characteristics of special relevance here are *long obliquity, comminution and segmentation*, which compromise stability. *Infection* in compound fractures also compromises fracture healing. In general, periods of immobilisation may vary from 6-8 weeks for a stress fracture or fractures in children to 24 weeks or more for infected, compound, comminuted or segmental fractures. Delayed union can be defined as one not occurring by 20 weeks.

METHODS OF TREATMENT OF COMBINED FRACTURE OF THE TIBIA AND FIBULA

NON-OPERATIVE METHODS

Immobilisation in an above-knee cast only.

This method is used for stress, undisplaced or minimally displaced fractures. The cast is a long-leg one and early weight bearing may be permitted if the fracture is stable.

Manipulative reduction plus immobilisation in an above-knee cast

This is still a suitable method of treatment of displaced fractures, despite increasing choice of intramedullary nailing or compression plating. Many orthopaedic departments in the developing countries are not able to support surgical treatment. Strong traction and countertraction achieve reduction by two assistants with the knee straight while the surgeon manipulates with the palm and digits. A long-leg cast is then applied with the knee in slight flexion (about 5-10 degrees). Wedging of the cast to correct angulatory deformity may be necessary later. The timing of when to start weight bearing depends on the stability characteristics of the fracture.

Initial traction followed by immobilisation.

This method can be used when fracture reduction cannot be achieved by any of the above mentioned methods. A Steinmann pin is inserted into the os calcis and a traction weight applied. After reduction has been achieved, immobilisation is effected using a cast - an ordinary above-knee, a Sarmiento cast or a cast-brace.

The cast-brace method (Fig.18.3)

The principle here is the same as in the treatment of femoral shaft fractures by this method and is similar to that of the Sarmiento cast. This method is particularly suitable for fractures in the proximal one-third of the tibial shaft. Manipulation or traction achieves reduction and initial immobilisation can be achieved with an above-knee cast or with traction for at least 2 weeks to allow the fracture to become "sticky". The brace is then applied with two hinges. Fig.18.3 shows the cast-bracing of a proximal tibial fracture using the author's metal hinges. Good results have been reported with this method of treatment.

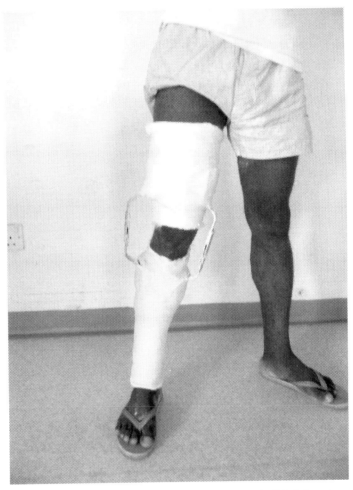

Fig.18.3. Cast-brace Treatment of proximal tibial fracture using two Zaria metal hinges designed by the author.

Use of the External fixator

The external fixator is used more frequently in the treatment of tibial shaft fractures than of fractures of any other long bone. The main indications are compound and segmented fractures as well as infected non-unions. The advantages claimed include fairly rigid fixation, easy access to associated soft-tissue injuries and early partial weight-bearing as soon as the wound has healed. There is a significant incidence of pin-track infection (10-15%) and non-union (10%).

OPERATIVE METHODS

Intramedullary nailing

This is the current treatment option of choice. In the past, Rush, Lottes or Ender's nails were advocated for transverse or short oblique fractures in the middle one-third of the shaft and for segmental fractures. *Interlocking nails* (Fig.18.4) have taken over because of the advantages of better stability and closed technique. They are suitable for all diaphyseal fractures in which there is enough room for the placement of two distal interlocking screws.

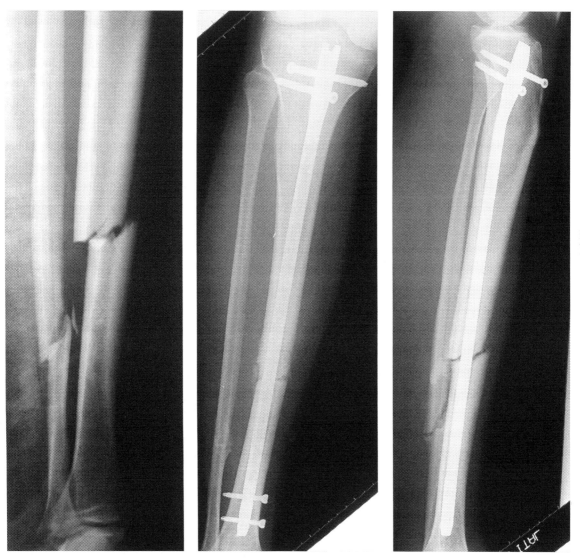

Fig.18.4. Operative Treatment of tibial shaft fractures: intramedullary nailing with interlocking screws is the method of choice.

Plating

The primary indication for plating is a displaced intra-articular fracture at either the knee or the ankle end. Mal-unions and non-unions are the others.

Plating is now less frequently used for diaphyseal fractures than in the past because of increasing mastery of and success with interlocking nails. Nevertheless, it remains a legitimate surgical option, especially in the developing countries. Good to excellent results have been reported in 85-90% of cases but the complications rate can be up to 30%.

Plating is applicable to many types of tibial shaft fractures but is probably best reserved for transverse and oblique fractures. In long oblique and spiral fractures, one or two inter-fragmentary screws may be required before a neutralisation plate is applied. Compression plating using a Dynamic Compression Plate (DCP) plate is the accepted type of plating. However, rigid fixation that will allow early weight bearing is seldom achieved by this method alone, so non-weight-bearing is recommended for the first 6 weeks. Non-weight-bearing is often difficult to achieve in the elderly, so this should be remembered in the choice of operative treatment option.

One or two points deserve mention here. The beginner needs to be cautioned not to regard plating of tibial fractures as a simple operation because the truth is that ***plating of tibial fractures requires mastery.*** What appears straight on the operating table may turn out to be bent on check X-rays the following day. This is usually due to the fact that an initially good reduction can be lost during the drilling of screw holes and placement of the screws. Furthermore, the use of ***aseptic technique is mandatory***.

TREATMENT OF OPEN TIBIAL FRACTURES

This is carried out according to the principles discussed in Chapter 10. Debridement is first carried out and then specific treatment is instituted according to the type of fracture. Types I, II and IIIA fractures can be treated conservatively or by intramedullary nailing (IMN). Types IIIB (the commonest, accounting for about 35% of cases) and IIIC are probably best treated by external fixation but some surgeons would consider IM nailing, using reamed or unreamed nails.

Union rates for Types I, II and IIIA are almost the same as for closed fractures. Delayed union is common with Types IIIB and IIIC fractures and bone grafting may be required to get them to heal. Compartment syndrome is reported in about 20% of cases. Acute amputation should be considered in Type IIIC fractures with posterior tibial nerve damage, severe ipsilateral foot injury or warm ischaemia time of more than 6 hours. Amputation rates for Type IIIC fractures exceed 50%.

CONSERVATIVE VERSUS OPERATIVE TREATMENT OF TIBIAL FRACTURES

The treatment of tibial fractures remains controversial in spite of the fact that a lot of experience has now been gained on the subject. As usual, there are proponents and opponents of either treatment method.

Arguments in favour of operative Treatment

- Accurate reduction and restoration of bone length.
- Rigid fixation and early mobilisation.
- Early weight bearing.

Arguments in favour of conservative Treatment

- Only in the hands of experts, working with ideal instruments and other facilities, can accurate and rigid reduction be guaranteed. The facts are, however, that most of these fractures are treated by non-experts. Furthermore, certain fractures e.g. comminuted ones, defy accurate reduction, even in the best hands.

- A certain degree of inaccurate reduction e.g. contact of only two-thirds of fracture surface or some shortening (of less than 1cm), is compatible with good gait and function.

- The risk of post-operative infection is real (1-12% of cases) and so, "to convert a closed fracture to an open one by operation" seems illogical.

- The delayed and non-union rates following operative treatment are higher than those following conservative treatment.

- A second operation is necessary to remove an implanted fixation device; this carries a certain amount of risk to the patient.

- Many fractures for which success is claimed for operative treatment can be equally successfully treated by conservative methods.

In the face of these points, the *absolute indications for surgical treatment* can be narrowed down to:

- Presence of compartment syndrome
- A floating knee
- Compound fractures.
- ORIF of fractures that cannot be reduced and held by closed methods.

ISOLATED TIBIAL SHAFT FRACTURES

An intact fibula connotes a less severe injuring force and a possible better prognosis because of this: the tibial fracture displaces less and the fibula imparts some stability. On the negative side, reduction of the tibial fracture is sometimes made difficult by an intact fibula, which acts as a strut. This strut action may also cause delayed or non-union by preventing compression at the fracture site during weight bearing. The same mechanism may cause valgus deformity of the distal fragment.

The treatment of isolated tibial fractures follows similar lines as discussed above for combined tibial and fibular fractures. An intact fibula causing delayed union can be osteotomised to allow compression at the fracture site with weight bearing.

ISOLATED FIBULAR SHAFT FRACTURES

These are almost always closed fractures. Local pain is controlled with a crepe bandage and analgesics. Specific treatment is not usually required.

FRACTURES OF THE DISTAL TIBIA AND FIBULA

These are discussed in Chapter 19 (ankle injuries)

DISTAL TIBIAL EPIPHYSEAL INJURY

Any of the Salter-Harris types of injury can occur. The treatment depends on the injury. The triplane epiphyseal injury must be borne in mind and excluded. Usually, closed reduction is stable but displaced fractures require open reduction and internal fixation with Kirschner wires or screws.

Distal tibial epiphyseal injury should be followed up for years during which possible deformity due to growth plate cartilage injury can be monitored and treated.

COMPLICATIONS OF TIBIAL FRACTURES

Early

Skin damage. Bruising is common with all tibial fractures. Breaching of the skin occurs with compound fractures. It may come from outside i.e. due directly to the injuring force or from within i.e. due to the sharp ends of the fracture fragments. The size of skin damage varies from just a puncture wound to frank skin loss with corresponding degrees of contamination and possible infection. Primary wound toilet is imperative; debridement is usually indicated and skin grafting (primary or delayed) may be necessary.

Vascular injury. Tibial fractures in the proximal one-third of the shaft are the most likely causes and the vessel concerned is the anterior tibial artery - usually at the point where it passes from behind to the front through the interosseous membrane. The anterior tibial artery can also be injured in distal-third tibial fractures. The posterior tibial artery is less frequently injured. Arteriography is necessary for the confirmation of clinical findings. Diagnostic exploration may be needed if arteriography is unavailable or cannot be performed on a patient strongly suspected to have suffered an anterior tibial artery injury.

The vascular surgeon must be involved as early as possible. Various treatment procedures are available for various injuries: decompression, anastomoses or vascular patch. Invariably these procedures are preceded by internal fixation of the tibial fracture. Severe vascular injury is the commonest indication for amputation following tibial (and fibular) fractures.

Fat embolism. This is rare but has been reported even in undisplaced fractures.

Compartment syndrome. This is seen in about 3-20% of cases. The anterior tibial compartment is the most commonly and severely affected; other compartments are occasionally involved (*please see Chapter 11*). The syndrome occurs more commonly in association with minor closed fractures than with the more severe ones or open fractures. This is because in the later injuries, the compartments are effectively decompressed. As with elbow and forearm fractures, the presence of a tight cast aggravates pressure increases in the compartments, with resultant ischaemia of contained muscles and other soft tissues.

The most consistent symptom of a compartment syndrome is pain. This may take up to 24 hours to build up. In an established case, splitting of the cast or its removal will usually not stop the pain and the presence of a distal pulse does not exclude or mitigate the effects of the syndrome. The best thing to do is to carry out a total fasciotomy i.e. decompress all four compartments. The clawing of toes seen in some patients following tibial fractures is probably due to minor degrees of undiagnosed compartment syndrome.

Infection is common with open fractures. Usually it is pyogenic but specific infections such as tetanus and gas gangrene sometimes occur. Prevention by good primary wound toilet, debridement and prophylactic antibiotics is far easier and cheaper than treatment. The treatment of tibial osteomyelitis is an arduous job and permanent cure is hard to achieve.

Late

Mal-union in the form of shortening, angulation or rotation of varying degrees of severity is common (2.5-11%). The degree of resulting functional disability will determine the treatment necessary. Raising the shoes can treat moderate degrees of shortening. Osteotomy may be indicated in angulatory or rotatory deformities.

Delayed union may be defined as union which has not occurred within 20 weeks of fracture. The incidence is reported as 16-30% following plating and 8-10% following IMN. It may be due to infection, severe displacement, or distraction, comminution, bone loss, an intact fibula, inadequate immobilisation or inadequate internal fixation . Treatment varies from more immobilisation, bone-grafting to osteotomy of an intact fibula.

Non-union. Quoted figures are about 2% with closed fractures treated by cast immobilisation, 4-8% after plating, 2-4% after IMN and 18% after external fixation. The causes of non-union are similar to those of delayed union. Depending on the characteristics of a given case, treatment may take the form of cancellous bone grafting only, bone grafting plus internal fixation (plating or intramedullary nail) or osteotomy of an intact fibula.

Joint stiffness. The knee, ankle and subtalar joints are susceptible to stiffness depending on the methods of treatment adopted. With this in mind, any joint not encased in a cast should be exercised as soon as possible following injury. A truly rigid internal fixation makes it possible to institute early movement of all the joints.

Further reading

Khoury A Liebergall M London E Mosheiff R. Percutaneous plating of distal tibial fractures. *Foot Ankle Int.* 23(9):818-824, 2002.

Russell T A. Fractures of the tibia and fibula. In: Rockwood CA, Green DP, Bucholz RW and Heckman ID eds. *Rockwood and Green's Fractures in Adults.* Philadelphia: Lippincott-Raven, 1996; 2127-2200.

Wiss DA Gibson T. IM nailing of the femur and tibia: indications and techniques. *Current Orthopaedics* (8): 245-254, 1994.

CHAPTER 19

INJURIES OF THE ANKLE AND FOOT

Injuries to the ligaments of the ankle

These are either sprains or ruptures (see also Chapter 12). They occur to a greater or lesser extent with ankle fractures but more often occur in isolation. Isolated ankle ligament injuries are an important cause of disability. They are more common in females than males and this probably has to do with the style of footwear. The ligaments most commonly injured are the lateral and medial collateral ligaments. Lateral collateral ligament injuries are much more common than those of the medial collateral ligaments.

Classification

Grade I injury - sprain consisting of microscopic stretching or tearing within the ligament substance
Grade II injury – gross macroscopic tear of the ligament
Grade III injury – complete rupture of the ligament

LATERAL COLLATERAL LIGAMENT INJURY

The lateral collateral ligament is a complex ligament consisting of three ligaments - the anterior talofibular, the calcaneofibular and the posterior talofibular ligaments. The usual **mechanism** of injury is an inversion strain during walking, running or jumping.

Diagnosis. The severity of injury varies, depending on whether one or more of the ligaments have been affected. There may be localised bruise or swelling and localised tenderness on palpation. Stressing the lateral ankle is usually uncomfortable.

X-ray investigation should include routine AP and lateral views as well as a mortise view. Stress views should include inversion stress and anterior drawer stress views. Ankle arthrography assesses ligament rupture by dye extravasation and is considered by some authors to be more accurate than the talar tilt test. Recently, stress tenography has been introduced; it is said to be more accurate in distinguishing between isolated anterior talo-fibular ligament ruptures and those combined with ruptures of the calcaneofibular ligament.

Treatment. The treatment of lateral ankle ligament injuries has been controversial. While all agree that Grades I and II sprains should be treated with rest, icing, elastic bandaging, elevation and early activity, there are two schools of thought in respect of the treatment of ruptures. One school advocates conservative treatment with below-knee cast immobilisation for 3-4 weeks followed by exercises, while the other advocates operative repair of the ruptured ligaments. However, there is now enough evidence that the results of operative treatment are no better than those of conservative treatment. Therefore, in view of the risks and costs of operative treatment (general anaesthesia, possible infection and the need for hospital admission), the initial treatment of choice should now be conservative. Should this fail, late repair or reconstruction is known to yield as good a result as primary repair.

Complications. Two main complications are recognised:

Recurrent subluxation of the ankle results if a severe injury involving the rupture of both the talofibular ligaments and the calcaneofibular ligament is inadequately treated.

Recurrent subluxation of the peroneal tendons is due to associated rupture of the superior peroneal retinaculum which is in intimate anatomical relationship with the calcaneofibular ligament. Diagnosis is easy: the patient can demonstrate anterior displacement of the peroneal tendons over the fibula during dorsiflexion and eversion. The treatment is operative and a number of procedures are available.

MEDIAL COLLATERAL LIGAMENT INJURIES

Injuries to this ligament are rarer than to the lateral ligament. The usual mechanisms are external rotation or abduction or both. Isolated injuries are rare; associated fractures of the fibula are common. Local symptoms and signs are located on the medial aspect of the ankle. Routine AP X-ray may show widening of the medial joint space, but stress abduction-external rotation films show this better. Both conservative treatment in a below-knee cast with the ankle slightly inverted and operative repair give good results. Conservative treatment should therefore be the treatment of choice since it avoids the risks and cost of operative treatment.

INFERIOR TIBIOFIBULAR JOINT INJURIES

This joint is stabilised by the anterior tibiofibular, interosseus and posterior tibiofibular ligaments which can be disrupted in different ankle injuries. The features and management are discussed below.

RUPTURE OF ACHILLES' TENDON

The injury is commonest among men past the middle age bracket. Squash, badminton and tennis are the commonest sources.

Diagnosis is usually easy; the history is typical - at the time of the injury, the patient feels as if he was sharply struck in the heel and thereafter he is unable to stand on his toes or actively plantar-flex the foot. On examination, a gap in the tendon may be seen or felt about 5 cm above the heel. Some active plantar flexion may be present due to the action of plantaris, flexor hallucis longus and tibialis posterior, all of which are usually intact. However, *Simmond's test* is positive: with the patient lying prone and the foot lying clear of the edge of the couch, the calf is squeezed - the foot does not go into plantar flexion. In a negative test, the foot is seen to passively plantar-flex, signifying an intact tendon. This test is described as *Thompson's test* in some texts.

An incomplete tear (i.e. a sprain) does exist but is perhaps over-diagnosed. A complete tear presenting after 24 hours often gets diagnosed as incomplete because the gap may get filled up by haematoma and the patient may be able to tiptoe for a short while. For this reason, an incomplete rupture can only be accurately diagnosed at exploration.

Treatment is with an below-knee cast with the foot in equinus, i.e. plantar flexion, for 6 weeks or by operative repair. An above-knee cast, though theoretically more appropriate, has not been shown to give better results. After 4 weeks, the initial cast is removed and a new cast is applied with the foot in as neutral a position as possible; this is retained for 2 more weeks. After the removal of the cast, a shoe raise may be needed a further 4-6 weeks.

Surgical repair is favoured in sporty people. The procedure consists of exposure via a posteromedial incision, approximation of the ruptured ends with a Bunnell-type suture augmented with simple interrupted sutures and repair of the paratenon. A below-knee cast is then applied. Arguments advanced in favour of surgical repair include a lower re-rupture rate and more rapid rehabilitation, compared with those treated by cast immobilisation alone. However, a complications rate of about 10% is reported with surgical repair and many studies have given results which are no better than those of non-operative treatment. Furthermore, non-operative treatment has a few advantages: it is associated with lesser mobidity and requires no hospital admission or general anaesthesia.

ANKLE FRACTURES

Introduction

These fractures have occupied the minds of surgeons for centuries. The fact that many of them bear the names of their original describers bears witness to this. Examples include *Pott's, Dupuytren's, Maisonneuve's, Tillaux's* and *Cotton's fractures.*

Ankle injuries are better understood now than before. Central to this is a better understanding of the anatomy of the region and of the importance of the ankle ligaments. As in the pelvis, the ankle mortise can be conceptualised as a ring, consisting (here) of three bones (the medial and lateral malleoli and the talus) and their uniting ligaments (Fig19.1). Of the three bones, the talus is the most important in the production of ankle injuries; it is its abnormal movement in the ankle mortise that puts the other components under stress, leading to possible disruption.

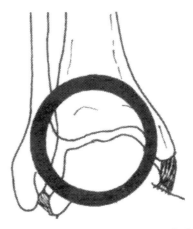

Fig.19.1. The ring structure of the ankle. As with the pelvis, the ankle can be conceptualised in the form of a ring. Similarly, a single break in the ring is a stable injury while a double break results in instability.

The ankle ring may be broken at one or more points. A break at one point only is a stable injury: there is no talar shift. Two breaks or more e.g. fracture of both malleoli or a fracture of one malleolus plus a rupture of one collateral ligament will constitute an unstable injury allowing a talar shift. It is important to emphasise the frequent co-existence of fractures and ligamentous injury. The presence of a ligamentous injury can be inferred if a single malleolar fracture is shown to be displaced since there must be another injury in the ring to permit such a displacement.

Classification

Classifications are another aspect of ankle injuries that usually pre-occupies the student. A number of them exist, one more complex (and perhaps more confusing) than the other. Try to learn one of the following:

- A simple classification based on the perceived mechanism of injury
- A classification based on the level of the fracture of the fibula is simpler (Weber classification)

CLASSIFICATION BASED ON THE PERCEIVED MECHANISM OF INJURY (Fig.19.2)

Abduction injuries

Abducting the foot puts the structures on the medial aspect of the ankle under tension. There is usually added rotation. The followings injuries may result:

1. Transverse fracture of the medial malleolus or rupture of the deltoid ligament.
2. Rupture of the syndesmotic ligaments or avulsion fracture of their insertions.
3. Short, transverse or oblique fracture of the fibula above the joint.

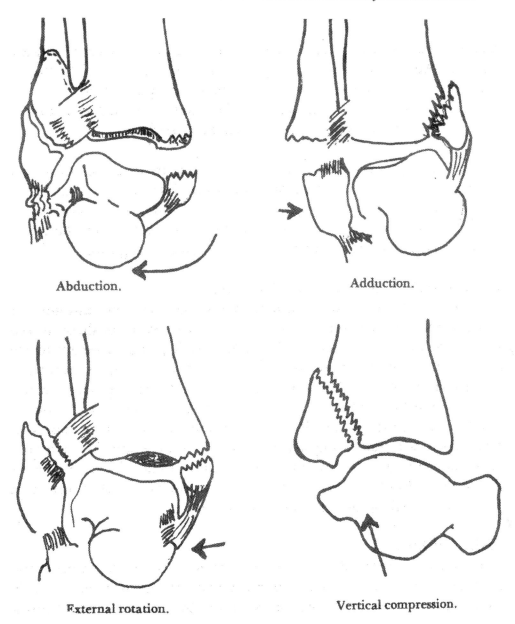

Fig.19.2. Mechanisms of ankle injuries – abduction, adduction, external rotation and vertical compression.

Adduction injuries

Adducting the foot puts the structures on the lateral aspect of the ankle under tension. There is usually added rotation. The followings injuries may result:

1. Transverse avulsion-type fracture of the fibula or lateral collateral ligament rupture.
2. Vertical fracture of the medial malleolus.

External rotation injuries

External rotation of the foot pushes the talus against the lateral malleolus. The following injuries may arise:

1. Transverse medial malleolar fracture or deltoid ligament rupture.
2. Disruption of the anterior tibiofibular ligament.
3. Short oblique fracture of the fibula above the syndesmotic joint.
4. Rupture of the posterior tibiofibular ligament or fracture of the posterior malleolus

Vertical compression injuries

Can arise from falls from a height or forced hyperextension of the foot. The following injuries can arise:

1. Fracture of the anterior margin of the tibia.
2. Supramalleolar fracture of the fibula.

THE WEBER CLASSIFICATION (Fig.19.3)

This classification is based on the level of the fibular fracture:

Type A: fibula fracture below the syndesmosis.
Type B: fibula fracture at the level of the syndesmosis.
Type C: fibula fracture above the level of the syndesmosis.

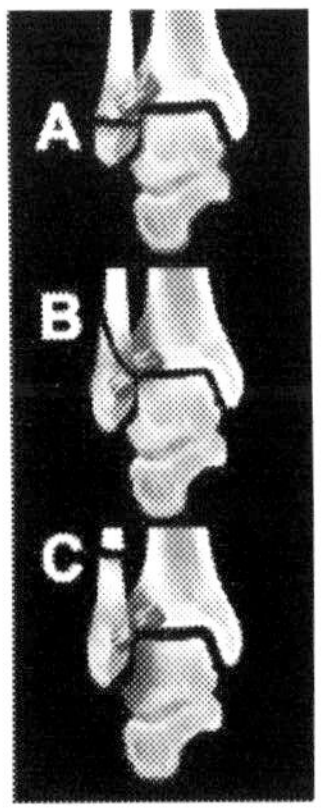

Fig.19.3. Weber classification of ankle fractures

DIAGNOSIS OF ANKLE FRACTURES

The history of the causative injury may suggest the mechanisms and through this the possible injuries to the ankle. Pain localised to one area or the other, bruising, swelling and inability to bear weight on the affected ankle are the main symptoms. Their severity varies according to the severity of the injury. For example, weight-bearing, albeit with a limp, is possible following a stable injury but absolutely impossible following an unstable one. Physical examination should be done with care, as pain is usually a marked feature. It is often made difficult by swelling which sets in quite quickly. Stability of the mortise should be tested and stress tests –anterior drawer, inversion, eversion and external rotation – may be indicated. If it is necessary to further elucidate a particular injury, examination can be done under local or general anaesthesia.

Routine AP and lateral X-rays should include a mortise view; stress views may be necessary to diagnose ligamentous injuries.

There could also be indications for conventional or computed tomography and MRI scanning is useful in elucidating tendon and ligament injuries as well as subtle fractures such as osteochondral fractures. Ankle arthroscopy can also be helpful in the diagnosis of intra-articular lesions and can be incorporated into a surgical treatment regime.

Treatment

What must be remembered here is that we are dealing with intra-articular injuries and as such we must strive for perfect reduction of displaced fractures. This can hardly be achieved closed, so open reduction and internal fixation is often resorted to.

- UNDISPLACED FRACTURES
  Treatment is with a below-knee (short-leg) cast (Fig.19.4). A period of immobilisation of 6 weeks usually suffices.

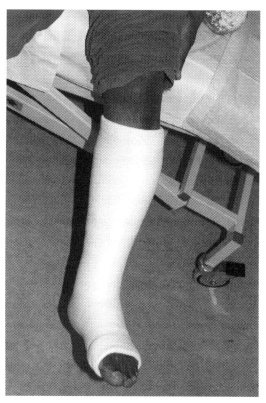

Fig.19.4. Treatment of undisplaced ankle fractures in a below-knee non-weightbearing cast

- DISPLACED FRACTURES: Conservative Treatment
  Closed reduction by manual traction and manipulation can be attempted. Here, a knowledge of the mechanism of a given injury is useful because a successful manipulation is best and most easily achieved by reversing the mechanism of injury. Most fractures of the medial and lateral malleoli can be reduced in this way. If *perfect reduction* is achieved, immobilisation is effected with an above-knee cast, with the knee flexed to 20 – 30 degrees. The cast is above-knee in order to prevent rotation of the tibia with possible re-displacement of the fractures. The patient is not allowed to weight-bear for the first 4 weeks, during which possible redisplacement is checked with X-rays. After this period, a new cast is applied with added walking heel or slipper for weight-bearing for another 2-4 weeks after which the cast is removed and ankle and foot exercises are commenced. In practice, perfect reduction is seldom achieved and open reduction and internal fixation is often resorted to.

OPERATIVE TREATMENT OF DISPLACED FRACTURES

Operative treatment is indicated in the following situations:

- failure of closed reduction
- closed reduction requires excessive force and abnormal positioning of the ankle/foot
- displaced fractures of either malleolus associated with talar tilt
- widening of ankle mortise > 1-2 mm
- some open fractures

After open reduction, internal fixation can be effected with a number of devices including screws, plates, Kirschner wires and cerclage wires (Fig.19.5). Fixation techniques applicable to individual injuries include:

Fractures of the medial malleolus

- One parallel cancellous lag screw
- Two parallel cancellous lag screws
- Tension-band wiring

Fractures of the lateral malleolus

- Interfragmentary compression screw (oblique fracture) plus semitubular plate and screws.
- Intramedullary long screw.

Fractures of the posterior malleolus

- One horizontal cancellous screw in the antero-posterior direction.

Diastasis of the inferior tibiofibular joint

- A diastasis cortical screw is inserted 2-3 cm above the syndesmosis from postero-laterally to anteromedially, transfixing the two cortices of the fibula and the lateral cortex of the tibia (3-point fixation).

POST-OPERATIVE CARE

If rigid fixation has been achieved, casting is unnecessary and early ankle exercises are instituted. Otherwise, a below-knee POP backslab is applied initially and completed later. Weight bearing (partial to begin with) is commenced at 4 weeks.

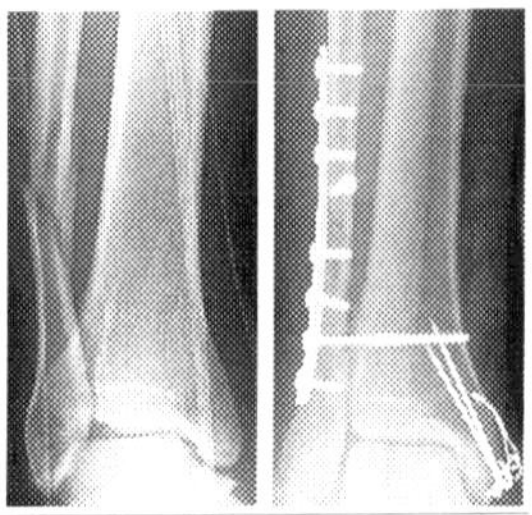

Fig.19.5. Internal fixation of a Weber Type C ankle injury.

Complications of ankle fractures

- *Osteochondral fractures*, especially of the talus, should be borne in mind.
- *Compartment syndrome* of the foot may occur after an ankle injury. Direct vascular injury is

rare but unreduced fracture or dislocation can cause vascular impairment. Early diagnosis and decompression are essential.

- *Infection* may complicate either open fractures or closed ones treated by operation.
- *Mal-union* is common with malleolar fractures.
- *Non-union* is seen mostly with medial malleolar fractures treated by closed reduction and cast immobilisation. It is rarely seen in the lateral malleolus.
- *Post-traumatic osteoarthritis* of the ankle joint will almost always result if there is malalignment of the talus, mal-union or non-union of a significant malleolar fragment.

DISLOCATIONS AND FRACTURE-DISLOCATION OF THE ANKLE

Posterior and anterior dislocations are distinguished. Fracture-dislocations are more common than pure dislocations and 50% of ankle dislocations are associated with open injuries. Unstable ankle injuries are invariably associated with varying degrees of ankle subluxation or dislocation.

Posterior dislocation

This occurs more often than anterior dislocation. The usual mechanism is a blow to the back of the lower tibia: the foot goes into plantar flexion with apparent shortening and the talus can be seen and palpated posteriorly. Urgent reduction is necessary in order to avoid neurovascular embarrassment. It is usually easily achieved by a longitudinal traction on the foot and then lifting the heel forward. Following this, most surgeons immobilise the area in a below-knee cast with the ankle in the neutral position for about 4 weeks. Others advocate open repair of the ruptured ligaments but the results are not better than those obtained with conservative treatment.

Anterior dislocation

This occurs when the tibia is forcible displaced posteriorly on the fixed foot. All the ligamentous and capsular attachments from the tibia and fibula are torn except, perhaps, the posterior talofibular ligament. The patient is in severe pain. The talus is prominent anteriorly, the foot is slightly dorsiflexed, the para-Achilles tendon grooves are obliterated and the dorsalis pedis pulse may be absent. Urgent reduction is indicated: firm longitudinal traction is applied while plantar-flexing the foot.

FRACTURES OF THE TIBIAL PLAFOND

These fractures are also called *pilon fractures*. Most of them are nasty and very difficult to treat and the outcome is seldom excellent. This stems from their complexity: there is a combination of bone, articular cartilage and soft-tissue damage. The usual mechanism is the action of the talus on the tibial dome in the course of high-energy road traffic accidents or falls from heights. They are also common in skiing accidents.

Classification

There are a few classifications of pilon fractures. The AO classification is simple and is described here:

Type A: Extra-articular fracture
Type B: Partial articular fracture with a portion of the tibial shaft intact
Type C: Complete articular fracture with no continuity between the articular surface and the tibial shaft.

Diagnosis

Swelling and deformity can be immense. Many of the fractures are open and the skin can easily be breached in closed fractures, so extra care should be taken during physical examination. Blisters are common and these can cause problems for both closed and open treatment.

AP, lateral and mortise views are essential but the CT scan, if possible with 3-D reconstruction, is the best modality.

Treatment

POP cast treatment: An undisplaced Type A fracture is treated with an above-knee cast as for a tibial shaft fracture. If displaced, it may yield to manipulative reduction and can be immobilised in the same way.

Calcaneal pin traction treatment: This can be used to treat Types B and C fractures – as a definitive treatment option or as initial treatment in patients in whom open reduction and internal fixation is planned but postponed because of skin or other problems. External fixation may be used in patients with open fractures or significant soft-tissue injuries.

Open reduction and internal fixation: This option is often used. It offers the best means of achieving early restoration of the anatomy of the ankle joint by achieving:

- Maintenance of the length and stability of the fibula
- Restoration of the articular surface of the distal tibia
- Restoration of bone defect and
- Buttressing of the medial tibia
- *Early ankle arthrodesis* may be indicated in joints so badly damaged that useful reconstruction is not possible.
- Complications of ORIF include delayed wound healing, infection, loss of reduction, delayed/non-union, joint pain and secondary osteoarthritis.

INJURIES OF THE FOOT

Introduction

Injuries of the foot consist of fractures of the bones of the foot and injuries to associated soft tissues, including blood vessels and nerves. Generally speaking, students do not find a study of trauma to the foot as exciting as a study of trauma to the femur, for example, one of the main reasons is a poor knowledge of the anatomy of the foot. My experience is that not all medical students in their fourth year can quickly and correctly name the bones of the foot. Be it as it may, we all need a working knowledge of the anatomy of the foot in order to be able to understand injuries to it.

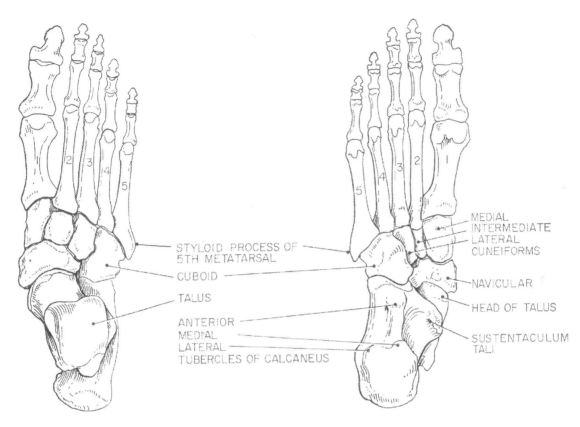

Fig.19.6. The bones of the foot and ankle.

Briefly, the foot is divided into the following parts (Fig.19.6):

- The hindfoot, consisting of the talus and calcaneum
- The midfoot, consisting of the navicular, cuboid and the medial, intermediate and lateral cuneiforms and
- The forefoot, consisting of the five metatarsals and the five toes. The big toe has two phalanges whereas the other toes have three each. These bones and parts have complex articulations between them, reinforced by complex ligaments, fascial strips and muscles.

The more important articulations are:

- The subtalar joint formed between the talus above and the calcaneum below
- The midtarsal (or Chopart's joint), formed by the talonavicular joint medially and the calcaneocuboid joint laterally
- The tarsometatarsal (or Lisfranc's joint), joining the distal tarsal bones to the bases of the five metatarsals
- The metatarsophalangeal joints and
- The interphalangeal joints.

A study of the tendinous and fascial origins and attachments of the foot is intriguing and instructive and a plea is made here to the student to check them up in an appropriate text.

The blood supply to the foot as a whole is also complex, but of particular popularity in orthopaedics is the supply to the talus. Like most bones of the foot, it receives blood from the branches of the anterior tibial, the posterior tibial and the perforating peroneal arteries. However, because about three-fifths of the surface is covered with articular cartilage, the area through which blood vessels can enter the bone is limited. In the event, they enter the bone in the region of the neck. In view of the anatomical relationship between the neck and the body, fractures through the neck constitute a danger to the blood supply to the body and avascular necrosis of the body is a real possibility in these fractures.

INJURIES OF THE TALUS

These injuries are rare. About 60% of the talar surface is articular, so the area available for vascular penetration is limited. Most of the blood supply is retrograde i.e. comes from distally to proximally, as with the scaphoid bone. Accordingly, displaced fractures of the neck pose a risk of avascular necrosis of the body.

Hawkin's classification

Type I: Undisplaced vertical fracture of the neck (most common).
Type II: Displaced fracture of the neck with subluxation or dislocation of the subtalar joint with the ankle joint remaining intact.
Type III: Displaced fracture of the neck with dislocation of the body from both the subtalar and ankle joints.

Other talar fractures include:

- Fracture of the lateral process – rare.
- Avulsion fractures.
- Osteochondral dome fractures.

The usual mechanism of fractures of the neck is hyperextension of the midfoot and ankle. The addition of compression of the talus by the inferior articular surface of the tibia results in fractures of the body. This mechanism is classically present when a motor vehicle driver suddenly and sharply marches on the brakes to avoid an accident. Talar fractures are also relatively common in pilots involved in airplane crashes where similar mechanisms are at play.

Diagnosis

This may be facilitated by a suggestive history. Intense pain in the ankle and foot and swelling are constant features. Where there has been marked displacement, the skin may be breached or be in danger of being breached easily. The circulatory status of the foot must be determined immediately.

X-rays are essential. AP, lateral and oblique views are needed to show the talus clearly and determine the site, and other characteristic of a given fracture. Associated fractures of neighbouring bones must be noted. The relationship of the talus to the tibia, calcaneum, navicular and other tarsal bones must be carefully assessed in order to be able to diagnose subluxations and dislocations.

Treatment

The treatment depends on the presenting injury:

Avulsion and osteochondral fractures

Tiny attached chips are treated as ankle sprains. Loose chips are best excised if they are small or fixed back if they are large enough.

Undisplaced fractures of the neck and body

These are treated in a below-knee cast for 6-8 weeks. Because of the marked tendency to swelling of the foot and ankle, high elevation is necessary in the first one week. Weight bearing is allowed thereafter for fractures of head; for fractures of the neck and body, this is delayed for about 4 weeks. Ankle and subtalar joint function is regained with normal use after the cast is removed. The prognosis is good.

Displaced fractures of the neck and body and fracture-dislocations

Reduction is imperative and should be carried out urgently because the integrity of the skin is often threatened. Closed reduction is first attempted; the key manoeuvre here is plantar flexion of the ankle and traction against counter-traction. X-ray control should be used. If reduction is achieved by either method, immobilisation is effected with an above knee cast with the knee in slight flexion and the ankle in equinus, if not, open reduction and internal fixation must be carried out.

Avascular necrosis of the body occurs in 40-100% of cases, depending on the degree of displacement. If painful post-traumatic arthritis of the ankle or subtalar joint (or both) develops, arthrodesis of the affected joint will be indicated.

Comminuted fracture of the body

In this case it is often difficult to obtain functional ankle and subtalar joints. Initial treatment should consist of immobilisation in a splint e.g. a P.O.P. backslab plus high elevation for 4-6 weeks to allow soft-tissue reactions to settle. Following this, one of a number of fusion procedures could be done:

- Pantalar fusion (i.e. fusion of the ankle and subtalar joints)
- Tibiocalcaneal fusion (after excising the talus)
- Blair's tibiotalar fusion (Fig.19.7).

The Blair fusion is the more physiological procedure: function is preserved in the talonavicular, calcaneocuboid and anterior talocalcaneal joints.

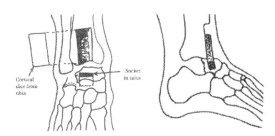

Fig.19.7a and b. Blair's tibiotalar ankle fusion

Complications of talar injuries

- Compounding is frequent because the skin in the area is frequently put under undue pressure by these injuries.
- Avascular necrosis of the body or whole of the talus is a frequent and serious complication.
- Non-union may occur.

FRACTURES OF THE CALCANEUM

Introduction.

The calcaneum is the most frequently fractured bone of the foot. The usual mechanisms is fall on the foot from a height. Two important features of the anatomy of the bone deserve mention here as they underlie the problems of management of the injuries:

- the calcaneum is essentially a cancellous bone. This structure suits its anatomical position and function as the weight-bearer of the body and springboard of the heel. However, beyond physiological levels of loading, it becomes a disadvantage: it is easily smashed.

- It contributes (with the talus) to the formation of the subtalar joint, the position of which is such that it is often involved in fractures of the calcaneum. Involvement of the subtalar joint always creates diagnostic and treatment problems and the prognosis is almost always bad.

- Associated injuries to other parts of the body is also worthy of mention in this introduction. Calcaneal fractures are associated with compression fractures of the thoracolumbar spine in over 10% of cases and with fractures of other bones of the lower limb in about 30% of cases.

Diagnosis

The diagnosis of calcaneal fractures is based on the history of the injury, the physical and the X-ray findings. Pain and swelling are intense, there is widening of the heel. Movement cannot be elicited in the subtalar joint in injuries involving this joint. AP and lateral X-ray views may show important features of a given injury but axial views are considered essential to elucidate the state of the subtalar joint.

Treatment

This depends on the type of fracture:

Fractures not involving the subtalar joint. These include the various chip Avulsion fractures (of the tuberosity, the sustentaculum tali, the anterior process) are usually treated conservatively with a crepe bandage plus elevation or in a cast moulded to effect reduction if there is displacement.

Occasionally, open reduction and screw fixation may be indicated.

Fractures involving the subtalar joint. These fractures are very difficult to treat because reduction, even though logical and desirable, is almost impossible to achieve by any method. Closed reduction and P.O.P. immobilisation for 6 weeks is practised by some. Other practices open reduction with bone grafting and fixation with Kirschner wires or slender pins. The results of both methods are poor. Subtalar or triple arthrodesis is available for the severe case or those complicated subsequently by stiffness and pain. Some surgeons recommend them as a primary procedure but this is hardly justifiable.

The complications of calcaneal fractures include chronic subtalar pain, entrapment of the peroneal tendons, shortening (following severe compression fractures) and sural neuropathy.

FRACTURES OF THE NAVICULAR

These are rare injuries. They may be stress or avulsion fractures, fractures of the body or fracture-dislocations. An undisplaced fracture can be treated with a below-knee plaster for 2-4 weeks, depending on its severity. A displaced fracture may require open reduction and screw-fixation.

TALONAVICULAR DISLOCATION

This may be associated with a fracture of the talus or of the navicular. Closed reduction is easily achieved and maintained with a below-knee cast for 4 weeks.

FRACTURES OF THE CUBOID AND CUNEIFORMS

These are rare. Conservative treatment usually suffices.

FRACTURE-DISLOCATION OF THE TARSOMETATARSAL JOINT

Injury to this joint, which is also known as *Lisfranc's joint* is rare. It is usually secondary to open injuries. Associated fractures are common. Closed reduction may fail if there is interposition of tendons, in which case open reduction may be resorted to. Associated fractures may need separate treatment. It is important to restore the transverse arch of the foot. Immobilisation in a non-weight bearing below-knee cast is required for 4-6 weeks.

FRACTURES OF THE METATARSALS

These fractures were recently popularised in the U.K. by David Beckham, the popular Manchester United midfielder and England captain, who sustained a fracture of the 2nd metatarsal (*David Beckham fracture*) six weeks before the start of the 2002 Football World Cup competition. They are fairly common injuries. Most are due to direct injury as in hits by heavy objects dropped on the foot. One metatarsal or more may be involved. The fracture line may go through the base, shaft or head and segmental fractures are not uncommon. An avulsion fracture of the tuberosity of the 5th metatarsal by peroneal brevis pull (*Jones' fracture*) is also a common injury usually from inversion sprains of the forefoot.

In all these fractures, wide displacement is unusual. Pain, swelling and disability may, however, be severe and immobilisation in a below-knee cast may be indicated for shaft fractures. Weight-bearing is uncomfortable for the first 2-3 weeks; thereafter partial weight bearing is encouraged. Rarely there may be indication for screw fixation or plating of a metatarsal fracture.

A rather characteristic fracture in the metatarsal region is the so-called *stress fracture*. It is seen most commonly in the 2nd metatarsal but sometimes also in the 3rd. The usual site is the shaft just proximal to the head. There is usually a history of a prolonged strenuous walk, not usually undertaken by the patient. It is common among army recruits and for this reason is called *'march' fracture*. There is pain, slight swelling and considerable local tenderness. Early X-rays (within 2 weeks) do not normally show any fracture. Because there is no 'dramatic' injury, the patient hardly considers the possibility of a fracture but when the symptoms increase rather than abate they are forced to see the doctor.

Classically, X-rays taken at this time (usually in the 3rd-4th post-fracture week) shows exorbitant callus. When suspected, the injury is best treated with a below-knee cast, rest and elevation. However, treatment with an elastic bandage and activity is acceptable in patients tolerant of pain.

DISLOCATIONS OF THE METATARSOPHALANGEAL JOINTS

Dislocation or subluxation of these joints occur rarely. Forced extreme dorsiflexion causing a rupture of the plantar capsule of the metatarsophalangeal joint is the usual mechanism. Closed reduction is usually easy but the injury may be occasionally irreducible due to interposition of the volar plate or a sesamoid bone. In such a situation, open reduction has to be carried out.

FRACTURES OF THE TOE PHALANGES

These are usually direct injuries, caused by dropped heavy object. They are very painful injuries. Minor fractures may be treated by garter strapping but more severe ones should be treated by immobilisation and non weight bearing. Some injuries require stabilisation with Kirschner wires.

DISLOCATIONS OF THE INTERPHALANGEAL JOINTS

Isolated dislocations or subluxation are very rare. Even in association with other foot injuries, they are still rare. Usually it is the proximal joints that are involved. Reduction should be carried out; K-wire stabilisation may be necessary.

Further reading

Schmolke S Wuelker N. Ankle fractures. *Current Opinion in Orthopedics (Ankle and Foot):* April 2000 - Vol 11 (2): 99-102, 2000.

Michelson J Magid D McHale K. Clinical Utility of a Stability-Based Ankle Fracture Classification System. *Journal of Orthopaedic Trauma Vol. 21 (5):* 307- 315, 2007.

CHAPTER 20

SPORTS INJURIES

Here, we will discuss bruises (contusions), sprains, knee cartilage tears, ruptures of muscles and tendons as well as dislocations. Fractures often result from sports but these have been previously discussed and will not be repeated here.

CONTUSION

A **contusion** is an area of skin discoloration caused by the escape of blood from underlying blood vessels following injury. It is synonymous with the word "**bruise**". The causative injury may be to soft tissues alone as is commonly seen in ankle sprains or may result from bleeding from a fractured bone.

The symptoms and signs of a contusion are *swelling* and *pain*. In white or fair-skinned people, the colour of a bruise changes with time from an initial red/pink colour to bluish, then greenish yellow before returning to normal. These colour changes are due to the chemical breakdown and absorption of the blood pigment, haemoglobin. A bruise is less obvious in dark-skinned people. Bruises heal quickly and normal skin colour is usually restored within six weeks.

SPRAINS

A *sprain* is illustrated below. It is a tear of the ligaments of a joint and could be *partial* or *complete*. There may not be a visible gap in a torn ligament. Common sites of sprains include the finger, wrist, ankle, and knee joints but no joint is exempt. The ligaments of the neck and lower back are also frequently sprained.

How long will a sprain take to heal?

If treated properly, most sprains will heal enough to allow reasonable use within six weeks. Poor treatment and non-compliance on the part of the patient can prolong the healing period.

COMMON SPRAINS

THE SPRAINED ANKLE

Ankle sprain is very common. It is the most common injury in sports and, in ordinary life, people sprain their ankles in the course of many activities of daily living, such as walking and running. In most cases, the ligaments on the outer aspect of the ankle are the ones torn but the ligaments on the inner aspect can also be torn. It has been estimated that one in 10,000 people sprains their ankle daily. This will give a figure of about 200,000 sprains in the world every day of the year!

Diagnosis

There is a history of injury, usually an inversion injury and there is pain and swelling around the ankle. Tenderness is elicitable by palpation, more on the lateral aspect. X-ray investigation is necessary to ascertain the degree of damage to the ligaments and rule out an associated fracture. An MRI scan may be indicated.

Treatment

Mild to moderate sprains

- Ice application at regular intervals, 4 times a day
- Supportive elastic bandaging of the ankle
- Elevation of the ankle higher than the hip level
- Pain-killing and anti-inflammatory drugs
- Physiotherapy to regain joint movement

Severe sprains

In addition to the above measures, severe sprains require immobilisation in a removable cast or brace for 2-4 weeks. Surgical repair is needed if the sprain has caused a disruption of normal alignment of the ankle joint.

GROIN SPRAIN

Groin strain is due to the detachment of some of the fibres of powerful muscles, the hamstring muscles, from their origin in bones in the pelvis. This usually happens during strenuous games, which put these muscles under intense pressure. X-rays may show the detached piece of bone. The treatment is mainly rest, taking pain-killers and physiotherapy. It may take up to eight weeks to heal.

THE SPRAINED KNEE

The knee has important ligaments both outside and inside, which can be sprained. Treatment follows lines similar to that of ankle sprains.

KNEE CARTILAGE INJURIES

Tears of the two cartilage shock-absorbers (the menisci) in the knee are common as a result of twist injuries during sports and day-to-day activities. They are usually investigated by MRI scanning and treated by key-hole surgery (arthroscopy): if torn, the torn portions are trimmed off and the knee is washed out.

KNEE CRUCIATE LIGAMENT INJURIES

The knee has two so-called *cruciate ligaments* connecting the femur to the tibia. They function as check reins, checking excessive sliding of the two bones on each other. They can tear if subjected to excessive disruptive forces, such as in an aggressive football tackle. This is a common sports injury, which causes the knee to become unstable in certain positions of knee bending.

Cruciate ligament injuries are diagnosed from the history of the injuries, special examination and an MRI scan. Treatment options can be non-operative (physiotherapy, knee bracing) or operative (cruciate ligament reconstruction).

THE SPRAINED WRIST AND FINGERS

Sprains of the wrist and fingers are common in cricket, baseball, other throwing games as well as in soccer. They also occur in the course of activities of daily living. As stated earlier, most cases are minor and heal well. A small minority may require further investigation and/or treatment. The outcome depends on the severity of the initial injury.

TENDON TEARS AND RUPTURES

You can imagine that there are very many tendons in the musculo-skeletal system. But only a few tend to tear or rupture often:

- **Achilles tendon**
  Achilles' tendon tears and ruptures are fairly common and were discussed in Chapter 19.

- **"Quadriceps mechanism" ruptures**
  The so-called "quadriceps mechanism" consists of the quadriceps muscle, which wraps round the front of the thigh and its main function is to straighten the bent knee. This muscle and its tendons can tear or rupture if their contraction is violently resisted, as in kicking hard against a stationary and hard object.

  The level at which it tears occurs has been observed to be related to the age of the patient: the older the patient the more proximal the rupture site is to the thigh. That is, it tears in the muscle belly in the very old, near the upper end of the knee cap in middle-aged people, through the knee cap itself in young adults and pulled out its lower attachment to the tibial tubercle in pre-adolescent or adolescent children.

The diagnosis is confirmed by physical examination, X-rays and scans, especially MRI scan.

Surgical repair is the treatment of choice. Following repair, the leg is put into an above-knee cylinder cast for 6 weeks. This is followed by quadriceps exercises. The regaining of function is slow and may not be full.

- **Biceps tendon rupture**
  The biceps muscle lies in front of the upper arm and has two tendons, the long and short heads, hence the "bi" in its name. Rupture of the long head near its scapular origin is more common in people past middle age in whom the tendon has begun to degenerate significantly. Rupture at its radial attachment is more common in sporty young people.

  The usual way a biceps rupture comes about is sudden and forcible flexion of the elbow against strong resistance such as is present during the lifting of a heavy object.

  The most characteristic sign is that resisted bending of the elbow makes the torn muscle to bunch up in front of the upper arm.

Treatment. Rupture of the long head near its origin from the shoulder blade is treated by immobilisation in a broad-arm sling or with a collar and cuff sling for a week or two. This usually suffices. With regard to rupture at the lower end, surgical re-attachment to bone is the preferred treatment.

- **Rotator cuff tears**
  The rotator cuff is a tissue sheet formed by tendons arising from the four muscles which envelope the shoulder joint, namely the supraspinatus, infraspinatus, subscapularis and deltoid. The adjective "rotator" derives from their function of rotating the humeral head.

  Tears of parts of the rotator cuff can occur as isolated injuries. Such a tear could be partial (with a better prognosis) or complete (with a worse prognosis). They can be caused by a direct blow as occurs in a fall on the point of the shoulder or by an indirect force such as is generated in a fall on the outstretched arm or during sudden pull of the arm. Most of the patients are elderly with pre-existing degeneration in the cuff.

Diagnosis: The symptoms and signs include muscle wasting and tenderness at the shoulder and inability to raise the shoulder due to pain (painful arc). The diagnosis can be confirmed with an ultrasound or MRI scan.

Treatment: Non-operative treatment consists of physiotherapy for partial tears. Recovery could be prolonged. Immediate surgical repair of an acute complete rupture is favoured by some surgeons. The results of repairs vary. Generally they are good for relief of pain but the painful arc persists in many patients.

DISLOCATIONS

A *dislocation* is a joint out of position. It may be complete or partial. When partial, it is called a *subluxation.* Most dislocations are probably partial and patients often describe this injury as "popping out and back again". The term **recurrent dislocation** is used to describe a situation in which a joint has dislocated three or more times. Recurrent dislocation is relatively common in the shoulder joint.

Diagnosis: The history and tell-tale symptoms and signs of a dislocation are – *pain, swelling, bruise, deformity and difficulty with movements* in the affected joint are diagnostic. X-rays are usually enough for the confirmation of the diagnosis but a CT or MRI scan may be needed to show the finer details of a complex fracture-dislocation.

Treatment: Many dislocations go back into place (reduce) spontaneously. Those that do not need to be put back into place as soon as possible, preferably under an anaesthetic. There is a choice of methods of reducing dislocations of various joints, without resorting to opening up the affected joint. In the shoulder, for example, Kocher's, Hyppocratic and Stimson methods are available and have been discussed in the relevant section. Only in a few cases is surgical intervention necessary. A reduced dislocation needs to be "immobilized" to rest it and allow it to heal.

NERVE AND TENDON INJURIES

Tendons, especially those in the hand and foot, and nerves can be injured directly or as part of fractures and other injuries. These can be complex and have been discussed elsewhere in this book.

Further reading

Textbook of Sports Medicine: Basic Science and Clinical Aspects of Sports Injury and Physical Activity. Editor(s): Michael Kjær, Michael Krogsgaard, Peter Magnusson, Lars Engebretsen, Harald Roos, Timo Takala, Savio L-Y Woo. Blackwell Science Ltd, 2003.

PART IV
MISCELLANEOUS BONE DISEASES

CHAPTER 21

SICKLE-CELL DISEASE AND THE SKELETON

Introduction

Sickle-cell disease is an inherited blood disease caused by an abnormal haemoglobin, HbS, which *"sickles"* in low oxygen environments to form blood clots. Such low oxygen environments are found in most tissues and organs of the body in the course of their everyday functions. *Sickling* is defined as "the assumption by red blood cells of peculiar shapes resembling that of the sickle". The vicious circle of *sickling* and *formation of blood clots* as a result lie at the root of most of the effects of sickle-cell disease on the various organs of the body, including the bones. Most of the patients with acute symptoms of the disease (chronic anaemia, sickle-cell crisis, hand-foot syndrome, chest pain, bone pain) are children.

Clotting blocks the blood vessels that feed tissues and organs. This blockage causes two levels of damage:

- *Tissue/organ ischaemia:* this is a temporary cut-off of the blood supply to the organ; the organ survives the attack without adverse effects.

- *Tissue/organ death*: this is otherwise termed *avascular necrosis* or *infarction*. This situation results from sustained cut-off of the blood supply to the tissues concerned. The affected organ or part of it dies and can only be replaced by a process of healing.

Avascular necrosis of bone tissue is the most important single adverse manifestation of sickle-cell disease on the skeleton. Virtually all bones of the body can be affected by this process, especially the ends and shafts of the long bones (humerus, radius, ulna, femur, tibia, fibula), the hand (metacarpals), the foot (metatarsals) and the backbone (vertebrae) (Table 21.1).

LESIONS ARISING FROM BONE INFARCTION

As can be seen from Table 21.1, virtually any bone may be affected.

Table 22.1. Location/Distribution of bone infarction in SCD

Humerus	Epiphysis (Humeral head)
	Metaphysis
	Diaphysis
Radius and ulna	Epiphysis; Metaphysis; Diaphysis
Metacarpals	Marrow; Diaphysis – not uncommon
Phalanges	Marrow; Diaphysis – not uncommon
Spine	Body
Pelvis	Rare
Femur	Proximal epiphysis/Metaphysis;
	Diaphysis
	Distal Epiphysis - rare
Tibia	Proximal Epiphysis/Diaphysis
	Diaphysis
	Distal Epiphysis - rare
Fibula	Rare
Metatarsals	Marrow; Diaphysis – not uncommon
Other bones	Seen but rare

COMMON BONE LESIONS

DACTYLITIS

Marrow infarction in metacarpals, metatarsals and phalanges give rise to dactylitis, which is also sometimes referred to as the *hand-foot syndrome*. Pathological studies reveal a complete necrosis of the bone marrow and the inner one-third of the cortex. Retention of the outer two-thirds of the cortex and an intact periosteum provides a capacity for healing and remodelling of affected bones, which are the usual outcomes of this condition. Secondary infection may occur and complicate the clinical picture and management.

Dactylitis occurs predominantly in children aged between 6 months and 7 years and about two-thirds of cases occur between the ages of 6 months and 2 years. It is seen mainly in HbSS disease patients in whom it is often the first presentation of the disease. The incidence is quoted as between 11% and 80%. The higher figures are from reports from Africa and it is postulated that the higher incidence of infections precipitating sickle cell crises in Africa may be to blame. Dactylitis has also been reported in HbSC and HbSThal patients but it has been noted that the affected patients are older than affected HbSS patients.

Clinically, the affected child presents with acute, non-pitting and painful swelling of the hands and feet, usually associated with fever. The swelling and pain usually subside within a week but repeated episodes are common. X-rays in the acute period show soft-tissue swelling only. After about two weeks, subperiosteal new bone can be seen. The metacarpals are most frequently involved, followed by the proximal phalanges. Radiolucent areas may be present and cortical destruction may be seen in the juxta-metaphyseal zone. Usually, there is multiple bone involvement but occasionally only one bone is involved. Rarely, most of a small bone may disappear. Simultaneous involvement of long bones e.g. the radius and ulna, in the infarction process is not uncommon.

Treatment consists mainly of rest and analgesia. If complicated by infection, antibiotics should be used based on blood culture studies.

LONG BONE DIAPHYSEAL LESIONS

These are essentially products of diaphyseal infarction, same as dactylitis, and are also characteristic of sickle cell disease in the young.

Diagnosis. Like dactylitis, it is most frequently seen in children aged between 1 and 10 years with HbSS disease and presents with fever, leucocytosis, soft-tissue swelling and marked bone and joint pain. The most commonly affected bones are the humerus, radius, ulna, femur, tibia and fibula. The lesions are often bilateral and symmetrical. The phenomenon is rare in HBSC patients under the age of 6 years.

The size/extent of diaphyseal involvement varies: the lesions may be *localised* or *extensive*. Three segment involvement is common in the very young (about 3 years of age). Generally, it appears that the younger the child, the more extensive the involvement. The x-ray appearance is characteristic and impressive: the involved segment presents the picture of a virtually destroyed bone, medulla and cortex, with a subperiosteal new bone envelope. Breaks in the continuity of the cortex may be seen at some points. In severe forms, all or a part of the old diaphysis may undergo avascular necrosis and become sequestrated, with an involucrum forming around it from periosteal new bone. In this situation, a characteristic *bone-in-bone picture* is produced(Fig.21.1), as in acute haematogenous osteomyelitis.

Beyond the age of 10 years, acute diaphyseal infarction is rare. Involvement takes the form of subacute and chronic ischaemia: there are little or no acute symptoms but signs of infarction are present on x-rays. The reasons for this difference are not clear but may have to do with anatomical differences in the two age groups: young children have more extensive marrow, less firmly attached periosteum and less well-developed periosteal circulation, compared with older patients.

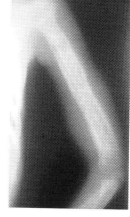

Fig.21.1. Diaphyseal infarction of the humerus with the classical bone-in-bone picture (Courtesy of Dr. Suleiman Giwa, Chief Consultant Orthopaedic Surgeon, LUTH, Lagos, Nigeria)

Treatment. Fortunately, the natural history of acute diaphyseal infarction is complete healing, with remodelling. The healing is surprising fast. There may be residual cortical thickening and narrowing of the medullary canal. Orthopaedic aspects of management focus on the *prevention and treatment of pathological fractures* that may occur in affected bones. As a point of fact, it must be mentioned that the incidence of pathological fractures is low, despite the alarming X-ray picture that suggests extreme fragility. This low incidence may be due to reflex protection of affected bones by the patients or to the affected bones managing to retain their structural strength or both.

The treatment/prevention of pathological fractures is usually non-operative, with appropriate splintage with casts or orthoses. Occasionally, *opportunistic infection of infarcted bones* occurs. The most common causative organism in this situation is *Salmonella*. The clinical course is more severe in younger children. Antibiotic treatment, preferably based on laboratory studies, is required.

EPIPHYSEAL LESIONS

The most commonly involved epiphyses are those of the proximal humerus, tibia and femur. Involvement of the proximal femoral epiphysis has the most devastating and long-lasting effect and is probably the most orthopaedically important manifestation of sickle cell disease.

Avascular Necrosis of the Femoral Head (Fig.21.2)

Avascular necrosis of the femoral head is probably the most important single bony complication of sickle-cell disease. It can lead to severe destruction of the hip, with serious and lasting consequencies. Most of the patients with hip disease that I have treated have been aged 12 years and above. The natural history of the disease is that it heals but the healing is rarely complete and residual femoral head deformity is to be expected. Therefore, treatment needs to be instituted early in order to improve the natural history of the disease.

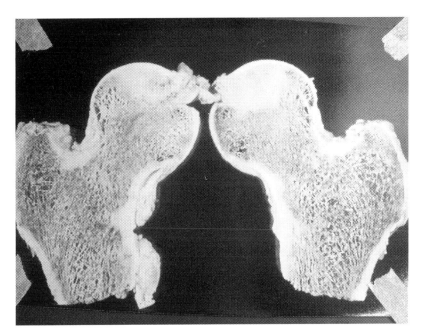

Fig.21.2. A pathological specimen showing avascular necrosis of part of the head of femur in a baby

DIAGNOSIS

The main complaints are pain, limp and restricted movement in the hip joint.

- *Pain.* Most patients have pain in the groin, front of the thigh or in the knee. It is sometimes reported that some patients with sickle-cell hip disease do not have hip pain. However, the very nature of hip disease makes hip pain inevitable but this may be masked by other more severe pain experienced by patients in crisis with vaso-occlusive attacks on the internal organs and other bones of the skeleton. Even if pain is not present at rest, the chances are that it would appear with weight-bearing or during examination.

- *Limp.* Limp is another important symptom and sign of hip disease. In early disease, it is caused by pain (*antalgic limp*), which makes the patient to automatically reduce the amount of body weight put through the affected hip – by limping. In late disease, limp may be due to both pain and limb shortening caused by destruction of the head of femur.

- *Deformity.* The leg on the affected side tends to turn outwards and the pelvis is tilted to compensate for leg shortening due to the damage done to the femoral head and also to adaptive contracture of the soft tissue around the joint. If both hips are affected, they may walk with a Charlie Chaplin gait. Multifocal affection can lead to severe crippling.

INVESTIGATIONS

- *Conventional x-rays* should always be requested first of all. They give significant information in most patients. This is the only investigative modality available in parts of the developing world where SCD is most prevalent. With experience and a high index of suspicion, doctors working in these environments manage to detect most lesions.

- *MRI scan.* Early disease cannot be reliably identified on conventional x-rays and the *MRI scan* is best in this situation.

- An *isotope bone scan* will provide information about the "activeness" of a lesion. It is not an essential investigation.

- *Bone biopsy (core decompression).* The bone obtained is used to stage the disease and the tunnel created by the drill used decongests the head of femur, *relieving* pain in the process.

TREATMENT

Non-surgical Treatment

Non-surgical management may be considered in all age groups and in all types of lesions, depending on the circumstances. It includes the use of analgesics and anti-inflammatory drugs, traction in the acute stage in children, weight-relieving walking aids, callipers, POP casts, braces and physiotherapy. However, patient compliance is low, making an aggressive operating policy more desirable.

Surgical Treatment

It is important to emphasise that surgery for hip problems in sickle-cell disease should be undertaken by an orthopaedic surgeon with special knowledge of and interest in the disease. The most frequently performed procedure in sickle-cell disease patients at the present time is total hip replacement, which is an operation designed mainly for old people. This should not be the case, as sickle-cell hip disease starts at an early age and most patients with hip disease are below the age of 40. I have argued for a long time that the most frequently performed procedures should be those that conserve the femoral head so that the salvage and the "final" operation of total hip replacement can be postponed for as long as possible.

Available femoral head conserving operations are:

- Core decompression (Fig.21.3)
- Bone grafting procedures (Fig.21.4)

Available salvage operations are:

- Bone cuts to contain a displaced head of femur
- Total hip replacement (Fig.21.5)
- Fusion (Arthrodesis) of the hip joint

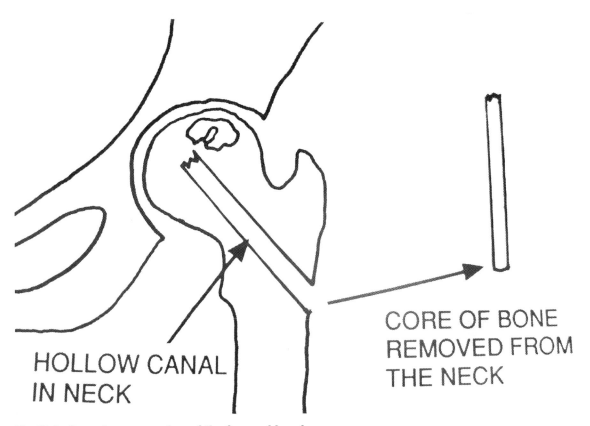

HOLLOW CANAL IN NECK

CORE OF BONE REMOVED FROM THE NECK

Fig.21.3. Core decompression of the femoral head.

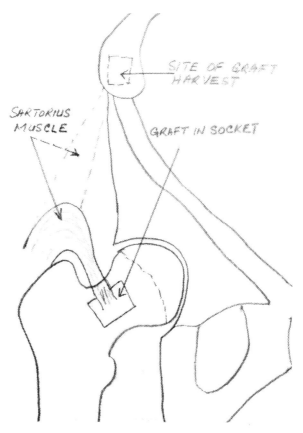

Fig.22.4. Bone grafting procedure invented by the author in 1983 aimed at getting the necrotic lesions to heal.

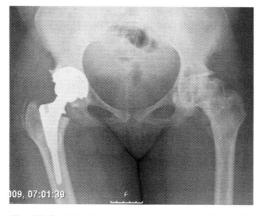

Fig.21.5. Total hip replacement of the right hip in a 28-year-old patient with severe bilateral involvement.

Further reading

Serjeant GR and Serjeant BE. *Sickle Cell Disease,* Third Edition, Oxford University Press, 2001.

Iwegbu, CG. *Orthopaedic diseases: Principles and Management,* 2nd Edition (Chapter 34), Authorhouse USA, 2006.

CHAPTER 22

SOME OTHER ORTHOPAEDIC DISEASES

Haemophilia

Haemophilia is a bleeding disorder resulting from a deficiency of either plasma factor VIII (Classical or Type A Haemophilia) or factor IX (Christmas or Type B Haemophilia). Both types are X chromosome-linked recessive disorders, affecting only males, and are clinically indistinguishable. Haemophilia A is said to occur in 1 out of 5,000 live male births and six times more common than Haemophilia B. It can be diagnosed pre-natally by linkage studies or direct gene analysis but more than a third of cases result from spontaneous mutations. Post-natal diagnosis can be made by direct assay of factor VIII or IX activity levels.

The severity of the disease is classified as follows:

- *Mild* – factor level between 5 and 30% of the normal
- *Moderate* – factor level between 1 and 5% of the normal
- *Severe* – factor level less than 1% of the normal

Orthopaedic aspects/complications of haemophilia include:

Acute

- *Bleeding into joints (haemarthrosis)*
- *Acute synovitis*
- *Bleeding into soft tissues (haematomas)*
- *Compartment syndrome*
- *Carpal tunnel syndrome*
- *Femoral nerve palsy*

Chronic

- *Chronic synovitis* secondary to repeated irritation/stimulation of the synovial membrane by blood and deposition of iron in it

- *Flexion contractures of joints* secondary to chronic swelling and pain in a joint

- *Angular deformities of long bones* secondary to asymmetrical growth plates growth

- *Secondary osteoarthritis of joints.* The joints most frequently affected are the knee, ankle and elbow. The x-ray picture is that joint destruction, with subchondral sclerosis, subchondral cysts and peripheral osteophytes, often against the background of osteoporosis.

The ***management of orthopaedic complications*** include:

- *Factor replacement.* This must precede any surgical intervention. To treat bleeding into soft tissues and joints, circulating levels of the deficient factor must reach 40-50% of normal. Surgical procedures require replacement to 100% of the normal level.

- *Prophylactic factor replacement.* Patients with factor levels greater than 1% rarely develop significant haemophilic arthropathy.

- *Correction of angular deformities* may be indicated.

- *Total joint replacement* may also be required, especially in the knee.

Achondroplasia

Achondroplasia is an autosomal dorminant disorder caused by a mutation in the fibroblast growth factor receptor type 3. However, most cases arise by spontaneous mutations, increased paternal age being a risk factor. Fibroblast growth factor regulates early chondrocyte development and causative mutations adversely affect this process. Abnormal development of the epiphyses, especially in the regions of greatest endochondral growth, results in characteristic shortening of the bones, with the more proximal bones being more severely affected than the more distal. Angular deformities may also result. The spine is also profoundly affected.

Affected children can be identified at birth by their characteristic physiognomy: frontal bossing; midface hypoplasia; short humerus and femur. Some of them are hypotonic. There may be foramen magnum stenosis and spinal affection includes *congenital spinal stenosis, kyphosis* and *narrowing of the interpedicular distances.* Surgery is occasionally performed for kyphosis and spinal decompression may be indicated. Deformities such as *genu varum* may require corrective osteotomies. *Short stature* is characteristic and generally not a problem for the patients but distractive osteogenesis to increase stature has been performed in some patients.

Spondylolysis and spondylolisthesis

Spondylolysis is a defect in the pars interarticularis and can occur in isolation or be a cause of *spondylolisthesis*, which is a slip of one vertebra on the one below. Although traditionally considered to be in the anterior direction, this slip can also be in the posterior or lateral directions. Spondylolisthesis is commonest in the lumbar spine. The most frequently affected level is L5/S1, followed by L4/L5 and then L3/L4. Aetiological factors include local congenital defects, certain pathological conditions (please see below), Scheuermann's disease, trauma, infection and bone tumours.

Classification of spondylolisthesis

The **Wiltse classification** is the most popular:

Type I (Dysplastic/Congenital)
There is a failure of formation of anatomic elements of the lumbosacral facet joint. There is a congenital defect in the inferior facets of L5 and/or superior facets of S1, along with elongation of pars interarticularis, but there have been no cases of spondylolisthesis observed in stillborn or newborn babies. Slippage is seen more commonly in saggitally-oriented facets than in axially-orientated ones. An intact par interarticularis usually limits slippage to 30-35% of the vertebral body dimension but instability may occur, so, patients should be followed up closely.

Type II (Isthmic)
The characteristic feature of this type is the presence of a defect in the pars interarticularis (also called the isthmus). In an oblique view of the lumbosacral spine, for example, elements of the transverse, ascending, descending and spinous processes of two adjacent vertebrae can be configured to represent a sketch of a Scottish terrier dog. In this sketch, the neck of the dog is formed by the pars interarticularis, which is seen to be cut across – the *"decapitated Scotty dog sign"*. There is a genetic/racial, as well as sex predisposition: Alaskan Eskimos have a high incidence (26%), compared to the general American population (6%); it is commoner in males than females and in whites than blacks. It is also more common in athletes than in non-athletes, pointing to a possible role of trauma in the aetiology. Sports involving cyclic flexion-extension activity have been positively linked with isthmic spondylolisthesis. Repetitive hyperextension is thought to shear off the posterior elements.

Type III (Degenerative)
Degenerative arthritis of the facet joints and intervertebral discs is associated with spondylolisthesis. Females are more frequently affected than males and the L4/L5 level is the most frequently involved.

Type IV (Posttraumatic)
This is associated with traumatic disruption of parts of the posterior arch and its articulations other than the pars interarticularis, e.g. fracture of the pedicles or articular facets.

Type V (Pathological)

This is spondylolisthesis resulting from systemic diseases such as osteogenesis imperfecta, osteopetrosis, arthrogryposis, bone tumours and infection.

Type VI (Postsurgical)

Spondylolisthesis can result from the removal of more than one facet joint at a single level during decompressive laminectomy for lumbar spinal disease.

Symptoms. Back pain is the most common presenting symptom in both children and adults. The pain is usually in the lumbar region and mild in severity but may radiate to the posterior thighs with increasing degrees of slippage.

Physical findings. Hamstring tightness is a common finding, with resultant stiff-legged gait and short stride length. Tenderness may be elicitable on palpation of the paraspinal muscles. Forward spinal flexion is limited. In severe slips, the sacrum and buttocks assume an elevated position and the abdomen is protuberant.

Investigations. Normal AP and lateral x-ray views can demonstrate significant slips but may not show a pars interarticularis defect; this can be shown by oblique views, which demonstrate the Scotty dog sign. The grade of slip is determined by the *Meyerding classification*, which measures the anterior translation as a percentage of the vertebral body dimension on a lateral X-ray (Fig.22.1):

- *Grade I.* Up to 25%
- *Grade II.* 26-50%
- *Grade III.* 51-75%
- *Grade IV.* 76-100%

The *slip angle* is the angle between a line drawn parallel to the lower endplate of L5 and a perpendicular to a line drawn along the posterior border of the sacrum (Fig.22.1).

Bone scan, CT scan and MRI scan have their places in diagnosis. A bone scan may show an increased isotope uptake, suggesting an unhealed or recent fracture. A CT scan provides a better view of the pars and the posterior elements whilst an MRI scan shows better the condition of the discs and the patency of the spinal canal.

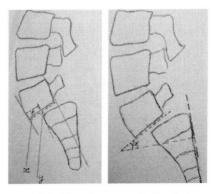

Fig.22.1. The degree of slip (x/y x 100%) and the slip angle (alpha).

Principles of management

- Treatment depends on the given pathology. Most patients do well with non-surgical treatment but some require surgery.

- *Non-surgical treatment options* include pain control with analgesics and nonsteroidal anti-inflammatory drugs, physiotherapeutic modalities such as muscle-strengthening exercises for the back and abdomen and bracing. These measures may be required by patients with all grades of slip.

- *Surgical treatment* The indications for surgical treatment include (a) slip greater than 50% (b) evidence of progression of grade II slip (26-50%) (c) failure of appropriate non-surgical treatment and (d) progressive postural deformity or gait abnormality. Surgical options include *primary repair, bilateral intertransverse fusion, bilateral postero-lateral fusion and segmental posterior instrumentation.*

Further reading

Dubousset J. Treatment of spondylolysis and spondylolisthesis in children and adolescents. *Clin Orthop 337: 77-85, 1994.*

Moller H and Hedlund R. Surgery versus conservative management in adult isthmic spondylolisthesis: A prospective randomized study. Part 1. *Spine 25: 1711-1715, 2000.*

Moller H and Hedlund R. Instrumented and nonintrumented posterolateral fusion in adult spondylolisthesis: A prospective randomized study. Part 2. *Spine 25: 1716-1721, 2000.*

Spinal stenosis

Spinal stenosis is narrowing of any part of the spinal canal or nerve foramen, usually with pressure on the spinal cord, spinal nerve or vessels supplying the nerve. Stenosis is considered absolute if the saggital diameter is 10-12 mm.

Types/causes of spinal stenosis include:

- *congenital type,* as seen in achondroplasia
- *post-traumatic,* as seen following fractures and spinal surgery
- *degenerative* spinal disease
- *in association with certain spinal diseases,* e.g. Paget's disease

The usual clinical presentation is back or leg pain or both, aggravated by exercise, and there may also be sensory disturbances and motor weakness. Increasing leg pain may force the patient to stop and rest after walking a short distance, as in intermittent claudication. However, unlike in intermittent claudication, leg pain in spinal stenosis is not relieved by standing still alone; the patient must sit or adopt a flexed position to obtain relief of pain. MRI and CT scans are the most helpful imaging investigations, especially if surgical treatment is planned. Both studies show the various stenosing factors: intraspinal masses, hypertrophic facet joints, hypertrophic ligamentum flavum and posttraumatic deformities.

Non-surgical treatment includes a physiotherapy programme emphasising postural exercises, stretching and strengthening of tight lumbar and lower limb muscles. Transcutaneous electrical nerve stimulation (TENS) is sometimes helpful. Epidural steroid injections are used by some surgeons. Surgical decompression can be achieved by laminectomy and excision of any stenosing structure, e.g. ligamentum flavum, medial facet or osteophytes. Relief of pain following this can be dramatic.

Frozen shoulder

Painful shoulder conditions, including trauma, have the effect of stiffening the soft tissue components of the joint, with resultant painful restriction of motion. The term *frozen shoulder* is used to describe a shoulder affected in this way. The more accurate pathological term is *Adhesive capsulitis of the shoulder joint*. Pain is the primary causative factor, restriction of shoulder motion is the result.

The pain may arise from the shoulder joint itself or be referred from neighbouring structures. Sources of such pain include dislocation, fracture, bicipital tenosynovitis, calcium deposit in the rotator cuff, rotator cuff tears, painful acromioclavicular joint lesions. Referred pain is seen following a myocardial infarction, radical mastectomy and surgery in the thoracic cage. The patient is unwilling to elevate the arm because of the pain and the shoulder gradually becomes stiff and more painful. Continued immobility allows the joint capsule to adhere to the proximal humerus.

Diagnosis. This is based on a history of pain in the shoulder followed by increasing restriction of elevation and other shoulder movements. An effort should be made to establish if any or some of the above-mentioned aetiological factors is/are present. On inspection, shoulder muscles are usually atrophic to some extent. On palpation, there is usually significant tenderness in the anterior shoulder capsule. On test of ranges of movement, elevation, flexion, extension and rotation are significantly limited. The patient is characteristically unable to scratch even the small of the back on the affected side.

Treatment. Most patients would gradually lose their pain and regain movements over a period of 18 -24 months but few are prepared to wait that long. An active treatment programme should be initiated as soon as the diagnosis is made:

- Analgesics and anti-inflammatory drugs should be prescribed.

- Physiotherapeutic pain-relieving modalities as well as range of motion exercises should be instituted.

- Injections of a mixture of local anaesthetic and steroid into the glenohumeral joint is known to be effective

- If the above measures do not bring about significant resolution of symptoms after six months, I have, over the years, practised having the patient put to sleep and injecting a mixture of 40mg of Depo-Medrone and 9 ml of 0.5% Marcain into the joint (4ml) and anterior capsule (6 ml), followed by gentle manipulation of the joint through the full ranges of movement. Adhesions can be felt and heard snapping during the procedure. This is followed by immediate physiotherapy to maintain the gained ranges of movement. The results have been very good.

Tennis elbow

The term *tennis elbow* is used to describe a common condition characterised by pain in the region of the common origin of the extensors of the wrist in the lateral humeral epicondyles. This pain characteristically radiates to the extensor surface of the forearm. The usual cause is activity requiring excessive pronation and supination of the forearm with an extended wrist. Thus, lawn tennis, table tennis, badminton or using a screwdriver are common causes.

The actual pathological process causing the pain is not clear but is thought to be inflammatory in nature. Possible causative pathologies include tendonitis of the common extensor origin, traumatic epicondylitis or periostitis of the lateral humeral epicondyle and radiohumeral bursitis.

Clinically, there is usually no visible abnormality. There is palpable tenderness over the lateral epicondyle and the radiohumeral joint and the pain is characteristically aggravated by forced dorsiflexion of the wrist against resistance, which puts tension on the common extensor origin. X-rays rarely show any pathology but calcium deposits are occasionally seen.

Treatment with moist heat, analgesics and anti-inflammatory drugs are helpful. Physiotherapeutic modalities are also helpful. A common treatment option is the injection of a mixture of steroid and local anaesthetic into the site of maximum tenderness. Such an injection can be repeated at a six-weekly interval to a maximum of 4-6 injections. The surgical option of release of the common extensor origin from the lateral epicondyles may be indicated in recalcitrant cases. The success rate is about 60%.

Golfer's elbow

Golfer's elbow is the term applied to a rare condition in which there is pain in the common flexor origin in the medial epicondyle of the humerus (*Medial epicondylitis*). There is palpable tenderness over the medial epicondyle and the pain is aggravated by resisted flexion of the wrist, which puts the common flexors under tension. The condition is quite similar to tennis elbow in its symptoms and course. The treatment also follows similar lines.

Olecranon bursitis

This condition results from repeated trauma to the point of the elbow. It is characterised by swelling of the olecranon bursa as a result of thickening of the bursal wall. Following trauma, the contained fluid may be blood-stained. Treatment consists of aspiration of the fluid and instillation of steroid, followed by pressure bandaging. Sometimes, surgical excision of the bursa is indicated.

Dupuytren's contracture

This term is applied to a disease of the hand characterised by contracture of the palm of the hand secondary to *hyperplasia and fibrosis of the palmar fascia*. Histologically, there is an abnormality of the fibroblasts of the palmar fascia; they develop contractile properties and are called myofibroblasts.

Aetiological factors include:

- *Age:* patients are usually over 40
- *Sex:* it is more common in males than females
- *Genetics:* there is a familial tendency and it is more common in people of northern European descent
- *Alcoholism*
- *Smoking*
- *Diabetes mellitus*
- *Antiepileptic drug intake* – Epanutin
- *Repetitive trauma* has also been blamed

Diagnosis. The first manifestation of the disease is a palpable hard nodular thickening of the palmar fascia overlying the head of one of the metacarpals. The nodule eventually disappears and is replaced by a cord-like band of contracted palmar fascia. The overlying skin is seen to be puckered and bound to the fascia. Flexion deformity is first seen at the metacarpophalangeal joint, where it may not cause functional disability for quite some time. As the disease progresses, the pretendinous bands of the palmar aponeurosis to the fingers shorten and pull the fingers into fixed flexion at the proximal interphalangeal joints. The fingers most frequently affected are the ring and little fingers, followed by the middle and index (Fig.22.2); the thumb is only occasionally involved.

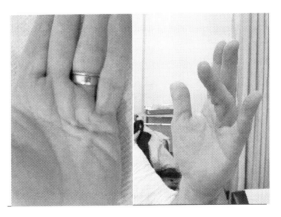

Fig.22.2. Dupuytren's contracture in a 65 year-old woman.

Treatment. No non-surgical treatment method has been of proven or permanent benefit. The indications for surgical treatment are:

- Palmar contracture and MP joint flexion contracture interfering with function (about 30-45 degrees) and
- Release of PIP joint flexion contracture. A wide exposure is needed for digital fasciectomy because the disease distorts the complex anatomy of the fingers.

The surgical options are:

- Simple fasciotomies in which the fascial cords are cut

- Total or subtotal fasciectomy
- Gross skin involvement may necessitate Z-incisions and the fashioning skin flaps to facilitate closure or even skin grafting

Recurrence of contracture to a greater or lesser extent is not uncommon.

De Quervain's tenosynovitis

This is stenosing tenosynovitis of the conjoint tendon sheath of abductor pollicis longus and extensor pollicis brevis tendons. It is commonest in adults aged between 30-50 years and women are more frequently affected than men in the ratio 10:1. It is almost always related to overuse, e.g. people who constantly work on the computer keyboard are frequently affected.

The presenting symptoms are usually pain and tenderness around the radial styloid. The sheath enclosing the two affected tendons may be thickened. *Finkelstein test* is regarded as the classical test for this entity: the thumb is adducted and flexed at the IP joint i.e. folded into the palm, and the hand is adducted "quickly" at the wrist to put the first extensor compartment under tension. In a positive test, "excruciating pain" is felt over the tip of the radial styloid.

Treatment. Rest in a splint and steroid injection may resolve the symptoms in early disease (first six months). About 10% of patients do not respond to this option and may require surgical decompression.

Trigger fingers and thumb

This clinical entity is characterised by the affected digit becoming flexed and stuck at the IP joint. This flexion deformity can be overcome by manipulating the digit into extension. A trigger thumb may be congenital or acquired; as a matter of fact, all the patients the author has seen with this condition have been infants and young children. Trigger fingers are more common and the ring and little fingers are the most frequently affected. Trigger digits are common in rheumatoid arthritis and multiple finger involvement is seen in collagen diseases. A partially lacerated tendon may heal with a blob big enough to cause triggering.

The pathological lesion is a nodule or fusiform swelling of the flexor tendon just proximal to its theca at the level of the metacarpophalangeal (MP) joint. When the nodule is on the proximal side of the annulus, the thumb or finger is flexed at the IP joint - *trigger position*. If it (the nodule) can be persuaded to go through the annulus to the distal side, the finger straightens and the flexion deformity is overcome. The main complaint is the deformity. There may be tenderness on palpation of the nodule. Local steroid injection may be effective but the definitive treatment is release of the proximal annulus.

Madelung's deformity

This is a growth disturbance involving the volar and inner portion of the distal epiphysis of the radius causing the radius to shorten and grow in a volar and ulnar direction. There is a volar and ulnar subluxation of the hand, with dorsal prominence of the distal ulna. There is an uncanny similarity between this condition and Blount's disease.

Ganglion

The term *ganglion* is used to describe a cystic swelling in the vicinity of a joint. Characteristically found in the region of the wrist, ganglia are thought to arise from the synovial membrane of the joint or from a tendon sheath. The swelling/cyst may be unilocular or multilocular and contains a viscous, colourless fluid. At the wrist, the most usual location is the dorsal aspect (Fig.22.3), where it is seen to lie just radial to the common digital extensors. Location on the volar aspect is the next most frequent and the favourite site here is between the tendons of flexor carpi radialis and abductor pollicis longus.

Clinically, a ganglion is usually painless but complaints of ache and discomfort are not uncommon, especially if "knocked". There is often a history of increase or decrease in size and there are anecdotal stories of cure of a dorsal ganglion by striking it with a book.

Treatment options include:

- *Aspiration* plus injection with steroid (Depo-Medrone) and pressure bandaging. Repeat injections may be needed.

- *Excision.* It is best to do this with the patient under general anaesthesia as local anaesthesia may not allow thorough dissection. The skin incision may be vertical or horizontal but should be large enough to give a good exposure. The mass is mobilised to its base and excised with a generous margin of the joint capsule. It is important that the joint capsule is not closed. Recurrence is rare following a good excision.

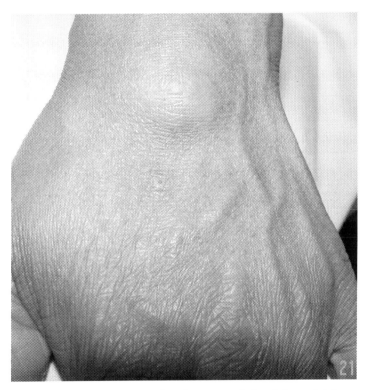

Fig.22.3. A ganglion on the dorsum of the left wrist in a 45-year-old lady.

Popliteal cyst (Baker's cyst) (Fig.22.4)

This a firm cystic swelling located along the medial border of the popliteal space. It is common in children but also occurs in adults, especially in patients with rheumatoid arthritis. It is thought that most popliteal cysts arise from distention of the bursal sacs at the origins of the gastrecnemius and semimembranosus muscle but some communicate directly with the knee joint cavity. Pain is not usually a factor. Parents of affected children and affected adults just want an explanation of the cause and possible effects, especially in the long term. However, some patients do complain of vague pain in the area and others complain of giving-way in the knee. Routine X-rays are usually negative but may show associated changes in the knee joint. If considered necessary, an MRI scan will show the cyst and its relationship with neighbouring sot-tissue structures. Symptomatic cysts may be surgically excised.

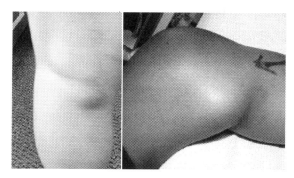

Fig.22.4. Popliteal cysts in two boys. The one on right is related to the semimembranosus tendon.

Hallux valgus and bunion (Fig.22.5)

The terms *Hallux valgus* and *Bunion* are used as synonyms. The entity consists of three elements:

- Valgus angulation of the big toe at the MP joint
- Bony enlargement of the medial aspect of the first metatarsal head at the MP joint (medial exostosis) and
- Bursal sac over the point the medial exostosis

In addition to the valgus angulation, the big toe also rotates medially on its longitudinal axis. The extensor hallucis longus tendon gradually displaces laterally, helping to maintain the deformity. *Metatarsus primus varus* of the big toe exaggerates the deformity. Hallux valgus is often bilateral; in severe deformity, the second toe overrides the big toe distally.

Bunions occur more frequently on women than in men; fashionable "pointed" shoes are blamed. The usual age group is middle-age or over but there is a significant group of patients with the *adolescent idiopathic hallux valgus* variety. Inflammation of the bursal sac (bursitis) from pressure from shoes is a common cause of complaint.

Useful quantitative assessments of hallux valgus (Fig.22.5b) include:

- *The Hallux valgus angle.* This is the angle between the axis of the first metatarsal and the axis of the proximal phalanx of the big toe
- *The intermetatarsal angle.* This is the angle between the longitudinal axis of the first and second metatarsals
- *The distal metatarsal articular angle.* This is the angle between the longitudinal axis of the first metatarsal and a perpendicular to a line joining the points of contact of the base of the proximal phalanx with the articular surface of the head of the first metatarsal.

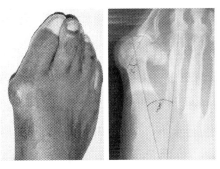

Fig.22.5. Hallux valgus deformity with moderate medial exostosis and overriding by the second toe (left picture). Angular measurements in hallux valgus: the angle "alpha" is the hallux valgus angle. The angle "beta" is the inter-metatarsal angle (right picture).

Treatment. Non-surgical options may suffice for mild deformities and include wearing wide-fronted shoes and the use of bunion pads to relieve pressure on the bursal sac. Surgical correction is the treatment of choice for moderate to severe hallux valgus.

Surgical options include:

1. For moderate medial exostosis with little hallux valgus:
   - *Simple medial exostosectomy (Silver)*

2. For moderate to severe medial exostosis and hallux valgus
   - *Distal metatarsal osteotomy, e.g. Wilson's osteotomy*
   - *Midshaft osteotomy, e.g. Mitchell's osteotomy*
   - *Proximal metatarsal osteotomy, e.g. Akin*

The author's preference is for **Wilson's osteotomy** (Fig.22.6), the details of which are as follows:

- *Medial exostosectomy during which the integrity of the medial capsule must be retained*
- *Oblique proximally-directed osteotomy of the metatarsal neck at 45 degrees, followed by proximal displacement of the distal (head) fragment*
- *Fixation with two K-wires from the proximal to the distal fragment*
- *Medial capsular repair, with overlapping and plication*
- *Routine closure*

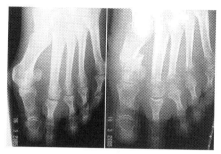

Fig.22.6. Left-sided hallux valgus before and after surgical correction with a Wilson's metatarsal neck osteotomy performed by the author.

Hallux rigidus

Hallux rigidus is a painful stiffness of the MP joint of the big toe secondary to osteoarthritis of the joint. The usual clinical presentation is that the patient experiences stiffness in the IP joint on walking and is unable to dorsiflex the toe at this joint. A relative enlargement of this joint occurs. Tenderness is present on palpation and X-rays show the classical features of osteoarthritis with narrowing of the joint space, subchondral sclerosis and peripheral osteophytes. Non-surgical treatment includes the use of analgesics and anti-inflammatory drugs, passive stretchings and other physiotherapeutic modalities as well as intraarticular steroid injections. Surgical treatment is by arthroplasty or arthrodesis.

Hammer toe

In this pathology, the toe lies in hyperextension at the MP joint and fixed flexion at the proximal interphalangeal (PIP) joint. The shape it assumes resembles that of a hammer, hence the term *hammer toe* (Fig.22.7). Painful callosities form over the PIP joint from footwear and under the tip of the toe. There is a congenital type but most patients are adults past the middle age bracket. Any of the lesser toes may be involved but the second and third toes are more frequently affected than the fourth and fifth.

Passive stretchings may help but the definitive treatment in an adult is extensor tenotomy and PIP joint fusion with K-wires.

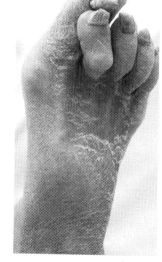

Fig.22.7. A hammer-toe deformity of the right 2nd toe

Bunionette

Bunionette or *Little bunion* is a bony enlargement (exostosis) of the lateral aspect of the head of the fifth metatarsal at the MP joint. It is usually associated with an overlying bursa and a medial deviation of the little toe. It causes pain or discomfort with footwear in some patients. Using pads may help relieve the pain. Surgical treatment may be indicated and takes the form of a lateral exostosectomy, oblique metatarsal neck osteotomy and capsular repair. The term *reverse Wilson's osteotomy* is sometimes used for this procedure.

Painful heel

Heel pain is fairly common in adults past middle age and is more common in women than in men. It has been seen in association with certain conditions, including the presence of a calcaneal spur, obesity, diabetes, gout, rheumatoid arthritis, gonorrhoea, Reiter's syndrome and ankylosing spondylitis. Entrapment of the first branch of the lateral plantar nerve to the abductor digiti minimi has also been suggested as a possible aetiological factor.

The pain is usually located on the anteromedial aspect of the calcaneal attachment of the plantar fascia/aponeurosis and the term *plantar fasciitis* is often used synonymously with *heel pain.* The pain is characteristically present on taking the first steps after rising from bed in the morning or after sitting for some time. It decreases after some walking but returns in the evening.

Non-operative treatment includes Achilles tendon and plantar fascia stretching, activity modification, control of weight gain, taking nonsteroidal anti-inflammatory drugs, using a heel cup or soft insoles and local injection of steroid. Rarely, operative treatment in may be indicated. Options include:

- Surgical release of the medial plantar fascia through a medial incision with release of up to 50% of the plantar fascia plus release of the abductor hallucis fascia to decompress the lateral plantar nerve
- Subperiosteal elevation of the entire heel pad, with release of all soft-tissue origins from the anterior aspect of the calcaneal tuberosity
- Osteotomy of the calcaneum
- Excision of the medial inferior tuberosity of the calcaneum
- Drilling of multiple holes in the calcaneum to decompress it
- Neurolysis of trapped branch of the lateral plantar nerve
- Recently, endoscopic release of the plantar fascia has been advocated but serious complications, including nerve injury, have been reported.

Ainhum (Fig.22.8)

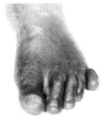

Ainhum is an acquired idiopathic progressive constrictive disease chiefly of the fifth toe, characterised by the presence of a fissure or groove. It is therefore to be distinguished from congenital constriction band conditions such as Streeter's syndrome (Streeter, **1930**; Pillay & Hesketh, 1965) and acquired constrictive conditions of known aetiology. The terms "pseudo-ainhum" and "atypical ainhum" are best avoided. It is not clear why the fifth toe is selectively affected and or why infection is at the level of the proximal phalanx. A strong genetic link is suggested by prevalence in non-Caucasians and by the presence of a familial history in many of the patients.

Fig.22.8. Ainhum of the left little toe

It appears that the constrictive process per se is painless and that pain, the usual presenting symptom, arises from tear and infection of the fissure. The histology shows that the blood vessels traversing the fissure to the distal portion of the toe remain patent even after fracture of the proximal phalanx. This shows that auto-amputation eventually occurs from lack of bony support rather than from lack of blood supply.

Infection of the torn fissure must be controlled before definitive treatment is embarked upon. The definitive treatment recommended is fissure excision with Z-plasty for stage I or II disease and disarticulation at the metatarsophalangeal joint for the stage III or IV disease. To shorten the period of morbidity, patients should be admitted at least postoperatively for elevation of the legs and for controlled use of prophylactic antibiotics.

Further reading

Cole GJ. Ainhum: An account of fifty-four patients with special reference to etiology and treatment. *J Bone Jt Surg 47B(1): 43-51, 1965.*

Iwegbu CG. Ainhum in Africa. In: *Foot* Helal BH and Wilson D (Eds). Churchill Livingstone, 1988, pp 703-709.

Kamalam A, Thambiah AS. Ainhum, trichosporosis and Z-plasty. *Dermatologica 162: 372-377, 1981*

Pillay VK, Hesketh KT. Intra-uterine amputations and annular limb defects in Singapore. *J Bone Jt Surg 47B: 514-519, 1965.*

Streeter GL. Focal deficiencies in foetal tissues and their relation to intra-uterine amputation. *Contrib Embryol 22:1, 1930.*

INDEX

A

Abdominal injury 175, 286
Acetabular fractures 153, 290, 292, 296–298, 297, 302, 303, 316
Acromioclavicular joint injuries 210
Adult respiratory distress syndrome 179
Ainhum 382, 383
Amputation 81, 118, 121, 124–127, 126, 183, 200, 201, 226, 229, 271, 330, 332, 382, 385
Anatomy of bone 4
Ankle injuries 168, 332, 336–339, 342, 343
    Weber classification 338, 340
Ankle joint 33, 49, 94, 144, 161, 192, 321, 343, 344, 346, 354
Ankylosing spondylitis 38, 45, 52, 53, 135, 382
AO classification of fractures 143, 144
Architecture of bone 5
Arterial injury 154, 158, 179, 183, 185, 223, 326
Arteriography 37, 154, 332
Arthritis 20, 36–38, 45, 46, 48–52, 53–56, 58, 67, 69–71, 77–79, 83, 106, 109, 135, 193, 218, 347, 371, 377, 379, 382
Arthroscopy 78, 192, 251, 263, 340, 355
ATLS 149, 155, 176, 275
Avascular necrosis 36, 41, 101, 104, 119, 173, 186, 195, 261, 263, 296, 299, 304, 305, 307–309, 319, 324, 346–348, 361, 363, 364
    Femoral head 364
Avulsion fracture 192, 221, 232, 250, 251, 255, 276, 283, 285, 287, 292, 338, 346, 349, 350
Axonotmesis 183, 195, 197, 200

B

Back pain 52, 60, 67, 82, 108, 124, 129, 130, 132, 133–135, 147, 283, 372
Bado classification 246

Baker's cyst 379
Bankart lesion 219
Barton's fracture 252, 253, 261
Bennett's fracture 142, 264–266
Biceps tendon rupture 356
Bisphosphonates 68
Blount's disease 97, 101, 102, 103, 378
Boutonniere finger 268, 270
Bow legs 26, 100, 101, 103
Brachial plexus injury 198, 199, 206
Brown-Sequard syndrome 279
Bunion 379, 380, 381
Bunionette 381
Bursa(e) 18, 46, 54, 119, 375, 381
Bursitis 375, 379
Burst fractures 276, 279, 283, 286

C

Calcaneal fractures 348, 349
Calcium 1, 9, 15, 20–22, 23, 38, 53, 55, 59–62, 64, 65, 124, 176, 182, 374, 375
Callus 65, 118, 143, 145, 146, 202, 350
Cardiac arrest 173, 174, 176
Carpal dislocation 262
Carpal tunnel syndrome 41, 369
Cast syndrome 189
Cavus foot 99
Centres of ossification 3, 292
Ceramic 36
Cerebral palsy 100, 109, 111, 113
Cervical fractures 160, 305, 307
Cervical rib 87
Cervical spine 51, 57, 86, 131, 154, 160, 275–277, 280–283, 286, 297
Cervical spondylosis 57, 130–132, 278
Chance fracture 287
Chondroitin 11

Chronic osteomyelitis 71, 74–76
Classification of fractures 143, 144
Clostridium tetani 181
Coccyx 129, 273, 274
Collagen 5, 8–12, 14, 18, 57, 65, 66, 146, 377
Colles' fracture 250, 251, 252, 254–256, 260
Compartment syndrome 99, 173, 184–187, 239, 321,
       323–325, 330, 331, 333, 342, 369
Complications of
    Chronic osteomyelitis 77
    Fracture healing 147
Compound fractures 188, 245, 316, 325–327, 331, 332
Compression plating 246–249, 327, 330
Conduction studies (nerve) 197
Congenital dislocation of the hip 26, 86, 87, 89, 95
Cord concussion 278
Cross-union 187, 246, 249
Cruciate ligament injuries 355
Crush syndrome 173, 182
Cytokines 46, 146

D

Deep vein thrombosis 37, 38, 154, 173, 177, 296, 308
Delayed union 147, 173, 187, 224, 246, 249, 327, 330,
       331, 333
De Quervain's tenosynovitis 377
Diaphysis 4, 15, 64, 120, 144, 169, 244, 256, 362, 363
Dinner-fork deformity 251, 254
Dislocation 26, 35, 67, 78, 86–88, 89, 95, 111, 112, 129,
       130, 154, 183, 190, 191–196, 201, 204, 211–216,
       218–221, 222, 232, 233–238, 241–244, 246,
       248, 249, 255–265, 272, 274–277, 280, 281, 284,
       286, 289, 293, 297, 299–305, 308, 313, 316, 319,
       343, 346, 347, 349, 350, 353, 357, 374
Dunlop traction 227
Dupuytren's contracture 375, 376

E

Ender's nails 312, 318, 329
Endochondral ossification 3, 5, 14
Epiphyseal injuries 169, 170, 211, 264, 318, 332
Erb's palsy 200, 201
External fixation 75, 167, 224, 242, 249, 252, 257, 293,
       324, 330, 333, 344

F

Facet dislocation 281
Fat embolism 173, 179, 180, 182, 316, 332
Femoral fractures 161, 171, 178, 306, 315, 319
Femoral head fracture 302
Femoral neck fracture 142, 143, 305–307, 309, 312
    Extracapsular 142, 305, 307
    Garden's classification 143, 306
    Intracapsular 77, 142, 305
Fibula, fracture 340
Finger injuries 268, 270
Finger joints 32, 49, 55, 57, 235, 236, 246, 272
Flatfoot 98
Foot injuries 330, 350
Forearm fractures 227, 255–257, 333
Fracture 5, 10, 14, 15, 20, 25, 27, 35, 40, 41, 57, 59–68,
       74–76, 101, 118–120, 122–124, 127, 129, 130,
       137, 139–147, 149–169, 173–190, 192, 194–196,
       199, 202, 203, 205, 208–214, 218, 220–232,
       236–251, 252–259, 264–268, 271–278, 279–297,
       299, 300, 302–308, 309, 309–319, 310, 321–344,
       346–351, 353, 354, 357, 363, 364, 371–374, 382
    Colles' 250, 251, 252, 254, 255, 256, 257, 260
    Compound 188, 245, 316, 325, 326, 327, 331, 332
    Crush 182, 290
    Displaced 155, 194, 208, 209, 213, 221, 222, 226,
       230, 232, 239, 241, 242, 247, 251, 252, 253,
       254, 256, 260, 266, 267, 296, 306, 319, 322,
       323, 324, 326, 327, 332, 341, 342, 346, 347,
       349
    Pathological 64, 65, 66, 68, 118, 120, 122, 123,
       124, 126, 127, 139, 152, 158, 187, 223, 224,
       363, 364
    Simple 245, 249, 295
    Stress 65, 142, 305, 327, 350
    Undisplaced 230, 231, 233, 240, 241, 242, 252,
       253, 256, 259, 267, 306, 311, 326, 332, 349
Frozen shoulder 26, 40, 374
Functional bracing 162

G

Gallows traction 317
Gamekeeper's thumb 266
Ganglion 198, 199, 378
Gangrene 87, 183, 226, 229, 333
Garden's classification 143, 306
Garter strapping 350
Gas gangrene 333
Golfer's elbow 26, 39, 375
Gout 38, 45, 54–56, 382
Greenstick fracture 142, 245
Groin sprain 354
Growth plate 1, 3, 10, 12–15, 41, 64, 66, 71, 101, 102,
       104, 120, 122, 143, 153, 168–170, 188, 229, 242,
       254, 318, 332, 370
Gustilo and Anderson classification 165

H

Haemarthrosis 192, 322, 369
Haemophilia 369
Hammer toes 381

Hand injuries 272
Haversian systems 5, 6, 146
Hawkin's classification 346
Head injury 180, 241, 313
Hip dislocation 299, 300, 302–305
Hip replacement 40, 58, 297, 303, 304, 308, 366, 367
Hormone replacement therapy 61
Hume fracture 237, 242
Humeral fractures 144, 190, 196, 221, 223, 225, 229
Hydroxyapatite 9
Hyperparathyroidism 23, 55, 65, 122

I

Imaging 34, 35, 36, 72, 153, 154, 166, 197, 212, 288,
        326, 373
    Arteriography 37, 154, 332
    Arthrography 37, 154, 192, 263, 335
    Magnetic Resonance Imaging 35, 154, 197
    Tomography 34, 36, 153, 322, 340
    Ultrasound 36, 39, 72, 89, 90, 94, 153, 168, 356
Implants 40, 75, 126, 127, 158, 165, 173, 189, 263, 308,
        312, 316
Infection 25, 26, 27, 35, 37–41, 46, 56, 69–71, 73,
        75–84, 86, 110, 111, 113, 118, 124, 135, 146, 154,
        158, 159, 162, 163, 166, 167, 173, 177, 180, 182,
        183, 187, 188, 189, 224, 268, 270, 287, 288, 293,
        296, 308, 314–316, 318, 324, 327, 329, 331–333,
        336, 343, 344, 362–364, 371, 372, 383
Inflammation 26, 27, 37, 45, 48, 49, 53, 55, 70, 72, 77,
        78, 81, 84, 104, 154, 180, 183, 379
Internal fixation 75, 83, 146, 157–159, 161, 165, 167,
        185, 189, 210, 213, 223, 224, 227, 230–233,
        237–241, 247–249, 252–254, 256, 260, 263,
        266–268, 292, 297, 302, 303, 309, 311, 318–320,
        323, 332, 333, 341, 342, 344, 347
Intramedullary nails 127, 224, 225, 315, 316, 318, 333
IWOT frame 156, 157, 292

J

Joint infections 69, 77, 79, 80, 84
Jones' fracture 350

K

Key-hole surgery 355
Kienbock's disease 261, 263
Klumpke's palsy 201
Knee replacement 40, 51, 57, 75
Knock-knee deformity 48, 103

L

Lamellar bone 5, 6
Letournel and Judet classification 295

Ligaments 1, 17–19, 45, 46, 48, 66, 130, 132, 153, 168,
        188, 191, 192, 207, 211, 213, 221, 229, 237, 239,
        249, 261, 264–267, 272, 274, 277, 280, 282,
        285–287, 291, 299, 313, 316, 322, 335–340, 343,
        345, 353–355
    Anterior cruciate 18
    Posterior cruciate 18
    Sprains and ruptures 191
Lumbago 132
Lumbar corset 134, 287
Lumbar spondylosis 57, 132
Lunate 259–263
    Dislocations 260, 262, 263
    Fractures 261

M

Magnetic resonance imaging 35, 154, 197
Mallet finger 268
Mal-union 147, 173, 187, 188, 209, 229, 232, 233, 246,
        249, 252, 255, 265, 293, 312, 316, 318, 330, 333,
        343
Marble bone disease 68
Marfan's syndrome 67, 110
Matrix 7, 8, 9, 11, 13, 14, 20, 26, 46, 66
Median nerve compression 255, 263
Metabolic bone diseases 20, 25, 26, 39, 59, 68, 97
Metals 126, 162, 165, 171, 243, 319, 328
Metaphysis 4, 12, 17, 70, 71, 77, 105, 117, 120–123, 126,
        170, 222, 362
Metatarsal fractures 350
Minerva jacket 160, 280, 282
Montaggia fracture-dislocation 238
Mycobacterium tuberculosis 79, 81, 84
Myositis ossificans 188, 195, 218, 220, 229, 236, 239,
        241, 304
Myotomes 277

N

Nerve compression 255, 263
Nerve conduction studies 197
Nerve injuries 130, 173, 183, 191, 195–197, 201, 202,
        204, 206, 209, 233, 239, 246, 249, 271, 293, 304,
        316, 318, 324, 326, 382
Neurogenic shock 175
Neurological examination 33, 232, 277, 285
Neurotmesis 183, 195, 197
Non-union 41, 147, 159, 167, 173, 187, 189, 210, 224,
        231, 232, 243, 246, 249, 255, 260, 282, 283, 293,
        305, 307, 308, 312, 315, 316, 318, 329, 329–331,
        333, 343, 344, 348

O

Olecranon bursitis 375

Olecranon fractures 237, 243

Open fractures 40, 75, 141, 154, 157, 158, 165–167, 181, 183, 188, 209, 223, 249, 256, 314, 318, 323, 333, 342–344

Ossification 3, 4, 5, 10, 12, 14, 120, 122, 218, 256, 292, 304
    Centres of 3, 4, 292
    Endochondral 3, 5, 14
    Intramembranous 3

Osteoarthritis 26, 38, 40, 45, 48, 55–58, 103, 130, 132, 173, 187, 188, 193, 195, 210, 220, 232, 233, 260, 263, 265, 296, 303, 304, 309, 318, 324, 343, 344, 370, 381

Osteoblasts 7, 8, 14, 20–22, 146

Osteochondroma 14, 27, 119, 121

Osteoclasts 7, 8, 20–22, 146

Osteocytes 7, 8, 20

Osteogenesis imperfecta 59, 66, 372

Osteomalacia 9, 26, 59, 62, 64, 65, 285, 305, 317

Osteomyelitis 26, 27, 36, 40, 69–74, 75–78, 102, 125, 189, 333, 363

Osteones 5

Osteoporosis 20, 22, 26, 48, 50, 53, 59–62, 64–67, 82, 83, 135, 188, 189, 221, 254, 284, 285, 305, 312, 317, 319, 370

Osteosarcoma 27, 35, 36, 117, 118, 121, 124, 126, 127

Out-toeing 98

P

Paget's disease 26, 37, 59, 67, 68, 147, 373

Painful heel 382

Paraplegia 82, 83, 152, 287, 297

Parathyroid gland 22, 55, 61, 65

Pathological fractures 63–66, 65, 68, 77, 118, 120, 122, 123, 124, 127, 139, 143, 146, 152, 158, 187, 223, 224, 363, 364

Pelvic fractures 153, 205, 289, 291, 293, 296, 297

Perilunate dislocation 262, 263

Peripheral nerve injuries 195, 196, 201, 206, 271

Peroneal nerve 196, 205

Perthes' disease 104, 106

Plastic 9, 40, 75, 165, 167–169, 268, 271

Plates 1, 3, 10, 12–15, 17, 41, 64, 66, 71, 101, 102, 104, 119, 120, 122, 143, 153, 159, 168, 169, 170, 188, 189, 222–224, 229, 231, 242, 252–254, 267, 296, 316, 318, 323, 324, 330, 332, 342, 350, 370

Pneumothorax 175

Polio 112, 113

Pott's fracture 143

Pseudogout 54, 55

Psoriasis 28, 55, 56

Pulled elbow 237

Pulmonary embolism 173, 175, 177, 178

Q

"Quadriceps mechanism" ruptures 355

Quadriplegia 283, 287

Quebec task force 284

R

Radial fractures 244, 247, 248–250, 254–257

Radial nerve injury 202

Radio-ulnar joint 248, 249

Rheumatoid arthritis 20, 37, 45, 46, 48–52, 55, 58, 71, 77, 80, 135, 377, 379, 382

Rickets 9, 14, 26, 59, 62–65, 102

S

Sacrum 129, 273, 274, 289, 290, 372

Salter-Harris classification 143, 169, 170, 254

Sarmiento cast 328

Scaphoid cast 259, 260

Scaphoid fractures 259, 261, 263

Scapular fractures 213

Schatzker classification 321, 322

Scheuermann's disease 106, 371

Sciatic nerve 99, 126, 132, 134, 183, 196, 204, 205, 293, 296, 304, 316

Scoliosis 26, 67, 86, 108–111, 116

Screws 143, 159, 167, 189, 222, 223, 224, 240, 242, 243, 253, 260, 265–267, 293, 296, 303, 306–309, 312, 315, 316, 318, 323, 324, 329, 330, 332, 342, 349, 350

Scurvy 65, 66

Secondary gout 53

Secondary osteoarthritis 56, 187, 193, 195, 220, 265, 309, 318, 344, 370

Secondary survey 149

Septic arthritis 36, 38, 69, 70, 78, 83, 193

Serpentine foot 96

Shock 11, 129, 152, 173, 173–175, 176, 178–180, 189, 219, 277, 278, 285, 291, 313, 316, 355

Shoulder dislocation 201, 213, 215, 218, 219, 220, 233

Skeletal traction 156, 163, 189, 226, 296, 314, 318, 323

Skin graft 76, 167

Skin traction 84, 156, 157, 163, 227, 292, 302, 308, 314, 317

Slipped disc 129, 130, 132–134

Slipped upper femoral epiphysis 83, 308, 309

Smith's fracture 252, 253

Spinal cord 1, 82, 99, 112, 154, 175, 181, 206, 273, 274, 277–281, 283–288, 373

Spinal fractures 35, 60, 277, 288

Spinal shock 277, 278, 285

Spinal stenosis 370, 373

Sports injuries 321, 353, 355, 357

Sprained ankle 354
Sprained wrist 355
Sprengel shoulder 86, 135
Still's disease 46, 52
Strain 9, 10, 79, 240, 322, 335, 354
Stress fracture 65, 142, 305, 327, 350
Strontium ranelate 61
Subluxation 191–194, 193, 195, 210, 211, 214, 219, 237,
    253, 255, 264, 265–267, 277, 280, 336, 343, 346,
    347, 350, 357, 377
Sudeck's atrophy 173, 188, 256, 260
Syndesmosis 17, 340, 342

T

Talar fractures 346
Tennis elbow 26, 39, 375
Tetanus 166, 173, 182, 219, 271, 333
Thompson's test 337
Thoracic spine 82, 106, 284
Tibial fractures 161, 205, 321, 325, 326, 328, 330–334
Toe walking 100
Total hip replacement 40, 58, 297, 303, 308, 366, 367
Total knee replacement 40, 51, 57
Toxicity 50, 176
Trapezium 261, 264
Trigger fingers 377
Trochanteric fractures 142, 307, 309, 319
Tuberculosis 79–85

U

Ulnar fractures 244, 246, 247, 249, 254
Ulnar nerve injury 204
Ultrasound 36, 39, 72, 89, 90, 94, 153, 168, 356

V

Vascular injury 165, 166, 173, 195, 209, 222, 249, 271,
    304, 313, 316, 323, 324, 332, 343
Vitamin D 21, 22, 53, 61, 62, 64
Volkmann's contracture 173, 186

W

Wallerian degeneration 195
Weber classification 338, 340
Whiplash associated disorders(WAD) 284
Wolff's law 9
Woven bone 5, 6, 68, 145
Wry neck 85, 86, 87, 135

Y

Yield point 9
Young's modulus 9, 10

Z

Zaria metal hinges 162, 328